W9-BMM-630

THE HEALTHCARE PROFESSIONAL'S
Guide to
Clinical Cultural
Competence

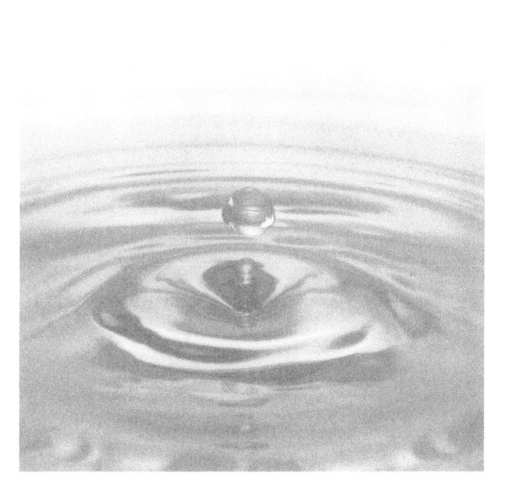

THE HEALTHCARE PROFESSIONAL'S

Guide to
Clinical Cultural
Competence

Edited by

RANI H. SRIVASTAVA, RN, MScN

Deputy Chief, Nursing Practice
Centre for Addiction and Mental Health
Lecturer, Faculty of Nursing
University of Toronto

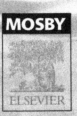

MOSBY

ELSEVIER

Copyright © 2007, Elsevier Canada, a registered business of Reed Elsevier Canada, Ltd.

All rights reserved. No part of this publication may be reproduced or transmitted in any form or by any means, electronic or mechanical, including photocopy, recording, or any information storage and retrieval system, without permission in writing from the publisher. Reproducing passages from this book without such written permission is an infringement of copyright law.

Requests for permission to make any copies of any part of the work should be mailed to: College Licensing Officer, access ©, 1 Yonge Street, Suite 1900, Toronto, ON, M5E 1E5. Fax: (416) 868-1621. All other inquiries should be directed to the publisher.

Every reasonable effort has been made to acquire permission for copyright material used in this text, and to acknowledge all such indebtedness accurately. Any errors and omissions called to the publisher's attention will be corrected in future printings.

Library and Archives Canada Cataloguing in Publication

Srivastava, Rani, 1960–
    The healthcare professional's guide to clinical cultural competence / Rani Srivastava.

Includes index.
ISBN 0-7796-9960-2

    1. Transcultural nursing. 2. Clinical competence.
3. Minorities—Medical care. 4. Nursing—Social aspects.
I. Title.

RA418.5.T73S74 2006   362.1'089   C2005-906419-6

Publisher: John Horne
Managing Developmental Editor: Martina van de Velde
Developmental Editors: Martina van de Velde and Adrienne Shiffman
Managing Production Editor: Lise Dupont
Copy Editor: Cheryl Cohen
Proofreaders: Susan Harrison and Scott Bryant
Cover, Interior Design: Teresa McBryan
Typesetting and Assembly: Jansom
Interior Printing and Binding: Sheridan Books, Inc.
Cover Printing: Phoenix Technology Park

About the cover: This design was chosen to exemplify the clinical implications of developing cultural competence. Much like the ripples caused by a drop of water, the impact of effectively practising cultural competence is far-reaching.

Elsevier Canada
420, Main Street East, Suite 636
Milton, ON Canada L9T 5G3
Phone: 416-644-7053

Printed in Canada

1 2 3 4 5   11 10 09 08 07

Working together to grow
libraries in developing countries
www.elsevier.com | www.bookaid.org | www.sabre.org

ELSEVIER   BOOK AID International   Sabre Foundation

DISCOVERING THE DIFFERENCE

We go looking for culture and cultural meanings
Only to find issues of equity and power
Our hidden expressions and lack of compliance
Are really a reflection of limitations
Imposed on us by a system, a society
That says it values difference and diversity
But what it really wants is conformity

The issue is racism, the challenge discrimination
The patterns are lost in processes of racialization
Being an "other" is to be inferior
Why can't it be equal or even superior

I do what I do because of who I am
But also what you have made me to be
"Different" can be strong or it can be weak
The answer, the choice is ours to seek

It's only when we embrace the difference
And deal with forces that impose conformity
That we will discover cultures
And the true value of diversity

Rani Srivastava

Contents

Preface, ix

SECTION III

Specific Cultural Considerations

Preface

This book marks a milestone in a journey that began nearly 25 years ago, when I first graduated from nursing school. Full of enthusiasm and committed to providing the best possible care for all my clients, I was also aware that my clients would reflect a range of ethnocultural and religious backgrounds and felt unprepared and uncertain as to how I would ever learn what was needed to provide care for all the different cultures I would encounter. So I started a project—to learn about as many cultures as I could. Before I knew it, the project had turned into a journey, with numerous twists and turns, each providing new insights but also raising more questions. The twists and turns were the varying perspectives on the "right" way to understand what culture really means, and while at times they added to the confusion and complexity, in the end they have been very useful. This book is an attempt to share the highlights of this journey—the insights and the questions that can be explored and debated still further.

This book is written mainly for students in the health professions and for health professionals who wish to develop a deeper understanding of cultural competence in clinical care. It is also designed for educators who desire to integrate the issues of culture and diversity into their healthcare curricula.

Like the concept of culture, the term "cultural competence" can mean different things to different people. A variety of theoretical perspectives underlie discussions about cultural diversity, and all of them need to be understood for their strengths as well as their limitations. Approaches to understanding and learning about culture and diversity have often tended to compete with each other—is culture about beliefs and traditions (patterns that exist within cultures), or is it about equity and social justice (power)? This book presents an integrated approach to cultural competence, highlighting some of the critiques as well as the strengths of the diverse approaches to learning about culture and cultural competence in health care.

Format and Style

The Healthcare Professional's Guide to Clinical Cultural Competence is divided into three sections: the first looks at the fundamentals of clinical cultural competence, the second at cultural knowledge across populations, and the third at cultural competence in working with specific populations. The three sections all reflect an application of both the fundamentals and generic cultural knowledge; where any overlap occurs in the chapters as a result, the intent was to illustrate how similar issues assume different guises among different populations.

The style of this book reflects an attempt to integrate theory into practice—through the use of learning tools labelled "Cultural Considerations in Care" and "Cultural Competence in Action." The purpose of these tools and exercises is to invite reflection. Developing cultural competence means developing new eyes, new ears, and new ways of thinking.[1] Readers are invited to use their new eyes, ears, and ways of thinking to challenge their own assumptions and to explore alternative meanings and opportunities within everyday occurrences. It will also be helpful to explore the reasons for your responses as this will strengthen insight into your own culture as an individual and as a member of various cultural groups. Pay attention to the emotions that may be invoked. Learning happens by engagement. Challenge the ideas in the book with what you see and experience in practice.

Providing culturally responsive care to individual clients, families, and communities requires knowledgeable healthcare providers as well as responsive organizations that support this practice. This book, however, focuses on the individual level and the practitioner, which reflects a belief that individual healthcare providers are at the heart of health care and that it is knowledgeable, committed healthcare providers who are providing, and will continue to provide, leadership for wider systems-level change. As you read through this book, consider what impact it has for your practice as a healthcare provider, but also as a colleague and as a member of committees, task forces, or workgroups in your educational or practice environment and community. As the College of Nurses has noted, quality healthcare services are a combination of competent professionals and a quality practice setting.[2] Healthcare providers are encouraged to challenge and develop not just their own practices but also the wider practices within their work setting.

Organization

The three sections of this book break down as follows:

Section I, "Foundation Stones," is presented in four chapters. Chapter 1 essentially examines what clinical cultural competence is and how Canadian healthcare perspectives have shaped this understanding. Chapter 2 discusses the concepts, preconceptions, misconceptions, and paradoxes associated with cultural diversity. It reflects a broader discussion of issues, complexity, and opportunity. Understanding the varying perspectives on diversity provides a frame of understanding for what we are attempting to do, where we may get stuck, and how we can move forward. Chapters 3 and 4 present the Culture Care Framework—an approach to integrating culture into health care that I developed as a way to integrate culture into my day-to-day practice and ongoing learning. This framework was developed to describe a way of understanding and thinking about cultural competence. It has been tested informally, and refined through numerous workshops with nurses and other health professionals from a variety of clinical areas.

---

[1] My thanks to Felix Munger and Diversity Level II: Clinical Cultural Competence Education Team at the Centre for Addiction and Mental Health, Toronto, for this metaphor.

[2] Mackay, G., & Risk, M. (2001). Building quality practice settings: An attributes model. *Canadian Journal of Nursing Leadership, 14*(3). Retrieved September 22, 2005, from http://www.cno.org/qa/pscp/building.html

Section II, "Universally Applicable Cultural Knowledge," examines the foundational knowledge that is relevant across cultural groups and clinical populations. Cross-cultural communication, caring for diverse families, and a fundamental understanding of what health and illness can mean across populations are all important to cultural competence. Regardless of the setting or the population that a healthcare provider might be working with, he or she is likely to encounter these issues.

Section III, "Specific Cultural Considerations," presents a discussion of cultural considerations in specific populations. The populations were chosen more for their availability than by design. The chapters in this section are the work of individuals with expertise and passion in specialized areas of practice, and each chapter reflects the individual authors' experiences as it highlights issues that are significant for the particular population under discussion. The intent is to illustrate how the basic understanding of culture and diversity needs to be combined with foundational cultural knowledge for the examination of issues and approaches involving specific groups. Readers are invited to consider what this could or would be like for the populations(s) with whom they may be working.

Scope

Like any book, this one is limited in its scope. Culture is a broad term, and during the course of a professional career, we can expect to encounter many cultural groups—some that are readily visible and others that are invisible on the surface. While the book discusses culture in broad terms, issues of ethnocultural diversity dominate. Readers are invited to develop their understanding of culture and reflect on its application to cultures that are not addressed explicitly in this book. The principles are the same—the approaches may be different. This book does not include an in-depth discussion of Canada's Aboriginal culture and the specific health issues that relate to this population; this limitation is acknowledged, and readers are referred to resources such as the Aboriginal Nurses Association of Canada (www.anac.on.ca) and National Aboriginal Health Organization (www.naho.ca) for more information.

The individual reader is asked to bear in mind that readers will approach this book with varying levels of familiarity and perspectives on culture and diversity. Developing a common ground for the dialogue means that at times information may seem too basic for some; the aim is not to insult any reader's intelligence, only to make explicit what may be obvious to some and difficult to see for others. There was another area, though, where finding a common ground was difficult, and that was in the treatment of the names of clients and healthcare providers mentioned in boxed features and in anecdotes sprinkled throughout the text. For various reasons, such as individual author preference, privacy and information available, first names are used sometimes and last names at other times—there is no hidden agenda behind the inconsistency.

Occasionally this book has used non-clinical examples to illustrate a point. The reason is to highlight that personal and professional boundaries are fluid; how we interpret behaviour in non-clinical settings influences how we interpret behaviour in clinical settings as well.

Assumptions and Bias of the Editor and the Contributors

There are different ways of knowing, and although all of the authors have drawn on literature that is theoretical and research based, and represents expert opinion, we have also drawn on our own lived experiences—in my case, as a nurse in a multicultural society, as an immigrant woman of colour, and as a bi-cultural child/youth developing my own identity in a Eurocentric multicultural society. Many of the examples used in the first two sections of the book are from my own experiences and practice. Where specific cultural groups are referenced, the intention is neither to stereotype nor to limit the example to that group only: a specific cultural group is used as a reference point and an illustration for the issue. It is the issue that needs to be understood in the context of culture. Readers are invited to use the examples as triggers for discussions that raise their own individual and collective awareness—not about just what is there but also about how it could be shaped differently in a different context.

Last, a note on terminology. Communication is not just about what is intended or said but also what is perceived or heard. Both the content and the words in the text are obviously reflective of the particular author's perspective. Language evolves over time and is contextual in its interpretation. The "correct" language changes and evolves. Over the years, the term "ethnocultural communities" has been replaced by "ethnoracial," "racialized communities," and, finally, "marginalized" or "underserved communities." There are also inconsistencies in how the terms are understood. For example, "multicultural health" can be understood superficially with respect to beliefs and rituals, or as a more complex concept that encompasses individual and systemic-level factors. Wherever possible, the terms have been defined (see Glossary); any readers who feel that there are glaring omissions or that terminology falls short are urged to forward their feedback.

Acknowledgements

Many people have contributed to this book and worked to see this dream become a reality. The biggest debt of gratitude goes to my family—Rajiv, Ratika, and Raman—for their unquestioned attitude of "Go for it!" even when that meant not having time for other activities, and "You can do it!" when I was feeling stuck, and for ensuring that this did not become all consuming for too long! You three have been my support, my motivation, and my inspiration, without which this book would not have been possible. To my parents, thank you for always being there, and to my many friends, thank you for your ongoing encouragement.

A special thank you to Jean Trimnell, a friend, mentor, and colleague who not only saw potential in my work on culture but also in my abilities to take it forward, long before I could—without her vision, this work and this book might have never been. Another mentor I have been privileged to call friend is Madeleine Leininger, and a very special gratitude is extended to her for the foundation on which this work is built, and for giving me time, opportunity, and encouragement to struggle with and explore these ideas further.

The experiences, insights, and knowledge that have contributed to this book have occurred over a considerable period of time. Thank you to the nurses and the students whose stories, comments, questions, ideas, and challenges shaped the ideas. In particular, I would like to recognize colleagues at Wellesley Hospital, College of Nurses of Ontario, and the Registered Nurses Association of Ontario, for their early support and development of the ideas. Also, a very special thank you to my colleagues at the Centre for Addiction and Mental Health, who have supported this endeavour in so many ways. I am grateful to my thesis committee and, in particular, Dr. Morton Beiser, for understanding what the book represented and for their patience and support amid competing academic priorities.

My deepest appreciation to all the staff at Elsevier Canada. I would especially like to thank Ann Miller (former Publisher) for getting this started; Adrienne Shiffman and Martina van de Velde (Freelance Developmental Editor and Managing Developmental Editor, respectively) for seeing this through; Lise Dupont (Managing Production Editor) for being there every step of the way; and Cheryl Cohen (Copy Editor) for bringing much needed clarity to what was often confusing.

The book would be incomplete without the valuable work of the contributors, who took on this task with enthusiasm and generously gave of their time. The same is true for the following reviewers, whose thoughtful expertise, as well as belief in and commitment to this project, have been critical to its completion:

John Atkins, Vanier College
Cynthia Baker, Queen's University
Barbara Carpio, McMaster University
Isolde Daiski, York University
Lisa Dutcher, President, Aboriginal Nurses Association of Canada
David Gregory, University of Manitoba
Sheila Heinrich, Lethbridge College
Marilyn Mardiros, Okanagan University College
Kathy Mitchell, Algonquin College
Elaine Mordoch, University of Manitoba
Esther Sangster-Gormley, University of New Brunswick
Sylvia Segal, Humber College
Marie Serdynska, McGill University
Riek van den Berg, University of Ottawa

Rani Srivastava
Summer 2006
Toronto

Foundation Stones

This opening section focuses on issues that help us understand and develop the set of behaviours, attitudes, and policies known as cultural competence. Chapter 1 examines the need for cultural competence and the meaning of the term. We consider disparities in the quality and outcome of health care, and discuss changing demographics. Understanding cultural competence begins with an exploration of associated terminology. We look at the various degrees of cultural competence (or lack of it), as well as the interdependence among the individual, organizational, and systemic levels of cultural competence. The chapter also discusses how clinical cultural competence differs from good clinical care.

Chapter 2 examines how our thinking about culture and diversity has developed over time, and looks at salient social issues that have contributed to that development. Multiculturalism, for example, has been a critical force influencing Canadian thinking and practice in this regard, so the chapter includes a discussion about phases of multiculturalism. As well, Chapter 2 discusses important theoretical perspectives that have been used to examine issues related to cultural diversity. Last, the chapter examines relevant common myths and misconceptions.

Chapters 3 and 4 present and discuss the Culture Care Framework, which is a practical approach to understanding cultural issues and blending cultural knowledge into health care. It is an integrated approach that builds on the perspectives presented in Chapter 2. Chapter 3 focuses on an overview of the framework and on the element of cultural sensitivity—the first step toward developing cultural competence. Self-awareness and understanding our own culture are crucial for cultural sensitivity. For too long, understanding cultural issues has generally meant learning about the "other" without examining our own impact on any cultural interaction; this is the focus of Chapter 3.

Chapter 4 completes the discussion of the Culture Care Framework, including a look at its application. Understanding cultural issues is one thing, but cultural competence requires that we apply that understanding. The chapter therefore ends with strategies and approaches aimed at bridging the gap across cultures.

CHAPTER 1

Understanding Cultural Competence in Health Care

RANI SRIVASTAVA

LEARNING OBJECTIVES

At the end of this chapter, the learner will be able to:

- Describe the cultural diversity that exists in Canadian society
- Recognize the need for cultural competence in health care
- Explain the concept of health disparity
- Define culture and cultural competence
- Differentiate between the concepts of culture, race, ethnicity, diversity, and minority
- Describe the Cultural Competence Continuum
- Discuss the interdependency between the levels of cultural competence

KEY TERMS

Biomedical	Ethnocentrism
Clinical cultural competence	Everyday racism
Cultural bias	Health disparities
Cultural blindness	Health inequity
Cultural competence	Lifeways
Cultural destructiveness	Marginalization
Cultural pre-competence	Minority
Cultural proficiency	Race
Cultural racism	Racism
Culture	Visible minorities
Diversity	Western cultures
Ethnicity	

Canada prides itself on being multicultural. Every aspect of society, including health care, is culturally diverse. However, our track record of caring for clients from a variety of cultures has been inconsistent at best.

The study of cultural issues has a long history in the field of anthropology. In the early 1970s, scholars Madeleine Leininger, an anthropologist and nurse theorist, and Arthur Kleinman, a psychiatrist and medical anthropologist, identified the need to integrate aspects of anthropology into health care, specifically nursing and medical practice. Leininger (1991) proposed the Theory of Culture Care Diversity and Universality and launched the field of transcultural nursing. Kleinman, Eisenberg, and Good (1978) highlighted the limitations of the **biomedical** model of traditional Western clinical practice (which is based on the biological and physiological sciences), making a case for applying social science to medical practice, and argued for the need to focus on the illness experience of the client. Since then, much has been written about the need for recognizing and addressing the importance of cultural issues in health care.

The purpose of this chapter is to discuss the role that culture plays in health, illness, and healthcare delivery. The chapter begins with a discussion of the need for cultural competence based on demographics and evidence of health disparities and health inequities in selected populations. An understanding of cultural competence requires familiarity with related terms such as "culture," "race," "ethnicity," "diversity," and "minority." As we examine the definitions of cultural competence and the Cultural Competence Continuum, the complex nature of cultural competence becomes clear. The chapter ends with a discussion about the levels of cultural competence and the implications for healthcare providers.

The Role of Culture in Health Care

Today, it is generally recognized that illness and health are inextricably linked to cultural issues. The impact of culture on health care is significant: it influences how illness is perceived and experienced, what symptoms are reported, what remedies are sought, and who is consulted in the process. However, the provincial health systems in Canada are largely built on a Western, biomedical model of health beliefs and healthcare delivery (including who is considered to be a legitimate provider of healthcare services); hence, it is difficult for healthcare providers to understand and/or accommodate all ethnocultural health beliefs and expectations (Kirmayer & Minas, 2000; Kleinman et al., 1978; Masi, 1988).

The culture clash between the Canadian healthcare system—with its roots in **Western culture**—and the individual client's values and beliefs, along with a failure on the part of the healthcare provider to recognize diverse ways of expressing distress, can lead to miscommunication, misdiagnosis, and inappropriate care (Beiser, 1985; Brach & Fraser, 2000; Burr, 2002; Flores, Abreu, Schwartz, & Hill, 2000; Kagwa-Singer & Blackhall, 2001; US Department of Health and Human Services, 2001). (For example, not recognizing that some Eastern cultures present psychological distress through physical symptoms can lead to an overtreatment of physical symptoms and a failure to recognize the root cause.) At the same time, the way health and illness is viewed in various cultural situations can pose a challenge to the biomedical model and the Western healthcare system. (For instance, in many cultures illness is seen as a sign from God and healing involves natural and spiritual connections as well as the use of plants and minerals.) Consequently, healthcare organizations struggle to provide culturally appropriate care to diverse communities, while communities struggle with issues related to access and ability to receive appropriate health care (Beiser, 1985; Camphina-Bacote, 1995; Health Canada, 2003; Leininger, 1991; US Department of Health and Human Services, 2001).

The healthcare system's initial approach to understanding culturally diverse communities was to focus on learning about the cultural stranger, whose ways were different from what was regarded as the mainstream norm. There was a desire to act in the client's best interest and also to minimize the problems associated with different cultural beliefs and values. In other words, cultural issues were perceived as a "problematic difference" (misconceptions and odd beliefs or practices), often viewed as an impediment to shared understanding and co-operation and regarded as belonging exclusively to clients (Kirmayer & Minas, 2000; Tripp-Reimer, Choi, Kelley, & Enslein, 2001). Cultural concerns were thus objectified and the healthcare providers could distance themselves from the whole matter. Addressing cultural diversity in the healthcare system was perceived as nice, but nonessential. Cultural sensitivity was seen as icing on the cake (Lock & Bibeau, 1993). The fact that healthcare professionals assumed that the problem lay in the client, without questioning their own values and assumptions, reveals both ethnocentrism and cultural bias. **Ethnocentrism** refers to the belief that one's own cultural values, beliefs, and behaviours are the best, preferred, and most superior ways. **Cultural bias**, a closely related concept, refers to the view that the values and beliefs of a particular culture must guide the situation or decisions (Leininger, 1995). To some extent, all individuals are ethnocentric and biased toward their own culture. We all have a preference for our own way of doing things, believing that to be the best way; however, problems arise when ethnocentrism and bias are so strong that we are unable to consider alternative viewpoints. Popper (1970) writes that "we are [all] prisoners caught in the framework of our theories . . .We tend to believe that others see the world as we do. And when we do acknowledge different perspectives, we normally form convenient notions about the differences that create little more than the illusion of understanding" (p. 52).

Over the years, there has been increasing recognition that cultural issues are important in relation not only to the client but also to the healthcare provider and the healthcare system. It is now widely acknowledged that cultural differences involve a recognition of the personal and professional background of the healthcare provider (Kirmayer & Minas, 2000; Leininger, 1991; US Department of Health and Human Services, 2001), as well as the social context of practice in terms of the "relative power, social position, and interaction of the local worlds of clinician and patient" (Kirmayer & Minas, 2000, p. 440). Cultural challenges arise from the differences between the client's and the healthcare provider's values, beliefs, and expectations regarding health, illness, and treatment. It follows, therefore, that strategies to develop cultural competence should include learning about other cultures as well as examining our own values and beliefs regarding health, illness, and other issues relevant to healthcare practice. This idea can be extended further to include critical examination of professional knowledge, healthcare dialogue, and the broader social, economic, professional, and political issues affecting healthcare provider–client relations and access to care (Browne & Smye, 2002; Kirmayer & Minas, 2000; US Department of Health and Human Services, 2001).

The role of culture in health care can be summarized in these key messages (US Department of Health and Human Services, 2001):

- Culture counts. It plays a pivotal role in health, illness, and both access to and outcomes of healthcare services.
- Culture is a concept associated with clients as well as the healthcare providers who treat them.

The cultural attitudes of the healthcare providers and the larger healthcare system affect the diagnosis, treatment, and organization of services, and have a noticeable impact on the quality and effectiveness of healthcare services.

Although the need for culturally sensitive and culturally appropriate health care has long been recognized in Canada (Anderson, 1987; Beiser, 1990; Ontario Ministry of Health, 1991; Tripp-Reimer, Brink, & Saunders, 1984), two trends have made this need increasingly urgent:

1. The changing demographics of the country, with respect to clients as well as the healthcare workforce, means that diversity is more visible and more frequently encountered.
2. An increasing amount of literature documents persistent and, in many cases, widening gaps in health outcomes for various cultural groups (Brach & Fraser, 2000; Institute of Medicine, 2002; Rorie, Paine, & Barger, 1996).

Thus, the need to address cultural competence in heath care has shifted away from being an "added" service to a necessary one.

Changing Demographics

Canadian society, by virtue of its First Peoples and immigration heritage, has been described as a kaleidoscope of cultures, languages, and nationalities. On a per capita basis, Canada accepts more immigrants annually than any other country in the world (Baeker, 2002). At the start of this century, statistics indicate, nearly 20 percent of the population in Canada was foreign born (Statistics Canada, 2003). The 2001 census data also identified over 200 groups with respect to ethnic ancestry, clearly validating Canada's identity as a multicultural society.

Although immigration has always been a part of Canada's heritage, the immigration patterns have shifted dramatically in the past few decades. Before 1961, 90 percent of the immigrants to Canada came from Europe and only 3 percent were Asian born. In contrast, only 20 percent of the immigrants in the 1990s came from Europe and 58 percent came from Asia and the Middle East (Statistics Canada, 2003). Even among European immigrants, the source countries have shifted from the British Isles, Italy, Germany, and the Netherlands to increasing numbers from Eastern European countries such as Poland, Romania, and the former Soviet Union. The shifting immigration and settlement patterns translate into considerable diversity across the nation. As noted by Galloway (2003), the concentration of new Canadians in big cities creates different Canadas. In Regina, Saskatchewan, for example, residents are largely descended from the first wave of settlers (Europeans and Aboriginal), while in Richmond, British Columbia, visible minorities—primarily Chinese and South Asians—account for more than 60 percent of the population (Galloway, 2003). The new arrivals also add to the growing diversity between urban and rural Canada as the majority of new immigrants,

TABLE 1-1

Diversity Across the Nation: Most Frequently Reported Ethnic Origins by Region

Atlantic provinces Nova Scotia, New Brunswick, Prince Edward Island, Newfoundland and Labrador	Long history of people from the British Isles and French ethnic origins. Canadian, English, Irish, Scottish, Acadian
Quebec	Canadian, French, Irish, Italian, English, Scottish, Native Americans, Quebecois, German, Jewish
Ontario	English, Canadian, Scottish, Irish, German, Italian, Dutch, Chinese, East Indian
Prairies (Saskatchewan, Alberta, Manitoba)	German, Ukrainian, Polish, Dutch, Canadian, English, Scottish, Irish, French, Aboriginal origins (including North American Indian and Métis)
British Columbia	English, Canadian, Scottish, Irish, German, Chinese, French, East Indian
Yukon	English, Canadian, North American Indian
Northwest Territories	North American Indian
Nunavut	Inuit

From *Canada's ethnocultural portrait: The changing mosaic,* by Statistics Canada, 2003, Ottawa: Minister of Industry (Catalogue no. 96F0030XIE2001008).

nearly 94 percent, settle in metropolitan areas (Statistics Canada, 2003). Table 1-1 reflects the diversity across the nation with respect to ethnic ancestry.

While immigration plays a big role in the diversity of the Canadian landscape, it is not the sole influence. In addition to ethnicity, diversity exists on the basis of gender, sexual orientation, disability, social class, and many other variables. The relationship between Aboriginal peoples and others in Canadian society is particularly complex. It needs to be understood in historical context. Cultural clashes are not limited to individuals from foreign lands; they can occur in regard to a wide number of communities who are perceived as minorities or as having differing needs and values. These include communities as wide-ranging as Aboriginal peoples and people who are deaf, gay or bisexual, or physically challenged.

Health Disparity

Increasing recognition of issues such as health inequity and disparity has made the need for cultural competence more compelling. **Health inequity** can be defined as the presence of

> systematic disparities in health (or in the major social determinants of health) between social groups who have different levels of underlying social advantage/disadvantage—that is different positions in a social hierarchy. Inequities in health systematically put groups of people who are already socially disadvantaged (for example, by virtue of being poor, female, and/or members of a disenfranchised racial, ethnic, or religious group) at further disadvantage with respect to their health. (Braveman & Gruskin, 2003, p. 254)

Inequities in health care are a result of complex interactions between clients, healthcare providers, healthcare organizations, and healthcare systems (King & Wheeler, 2004).

Recently, a large body of literature has documented significant and staggering racial and ethnic disparities in both health care and health outcomes (Adelson, 2005; Amin, Kuhle, & Fitzpatrick, 2003; Brach & Fraser, 2000; Geiger, 2001; Gerrish, 2000; Institute of Medicine, 2002; Kendall & Hatton, 2002; Long, Chang, Ibrahim, & Asch, 2004; Rorie et al., 1996; Smedley, Stith, & Nelson, 2002). **Health disparities** can exist with respect to either health outcomes and healthcare equality, or both. Disparities in healthcare outcomes refer to the differential burden of diseases, death, and morbidity in ethnic and racial minority groups compared with that of non-minorities. Disparities in health care refer to the lower-quality care provided to minority populations, even when access-related factors are controlled (Smedley et al., 2002). Health inequities point to the underlying causes of disparities, many of which are largely outside the typical domain of health. These include social, economic, cultural, and political inequities that directly and indirectly contribute to the disproportionate burden of ill health and social suffering on selected populations (Adelson, 2005).

While addressing health inequities may be beyond the scope of individual healthcare practitioners, healthcare providers must recognize the individual effects of inequity. Health disparities should be understood as social, political, and cultural inequities, rather than as cultural traits. In other words, when an illness is prevalent in a culture, neither the individual nor his or her cultural background is the cause of illness; the broader social and political factors must be examined and understood in order to address the disparities (Adelson, 2005).

Health disparities are becoming a critical issue in health care around the world. US research indicates that members of minority groups are less likely than Whites to receive needed services, including medically necessary procedures. Further, these disparities exist in a number of disease areas, including cancer, cardiovascular disease, HIV, AIDS, diabetes, and mental illness, and are found across a range of procedures, including routine treatments for common health problems (Brach & Fraser, 2000; Institute of Medicine, 2002). Although the Institute of Medicine studies are based on US health outcomes, evidence of inequality and exclusion also exists in Britain (Mir & Tovey, 2002) and in Canada. In Canada, potential differences in quality of care for culturally diverse groups have received less research attention, but the disparities are remarkably similar to those reported in the United States, where variables such as income, age, geography, and insurance status were controlled (Villeneuve, 2002). There is also compelling evidence of the poorer health status of Aboriginal people (Adelson, 2005; Health Canada, 2003). While immigrant populations are found to be healthier on arrival than people born in Canada, the effect does not last. Immigrants are more likely to develop tuberculosis during their first decade in Canada, and, over their total lifespan, some immigrant groups experience a particularly high risk for cardiovascular disease, obesity, and colon cancer (Beiser, 2005). In addition, research indicates that immigrant and refugee populations encounter difficulties accessing health services and that they underutilize mental health services as well as such preventive services as cancer screening (Health Canada, 2003).

Health disparities also have been noted in relation to gender, sexual orientation, and health literacy. Canadian women are more likely than their male counterparts to suffer from chronic conditions, and the disparities are further configured by ethnicity and the potentially corresponding discrimination that ensues from it (Spitzer, 2005). Lower levels of health literacy also have been associated with lower health status and increased rates of hospitalization (Rootman & Ronson, 2005). Homosexual orientation has been linked to increased risk for depression and suicide (Health Canada, 2003), as well as decreased usage of preventive services (Rorie et al., 1996).

Understanding and providing culturally competent care is now seen as a strategy to reduce health disparity and enhance the health outcomes of many cultural groups (Brach & Fraser, 2000; Canadian Nurses Association, 2004; King & Wheeler, 2004; Mir & Tovey, 2002). While disparities in health care arise from a broad range of factors at several levels—those of the client, the healthcare provider, and the healthcare system—healthcare providers, "as the more powerful actors in the clinical encounter" (King & Wheeler, 2004, p. 815), bear the most responsibility for disparities in healthcare quality.

Understanding Cultural Competence

The need for cultural competence in health care is clearly recognized, but the term itself is poorly understood. The term **cultural competence** evolved from older terms such as "cultural sensitivity," "cultural awareness," and "cultural skills." Sensitivity and awareness refer to requirements on the part of the healthcare professional and imply a need for specific knowledge and skills (Smith, 1998). Cultural competence takes the concept one step further: it refers to the ability of healthcare providers to apply knowledge and skill appropriately in interactions with clients. "Cultural" is the adjectival component of the term, while "competence" refers to the performance aspect (Burchum, 2002). The next section will explore the definitions of terms associated with cultural competence.

Exploring the Concepts: Definitions and Meanings

One of the greatest difficulties associated with developing cultural competence in health care has been a lack of clarity regarding the meaning of the terms "culture" and "cultural competence," as well as related terms such as "diversity," "minority," "ethnicity," and "race." Some discussions about culture use the terms "culture," "race," and "ethnicity" interchangeably, while others argue for greater specificity and advocate using terms such as "ethnocultural" and "ethnoracial." The terms "diversity" and "minority" also are being used with increasing frequency as alternative concepts that transcend culture, race, and ethnicity. In order to develop an understanding of a concept, we have to understand both the definition of the term and its associated meaning. Cultural competence requires a basic understanding of core concepts such as culture, race, ethnicity, diversity, marginalization, and minority. Each of these concepts is examined briefly in the discussion that follows. The intent is to present the meaning of the terms so that readers can compare and challenge their own assumptions and interpretations, while recognizing where meanings are basically similar or different.

CULTURAL COMPETENCE IN ACTION

What's Your Take on These Terms?
What comes to mind when you hear the following terms: "race," "ethnicity," "diversity," and "culture"? Note the descriptors you think of as well as your feelings or emotions. What were some of the feelings—fear, confusion, frustration, anger, challenge, or excitement? Are there terms that you are more comfortable with or have a preference for? What are they? Are there related terms that you prefer? If so, what are they?

The first step toward developing cultural competence is to increase our own awareness of what the various terms mean to us and the emotions they generate. As you compare your answers with those of a colleague, note the similarities and differences in your perspectives.

Race

The American Heritage Stedman's Medical Dictionary defines the term **race** as a "local geographic or global human population distinguished as a more or less distinct group by genetically transmitted physical characteristics." The physical characteristics referred to are observable characteristics such as skin colour, hair type, and body proportions. The physical attributes are then linked to social behaviour and status (Holland & Hogg, 2001). Race has been used to denote superiority and inferiority, and colour has been an important determinant in such classifications. In societies dominated by White Caucasians, for example, Black people were generally defined as inferior and White people viewed as superior and progressive. However, whether race is a biological category or a social category is debatable. Anthropologists such as Margaret Mead challenge the assumption of race as a culture, a scientific construct, or a brute fact. They argue that race has been established mainly as a social category that groups people by skin pigmentation or other physical characteristics such as hair type and body proportions (O'Bryne, 2004).

In recent years, the biological basis of race has come under increasing challenge. Children of mixed-race couples can have varying degrees of skin pigmentation and shared physical characteristics, yet share similarity in genetic makeup and social culture. With increasing numbers of White people with Black ancestry and Black people with White ancestry, the term "race" can no longer be used to describe culture (Fernando, 2003). As a result, the term "ethnicity" has become more prevalent as a concept for categorization and a way of ascribing identity.

Despite the fact that race is now considered to be more of a social or mental construct than an objective biological fact (American Heritage Dictionaries, 2000), it continues to be used as a variable within the context of research. Such usage is controversial, though. Opponents argue that racial categorization is biologically outdated and does not reflect biological variations. Furthermore, they argue that the concept is inconsistently applied and that the classification system itself may be rooted in racist beliefs. Proponents argue that although the concept of ethnicity (often used to replace race) offers a broader contextual description, it does not denote basic inequities, racialized structures, and social practices. "If race is allowed to take a back seat in favour of ethnicity, discriminatory practices could be more easily overlooked and [researchers] become blind to the role racism plays in health care" (Kendall & Hatton, 2002, p. 24). North American literature on Black Americans and other people of colour indicates that race continues to be a greater barrier to improved health than social class, socio-economic status, and lifestyle choices. For example, African Americans are more likely than Whites to receive inadequate treatment for pain, curative surgery for some cancers, referral to renal transplant centres, and diagnostic evaluation for life-threatening coronary artery disease—"findings that are more related to racial bias, however subtle and unintentional, than to social customs" (Kendall & Hatton 2002, p. 27) or genetics.

Where race is used as an identifying variable, it is important to explore the meaning and intention behind the term, in order to determine its utility and appropriateness.

Racism

The term **racism** has also come to mean many different things. Essentially, racism results when preconceived, adverse judgement or opinion (prejudice) is formed on the basis of racial characteristics. The addition of power to racial prejudice leads to the exclusion of groups of people (based on their race, colour, nationality, ethnicity, or religion) from decision-making processes, leadership, and economic opportunities. The effect is to marginalize or exclude and oppress some people and to sustain advantages for those belonging to other social groups (Registered Nurses Association of Ontario [RNAO], 2002a).

Racism can take many forms. It is considered to be both an attitude and a behaviour resulting from that attitude. While individual racism can be seen in the actions and attitudes of individuals, systemic or institutional racism is less visible and manifests itself in organizational policies and practices. Cultural racism is subtler and forms the basis of both individual and systemic racism. **Cultural racism** has been defined as "prejudice by those with power against another racial, religious, or social group demeaning their culture, at times attempting to change it, substitute their own over another or eradicate it" (Yagniza, 2004). It is the value system, embedded in society, that supports and allows discriminatory actions based on perceptions of racial and/or cultural superiority and inferiority (RNAO, 2002a). The minority group culture is seen as flawed, primitive, and standing in the way of progress. Members of minority groups may be encouraged to turn their backs on their own cultures and to become absorbed by the majority culture (Yaginza, 2004).

Although overt forms of racism are easier to see and understand, systemic racism is reproduced largely through routine and taken-for-granted practices and procedures in everyday life. **Everyday racism** is a concept introduced by Essed (2000) to highlight this particular meaning. The everyday injustices are reflected in unconscious assumptions (such as believing that particular groups are lazy, promiscuous, or lack ambition) and practices that systematically exclude individuals from particular events or opportunities (Essed, 2000). The persistent injustices can be difficult to pinpoint and are thus hard to address, but the persistent nature of such events can have a negative impact on mental and physical health.

Reviews of research into the effects of racism on identity, health, and well-being indicate that perceived racism jeopardizes the health of those who experience it and continues to compromise access to and effective use of public institutions (Baker, 2001; Spitzer, 2005).

Marginalization

Hall, Stevens, and Meleis (1994) identified marginalization as a guiding concept to understanding diversity. To marginalize people is to confine them to an outer limit or edge (the margins), and thus view them as somehow different from the norm. The social process of **marginalization** refers to the "process through which persons are peripheralized on the basis of their identities, associations, experiences, and environments" (Hall et al., 1994, p. 25). Marginalization is closely related to disadvantage through low income, culture, gender, ability, or geography and can have harmful health effects. In Canada, references to marginalized groups include members of visible minority communities, immigrants, refugees, Aboriginal peoples, the homeless, sexual minorities, and persons with physical or mental disabilities (Beiser, 2005; Spitzer, 2005). Marginalized groups also are referred to as "vulnerable populations," as they are more likely to be exposed to, or unprotected from, health-damaging environments and less likely to receive appropriate care (Beiser, 2005; Hall et al., 1994).

Minority

The term **minority** means existing in proportionally smaller numbers; however, this simplistic definition can be misleading. Within the healthcare context, minority group status is associated with marginalized status, meaning that such groups have limited access to opportunity, power, and resources including healthcare services. Minority group status, then, is not about the mathematical percentage of the population; rather, it is about being disadvantaged, underprivileged, discriminated against, exploited, or disempowered in the governing structures of the dominant society (American Academy of Nursing, 1995). Even in instances where the actual number of individuals with minority group status reaches 50 percent or more of the population, they are still likely to experience systemic inequities within the dominant social systems. Although minority group status can be conferred on the basis of any social characteristic, it most often refers to race, ethnicity, religion, gender, or sexual orientation.

Ethnicity

The term **ethnicity** also means different things to different people. The *Oxford Dictionary of Current English* defines the term "ethnic" as an adjective used to "denote origin by birth or descent" or "to refer to a social group having a common national or cultural tradition" (Thompson, 1998, p. 296). The traditional characteristics include kinship, family rituals, food preferences, special clothing, and particular celebrations.

Leininger (2002a) describes ethnicity as a term used to refer to the racial or skin-colour identity of particular groups related to features based on national origins. Fernando (2003) notes that the term "ethnicity" acknowledges the place of history, language, and culture in the construction of identity. In Britain, ethnicity is taken to mean a mixture of cultural background and racial designation, the significance of each being variable (Fernando, 2003). Whereas race generally denotes physical attributes, ethnicity is related to the common national and cultural traditions, and is used to describe group identification with a particular country or heritage. Although shared ethnicity may reflect shared culture, the terms "ethnicity" and "culture" cannot be used interchangeably (Leininger, 2002a).

Diversity

Diversity is a broad term with multiple meanings. For some, the term simply refers to differences or variations across individuals and social groups, while for others, it represents differences that make a difference, usually with respect to unequal access to social, political, and economic power, as well as privilege and prestige (Rummens, 2004). In discussions about health care, then, diversity does not simply refer to difference but rather implies difference from the majority, which is assumed to be the norm. Diverse groups and communities, in this context, refer to a marginalized status within society, and diversity initiatives become almost synonymous with protection of human rights, freedom from discrimination, and social justice. The problem is not difference in itself, rather that individuals and groups that are considered "different" are more likely to encounter oppression and exclusion (Cooke, 1999). In Canada, equality rights within the federal *Charter of Rights and Freedoms* specifically prohibit discrimination on the basis of race, national or ethnic origin, colour, religion, sex, age, or mental or physical disability (Department of Justice Canada, 1982). Most scholars further expand this definition to include other variables such as sexual orientation, immigration status, and language abilities (Bowen, 2004; Frusti, Niesen, & Campion, 2003; Green, Lopez, Wysocki, & Kepner, 2002).

Diversity can be both visible and invisible (Clair, Beatty, & MacLean, 2005). Visible diversity refers to characteristics such as race, age, ethnicity, physical appearance, speech patterns, dialect, and gender. Invisible diversity characteristics usually include differences that may not be readily evident, such as sexual orientation, social class, religion, illness, national origin, and occupation. The visible or invisible nature of difference can have very real advantages and disadvantages. Visible differences are always evident; thus, members of visible minorities have no choice in either concealing or revealing them. The fact that the differences are always present increases the risk of stereotyping, discrimination, and marginalization. Invisible differences, on the other hand, are not always apparent, and those who bear invisible differences are continually faced with the choice of whether or not to expose the differences. Clair et al. (2005) describe this as a choice to pass (hide) or disclose (reveal) the difference. Some people believe that those with invisible or concealable differences are "better off" because the stigma is based on the reaction of others; however, invisible differences create their own challenges. Although the inconspicuousness may help avoid some problematic interactions and automatic judgements, the fact that the person is a member of a minority group often is unacknowledged and thus not taken into consideration. Invisible differences also can cause people to live double lives, as individuals anticipate and manage risks associated with being stigmatized as a result of revelations (Clair et al., 2005).

A broad view of diversity can be problematic. As the definition expands to include "all kinds of difference," the list becomes so long that it can become unmanageable and lose its impact (Cooke, 1999). Another challenge involved with associating all marginalized groups under the diversity umbrella is that the actual diversity within diverse groups can easily be overlooked. For example, in North America the terms **visible minorities** or "people of colour" collapse a broad, heterogeneous group of non-White persons into a single category, thus masking class and ethnic differences. Similarly, while diverse communities may be similar in that they share a marginalized status, they continue to differ in terms of history, traditions, beliefs, and values. In other words, each community has its own culture and it is equally important to understand the similarities as well as differences across the communities. The term "diversity," then, also cannot serve as a substitute for the term "culture."

Culture

Culture is a difficult term to define simply and without ambiguity. The concept consists of several elements, some of which are explicit, others implicit. Most often these elements are described in terms of behaviours, values, norms, and basic assumptions. Culture is said to constitute several layers. The shallow first layer reflects behaviour and represents the explicit culture. It is what is seen and interpreted by others. The second layer, deeper and more implicit, is that of values, and the core of culture is formed by basic assumptions that often are hidden, even from those who belong to the cultural group (Groeschl & Doherty, 2000).

Classic and current definitions of culture include the following:

- "The learned, shared, and transmitted knowledge of values, beliefs, norms, and lifeways of a particular group of people that guides an individual or group in their thinking, decisions, and actions in patterned ways." (Leininger, 1995, p. 60)

- "Any group of people who share experiences, language, and values that permit them to communicate knowledge not shared by those outside the culture." (American Medical Association, 1999, p. viii)

- "Shared patterns of learned behaviour and values that are transmitted over time, and that distinguish the members of any one group from another. In this broad sense, culture can include ethnicity, language, religion, and spiritual beliefs, gender, socio-economic class, age, sexual orientation, geographic origin, group history, education, upbringing and life experiences." (Canadian Nurses Association, 2004, p. 2)

Some authors equate culture with ethnicity, but the above definitions are broader, referring to patterns within groups without specifying whether those involved are part of a minority group at all. "Culture," then, is a term that applies to any group of people where there are common values and ways of thinking and acting that differ from those of another group. The concept of culture will be discussed in greater depth in Chapter 2.

Cultural Competence

Just as there are many definitions of culture in healthcare literature, so, too, are there many descriptions and definitions of cultural competence. Leininger talked about the need for culturally competent care in the late 1960s and called on nurses and other healthcare providers to develop a comparative focus to illustrate patterns, expressions, values, and "lifeways" within and between cultures (Leininger, 1991). (**Lifeways** is a term used to describe a cultural group's way of life with respect to customs and practices.) Culturally competent nursing care was defined as the "explicit use of culturally based care and health knowledge in sensitive, creative, and meaningful ways" (Leininger, 2002b, p. 84). Within the medical domain, the term was first defined by mental health researchers over a decade ago as a set of congruent behaviours, attitudes, and policies that come together to work effectively in cross-cultural situations (Cross, Bazron, & Issacs, 1989).

The concept of cultural competence includes respect, as well as knowledge and skills and the ability to use them effectively in cross-cultural situations (Brach & Fraser, 2000; Sue, 2001). Table 1-2 provides a range of definitions for cultural

TABLE 1-2

Definitions of Cultural Competence

- A continuous, evolutionary process of pursuing cultural awareness, knowledge, skill, and encounters. (Camphina-Bacote, 1995)
- The ability to effectively deal with persons and groups of diverse backgrounds. (Capers, 1994)
- Care that is sensitive to issues related to heritage, sexual orientation, socio-economic situation, ethnicity, and cultural background, and is provided with an understanding of how those differences may inform the responses of the people and the care processes. (Meleis, 1999, p. 12)
- Care that is free of stereotypes and assumptions or demonstrated awareness. (Wilson, Sanner, & McAllister, 2003, p. 8)
- Simply the level of knowledge-based skills required to provide effective clinical care to clients from a particular ethnic or racial group. (US Department of Health and Human Services, 2001)
- Application of knowledge, skill, attitudes, and personal attributes required by nurses to provide appropriate care and services in relation to the cultural characteristics of their clients. Cultural competence includes valuing diversity, knowing about the cultural norms and traditions of the populations being served, and being sensitive to these while providing care to individuals. (Canadian Nurses Association, 2004, p. 1)
- Integration of three population-specific issues—health-related beliefs and cultural values, disease incidence and prevalence, and treatment efficacy—that must be addressed in an integrated fashion. (Lavizzo-Mourney & Mackenzie, 1996, p. 919)

competence. Hudecek (2002) cites five essential elements of cultural competence that healthcare providers need:

1. Valuing cultural diversity
2. Having the capacity for cultural self-assessment
3. Being conscious of the "dynamics" inherent when cultures interact
4. Having institutionalized cultural knowledge
5. Developing adaptations in service delivery that reflect an understanding of cultural diversity

Rodriguez (1999) notes that being culturally competent does not mean knowing everything about every culture or needing to abandon our own cultural identity; rather, it means a respect for differences and a willingness to accept the idea that there are many ways of viewing the world.

Regardless of the specific definition, underpinning the concept of cultural competence is the assumption that competence transforms knowledge and understanding into effective healthcare responses or interventions. Also, there is general agreement that cultural competence includes attitude (awareness), knowledge, and skill, and represents a lifelong process. In this respect, cultural competence is regarded as a verb, not a noun.

The Cultural Competence Continuum

Cultural competence has been described as a continuum that ranges from cultural destructiveness to cultural proficiency (Cross, 2001; Kerr, Struthers, & Huynh, 2001; National Alliance for Hispanic Health, 2001) (see Figure 1-1). Unlike other approaches that advocate cultural competence as a method of enhancing the quality and effectiveness of care, the Cultural Competence Continuum clearly highlights that a lack of competence can actually be destructive. In other words, cultural competence is a necessary ingredient for effective care and cannot simply be equated with icing on the cake. Although the continuum is presented in a linear fashion, it should not be interpreted as a series of predetermined, rigid phases; rather, it presents possible ways to respond to cultural differences and the steps outline developmental tasks that reflect growth toward a goal of cultural proficiency.

The extreme negative end of the continuum, **cultural destructiveness**, refers to attitudes, practices, and organizational policies that focus on the superiority of one culture to the extent that other cultures are dehumanized and destroyed. Historical examples of cultural destructiveness can be found with respect to Canadian Aboriginals whose children were removed from their homes and placed in residential schools run by non-Aboriginal people (Industry Canada, n.d.). An example from the United States is the Tuskegee, Alabama, experiments, in which Black men with syphilis were observed but not treated for a number of years because researchers were interested in studying the disease progression (Cantwell, n.d.). Cultural destructiveness can occur in individual healthcare provider–client encounters as well. Rorie and colleagues (1996) note that when the insensitivity or prejudice of the healthcare provider impedes health care, it crosses the line from cultural incompetence to destructiveness.

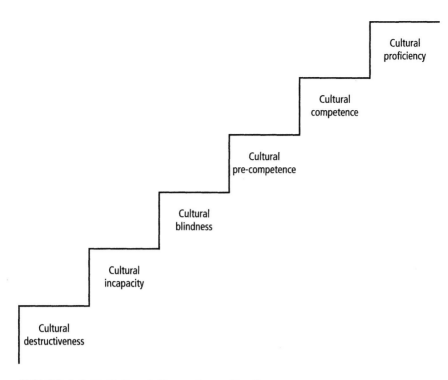

FIGURE 1-1 ■ **Cultural Competence Continuum**
Based on *Cultural competence continuum,* by T. Cross, 2001, New York State
Citizens' Coalition for Children. Retrieved October 10, 2004, from
http://www.nysccc.org/T-Rarts/CultCompCont.html

Cultural incapacity refers to the inability of healthcare providers and institutions to help clients from different cultures. The dominant client group serves as the norm for all care, and systemic biases lead to paternalism or exclusionary approaches for diverse communities. The subtle and not-so-subtle messages are that members of communities that are different are not welcomed, valued, or able to fit into the systems of care. The expectation is that the minority culture will adapt to, accept, and even be grateful for, the care provided. Cultural incapacity is said to exist when healthcare providers are aware of the need to do things differently but do not recognize the significance of cultural competence or see it as their role, or else feel powerless against the "system" (Rorie et al., 1996). The lack of language interpretation services may be one example of cultural incapacity.

Cultural blindness occurs when the existence of cultural differences is denied in a desire to be unbiased and treat all clients identically. Cultural blindness prevents us from examining the longstanding systemic biases that exist in our clinical practices and in ourselves, and thus prevents us from developing ways of enhancing the safety and quality of healthcare experiences for all communities. Healthcare providers who feel it is critical to approach all their clients the same way are at risk for cultural blindness. There are numerous examples of cultural blindness in clinical practice. For example, Canadian hospital settings have long had a tradition of giving clients cold water with their medications, even though many cultures avoid cold foods and liquids during times of illness. Similarly, healthcare providers who allocate the same amount of time for each client's visit and ask the same questions as part of the initial assessment fail to recognize differential needs and thus may exhibit culturally blind behaviours.

Cultural pre-competence refers to the recognition of needs based on culture and some movement toward meeting those needs. Examples of cultural pre-competence include:

■ The desire to deliver high-quality, cost-effective services
■ A commitment to civil rights and social justice
■ Engagement with individuals and communities to ask, "What can we do?"
■ Development of inclusive policies and workforce diversity initiatives

At the individual level, healthcare providers often desire to seek out learning experiences by working with diverse communities. However, one of the dangers of cultural pre-competence is a false sense of accomplishment or tokenism. Often healthcare providers believe that engaging in one or two initiatives makes them culturally competent, and thus further progress along the continuum is compromised. Demoralization is another potential difficulty that can arise when healthcare providers encounter challenges during activities and initiatives at this stage. Lack of progress is regarded as failure, which in turn can lead to reluctance to make subsequent efforts, and again progress on the continuum is compromised (Cross, 2001; National Alliance for Hispanic Health, 2001).

Cultural competence is characterized by a recognition of, and respect for, difference and an ongoing effort toward self-assessment and working with diversity. Cultural competence requires an understanding of the relationship between policy and practice and a commitment to policies that enhance services to culturally diverse communities (National Alliance for Hispanic Health, 2001). Cultural competence, then, is "a set of behaviours and attitudes . . . that takes into account the person's cultural background, cultural beliefs, and incorporates it into the way health care is delivered to that individual" (Betancourt, Green, & Carillo, 2002, p. 3).

The last stage of the Cultural Competence Continuum is described as **cultural proficiency.** Practitioners and organizations in this stage value diversity and seek out the positive role that culture can play in health and health care. Rather than just providing unbiased care, culturally proficient healthcare providers and agencies look for opportunities to create new knowledge and innovative practices to ensure high-quality health care for all (Rorie et al., 1996).

Along the same lines as the Cultural Competence Continuum, Tripp-Reimer et al. (2001) describe a four-stage continuum of culturally responsive interventions: culturally neutral, culturally sensitive, culturally innovative, and culturally transformative. Culturally neutral interventions are described as those that represent standard practice. However, in reality, these interventions are not culturally neutral because, as the authors note, they are "generally developed by Anglo practitioners and tested for efficacy with Anglo clients" (p. 18). Culturally sensitive interventions modify standard approaches by using bilingual/bicultural materials

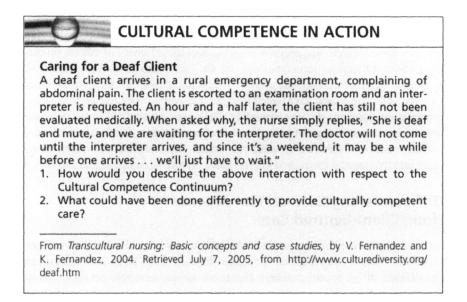

CULTURAL COMPETENCE IN ACTION

Caring for a Deaf Client

A deaf client arrives in a rural emergency department, complaining of abdominal pain. The client is escorted to an examination room and an interpreter is requested. An hour and a half later, the client has still not been evaluated medically. When asked why, the nurse simply replies, "She is deaf and mute, and we are waiting for the interpreter. The doctor will not come until the interpreter arrives, and since it's a weekend, it may be a while before one arrives . . . we'll just have to wait."

1. How would you describe the above interaction with respect to the Cultural Competence Continuum?
2. What could have been done differently to provide culturally competent care?

From *Transcultural nursing: Basic concepts and case studies*, by V. Fernandez and K. Fernandez, 2004. Retrieved July 7, 2005, from http://www.culturediversity.org/deaf.htm

(e.g., food or prayer) and address issues of access (e.g., hours of operation). Culturally innovative interventions involve the intentional and active use of cultural elements to develop interventions using cultural themes, metaphors, or key cultural institutions such as ethnic media. Last, culturally transformative interventions mean change in the structural elements involving power and oppression. Examples of transformative interventions include programs that involve cultural communities in the design and delivery of health care, with a plan for sustainability driven by the cultural groups.

Communication and Intercultural Sensitivity Continuum(s)

Other models that can be applied to the development of cultural competence include Howell's Levels of Communication Competence and Bennett's Model of Intercultural Sensitivity (Crandall, George, Marion, & Davis, 2003). Howell describes a communication continuum of five levels that learners undergo when developing empathic communication skills. The first level is that of unconscious incompetence, in which a person does not recognize that she or he is miscommunicating. In the second level, learners recognize their mistakes but are generally unable to correct the problems. The third level adds a layer of understanding with respect to what strategies are useful. The fourth and fifth levels are those of unconscious competence and unconscious "supercompetence," respectively, where learners function at a proficient or expert level, modifying their interactions with others as needed without conscious thought and/or pronounced effort to interact (Crandall et al., 2003).

Similarly, Bennett proposes a six-stage model of intercultural sensitivity that begins with denial and evolves through the stages of defence, minimization, acceptance, adaptation, and integration. Bennett's model has subsequently been revised and collapsed into five stages: stages one and two reflect complete lack of, or minimal, healthcare provider insight about the influence of culture on care; stage three reflects an understanding, on the healthcare provider's part, of the influence of culture in care and a belief in negotiating with the client with respect to care; and stages four and five reflect an inclusion of cultural awareness into professional practice by incorporating "help me understand" questions and adjusting to a wide range of cultural beliefs (Crandall et al., 2003). Regardless of which model or framework is used, it is critical that healthcare providers recognize that they need to learn and exhibit more culturally competent behaviours.

Differentiating Cultural Competence from Client-Centred Care

A question that healthcare providers often ask is how clinical cultural competence is different from "client-centred" or "client-focused" care. Client-centred care can be defined as "an approach where clients are viewed as whole persons; it is not merely about delivering services where the client is located. Client-centred care involves advocacy, empowerment, and respecting the client's autonomy, voice, self-determination, and participation in decision making" (RNAO, 2002b, p. 12). Fundamental components of client-centred care include identifying client preferences for health care, hearing and respecting client choices, and involving clients in decision making. In theory there is significant overlap between client-centred care and cultural competence, but in practice the client-centred approach has not yet demonstrated adequate attention to cultural issues (Bowen, 2004). In fact, it can be argued that literature on healthcare disparity indicates that clinically competent, caring healthcare providers unknowingly provide care that is culturally ineffective or unsafe.

Clearly, **clinical cultural competence** is not just about understanding client cultural values, but also about understanding our own limitations; valuing diversity; and managing the potential dynamics of systemic bias, racism, prejudice, and exclusion within client–health provider relationships. Discussions of cultural dynamics need to include consideration of ways in which culture intersects with issues of power and equity. In other words, clinical cultural competence can be re-defined as the ability to provide care with a client-centred orientation that both reflects the client's cultural values and beliefs and recognizes the impact of marginalization in healthcare interactions and responses.

Levels of Cultural Competence

Within the healthcare literature, cultural competence largely has been addressed at three levels: individual, organizational, and systemic.

Individual Cultural Competence

The majority of literature on cultural competence is either explicitly or implicitly aimed at the individual healthcare provider operating within the broader context of professional practice. For example, nursing literature talks about the importance of the nurse understanding cultural issues with the aim of strengthening nursing practice. Similarly, social work, psychology, and psychiatry highlight issues and strategies for the respective practitioners with implications for the profession as a whole (Kirmayer & Minas, 2000; Leininger, 2002a; Masi, 1988; Sue, 2001; Tsang & George, 1998). The underlying theme is that healthcare providers need to understand the issues and apply the knowledge in order to enhance their own practice and help develop the profession. The focus is on enhancing healthcare providers' awareness of cultural issues and health beliefs and providing tools and strategies to elicit, negotiate, and manage this information. In some ways, the healthcare provider's role becomes that of a cultural broker who serves as a bridge between the culture of the client and that of the healthcare system. Cultural brokering in health care has been described as "the act of bridging, linking, or mediating between groups or persons of differing cultural backgrounds for the purpose of reducing conflict or producing change" (Jezewski, 1995, p. 16). It involves the healthcare provider using cultural and health science knowledge and skills to negotiate a healthcare plan that is relevant and effective for the client (Wenger, 1995).

Organizational Cultural Competence

Literature on organizational cultural competence focuses on systems within the healthcare delivery process and emphasizes the need for organizational change by zeroing in on organizational structure, governance, policy, and programs (Bowen, 2004; Srivastava, in press). Although considerable literature exists on frameworks and guidelines regarding institutional or organizational diversity, there is a general lack of empirical research on organizational diversity, and the literature relies on theoretical and anecdotal reports (Bowen, 2004).

Organizational interventions address systems issues for two main reasons:

1. To increase access, by trying to reduce barriers such as hours and location of service availability, and by providing language support and reducing financial burden through support for transportation and treatment costs
2. To increase the organization's capacity to serve a diverse population, through initiatives such as education and training, enhancing workforce diversity, and outreach activities involving community partnerships

Brach and Fraser (2000) identify nine cultural competency techniques at the organizational level that can reduce health disparities:

- Interpreter services
- Recruitment and retention policies (of minority group members)
- Training
- Coordination with traditional healers
- Use of community healthcare workers (to serve as culture brokers and liaisons)
- Culturally competent health promotion
- Inclusion of family and community members
- Immersion into another culture (to overcome one's own ethnocentrism)
- Administrative and organizational accommodations (including altering physical environments and written materials, which influences access and utilization)

Brach and Fraser propose that interventions at the organizational level will lead to changes in the behaviour of the healthcare provider and the client, thereby resulting in overall improved communication, enhanced trust, greater healthcare provider knowledge of differential epidemiology and treatment efficacy, and expanded understanding of clients' cultural behaviours and environment (2000).

System-Level Cultural Competence

Literature in this category addresses systems issues beyond the healthcare organizations and health services delivery system, and reflects a focus on such steps as recruiting minority students to health professions and examining curricular content, professional standards, accreditation standards, rights legislation, and research agendas and funding (Bowen, 2004). Examples of such initiatives include the Canadian Institutes of Health Research (CIHR) Reducing Health Disparities Initiative, which has built tremendous research capacity; generated alliances between researchers, practitioners, policymakers, and the public; and translated research knowledge into information that can be used to develop programs, policies, and practices in health care (Beiser, 2005).

Team-Level Cultural Competence

This fourth level of cultural competence is a recent proposal (Srivastava, in press). Cultural competence at the team level means creating an environment that promotes healthy dialogue on differences by setting up mechanisms in the care process that allow for the exchange of diverse viewpoints and knowledge, in order to develop innovative and transformative interventions (Dreachslin, Sprainer, & Jimpson, 2002; Rosenzweig, 1998). Team-level competence is seen as necessary to link the organization's espoused values to day-to-day care practice. Putting policy in place is often hampered by differing priorities of individual staff, particularly those in senior or more authoritative and leadership positions. For example, an individual's attempts at cultural assessment may not be valued or seen as legitimate if this is not part of the usual protocol or if the process will take too long and thus be considered impractical. Team-level cultural competence makes the group values explicit, establishes and/or clarifies group norms, and draws on the strength of the collective to support the group's culture.

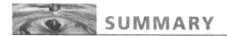 SUMMARY

There is agreement that clinical cultural competence means having the requisite awareness, knowledge, and skills to address diversity. However, vagueness, inconsistencies, and variations in definition, content, and approaches to care have made it difficult to put the concept into operation and have led to a wide range of practices related to culture and diversity. Cross-cultural encounters entail differences in beliefs and approaches to health care and also reflect the dynamics of difference itself in the form of ethnocentrism, racism, prejudice, and exclusion at the individual level as well as systemically.

For good outcomes in health care, cultural competence is needed at the individual, team, organizational, and systemic levels. While each level can be developed in isolation, all levels need to work together to be effective (Srivastava, in press). The synergy that comes from all levels working together further strengthens each level. Cultural competence involves more than accepting diversity; it also means challenging systemic barriers and changing the existing structures and practices that perpetuate intolerance, oppression, and inequity (Carter, 2001; Cortis, 2003).

This chapter has discussed the need for cultural competence in light of changing demographics and the evidence that health disparities exist across selected populations both in Canada and internationally. Culture plays a pivotal role in health; however, there is much confusion about the meaning of terms such as "culture" and "cultural competence" and the related terms of "ethnicity," "diversity," "minority," and "marginalization." Discussion of the Cultural Competence Continuum and of the levels of cultural competence further illustrates the complexity of the issues surrounding cultural competence in clinical care.

REFERENCES

Adelson, N. (2005). The embodiment of inequity. *Canadian Journal of Public Health, 96*(Suppl. 2), 45–61.

American Academy of Nursing. (1995). *Promoting cultural competence in and through nursing education: A critical review and comprehensive plan for action.* Washington: Author.

American Heritage Dictionaries. (2000). *The American heritage dictionary of the English language* (4th ed.). Boston: Houghton Mifflin Company. Retrieved February 10, 2005, from http://dictionary.reference.com/search?q=race

American Medical Association. (1999). *Cultural competence compendium.* Chicago: Author.

Amin, S., Kuhle, C., & Fitzpatrick, L. (2003). Comprehensive evaluation of the older woman. *Mayo Clinic Proceedings, 78,* 1157–1185.

Anderson, J. (1987). The cultural context of caring. *Canadian Critical Care Nursing Journal, 4*(4), 7–13.

Baeker, G. (2002). Sharpening the lens: Recent research on cultural policy, cultural diversity, and social cohesion. *Canadian Journal of Communication, 27,* 179–196.

Baker, C. (2001). *Service provision by representative institutions and identity.* Halifax: Department of Canadian Heritage.

Beiser, M. (1985). The grieving witch: A framework for applying principles of cultural psychiatry to clinical practice. *Canadian Journal of Psychiatry, 30,* 130–141.

Beiser, M. (1990). Towards culturally sensitive health care. *Santé Culture Health, 7*(2–3), 125–137.

Beiser, M. (2005). Reducing health disparities: A priority for Canada. *Canadian Journal of Public Health, 96*(Suppl. 2), 4–5.

Betancourt, J., Green, A. R., & Carillo, J. (2002). *Cultural competence in health care: Emerging frameworks and practical approaches.* New York: The Commonwealth Fund. Retrieved August 9, 2005, from http://www.cmwf.org/usr_doc/betancourt_culturalcompetence_576.pdf

Bowen, S. (2004). *Assessing the responsiveness of health care organizations to culturally diverse groups.* Winnipeg: University of Manitoba, Department of Community Health Sciences.

Brach, C., & Fraser, I. (2000). Can cultural competency reduce racial and ethnic health disparities? A review and conceptual model. *Medical Care Research and Review, 57*(Suppl. 1), 181–217.

Braveman, P, & Gruskin, S. (2003). Defining equity in health. *Journal of Epidemiology and Community Health, 57,* 254–258.

Browne, A. J., & Smye, V. (2002). A post-colonial analysis of health care discourses addressing Aboriginal women. *Nurse Researcher, 9*(3), 28–41.

Burchum, J. L. (2002). Cultural competence: An evolutionary perspective. *Nursing Forum, 37*(4), 5–11.

Burr, J. A. (2002). Cultural stereotypes of women from South Asian communities: Mental health care professionals' explanations and patterns of suicide and depression. *Social Science and Medicine, 55,* 835–845.

Camphina-Bacote, J. (1995). The quest for cultural competence in nursing care. *Nursing Forum, 30*(4), 19–25.

Canadian Nurses Association. (2004). *Promoting culturally competent care.* Ottawa: Author.

Cantwell, A. (n.d.) The CDC Tuskegee experiment. Retrieved June 14, 2005 from http://www.whale.to/p/tuskagee.htm

Capers, C. (1994). Mental health issues and African-Americans. *Nursing Clinics of North America, 29,* 57–64.

Carter, R. T. (2001). Back to the future in cultural competence training. *The Counseling Psychologist, 29*(6), 787–789.

Clair, J., Beatty, J., & MacLean, T. (2005). Out of sight but not out of mind: Managing invisible social identities in the workplace. *Academy of Management Review, 30*(1), 78–95.

Cooke, A. (1999). Oppression and the workplace: A framework for understanding. *Diversity Factor, 8*(1), 6–11.

Cortis, J. (2003). Managing society's difference and diversity. *Nursing Standard, 18*(14–16), 33–39.

Crandall, S., George, G., Marion, G., & Davis, S. (2003). Applying theory to the design of cultural competency training for medical students: A case study. *Academic Medicine, 78*(6), 588–594.

Cross, T. (2001). Cultural competence continuum. New York State Citizens' Coalition for Children. Retrieved February 16, 2005, from http://www.nysccc.org/T-Rarts/CultCompCont.html

Cross, T., Bazron, D. K., & Issacs, M. (1989). *Towards a culturally competent system of care.* Washington, DC: Georgetown University Child Development Center.

Department of Justice Canada. (1982). *Canadian Charter of Rights and Freedoms.* Ottawa: Author.

Dreachslin, J., Sprainer, E., & Jimpson, G. (2002). Communication: Bridging the racial and ethnic divide in health care management. *Health Care Manager, 20*(4), 10–18.

Essed, P. (2000). Towards a methodology to identify converging forms of everyday discrimination. EuroWrc. Retrieved December 6, 2004, from http://www.eurowrc.org/06.contributions/1.contrib_en/46.contrib.en.htm

Fernandez, V., & Fernandez, K. (2004). Promoting cultural diversity in nursing. Retrieved July 7, 2005, from http://www.culturediversity.org

Fernando, S. (2003). *Cultural diversity, mental health, and psychiatry: The struggle against racism.* New York: Brunner-Routledge.

Flores, G., Abreu, M., Schwartz, I., & Hill, M. (2000). The importance of language and culture in pediatric care: Case studies from the Latino community. *The Journal of Pediatrics, 137*(6), 842–848.

Frusti, D., Niesen, K., & Campion, J. (2003). Creating a culturally competent organization: Use of the diversity competence model. *Journal of Nursing Administration, 33*(1), 31–38.

Galloway, G. (2003, January 22). Toronto most ethnically diverse in North America. *The Globe and Mail*, p. A6.

Geiger, H. J. (2001). Racial stereotyping and medicine: The need for cultural competence. *Canadian Medical Association Journal, 164*(12), 1699–1700.

Gerrish, K. (2000). Individualized care: Its conceptualization and practice within a multi-ethnic society. *Journal of Advanced Nursing, 32*(1), 91–99.

Green, K., Lopez, M., Wysocki, A., & Kepner, K. (2002). *Diversity in the workplace: Benefits, challenges, and the required managerial tools.* Gainesville, Florida: Institute of Food and Agricultural Services, University of Florida. Retrieved June 15, 2004, from http://edis.ifas.ufl.edu/pdffiles/HR/HR02200.pdf

Groeschl, S., & Doherty, L. (2000). Conceptualising culture. *Cross Cultural Management, 7*(4), 12–17.

Hall, J., Stevens, P., & Meleis, A. (1994). Marginalization: A guiding concept for valuing diversity in nursing knowledge development. *Advances in Nursing Science, 16*(4), 23–41.

Health Canada. (2003). *Access to health services for underserved populations in Canada.* Ottawa: Author.

Holland, K., & Hogg, C. (2001). *Cultural awareness in nursing and health care.* London: Arnold.

Hudecek, N. (2002). Cultural competence: Reflect elements of cultural diversity in attitudes, policies, and services. *Inside Case Management, 9*(9), 1–3.

Industry Canada. (n.d.). First Nations SchoolNet, residential schools. Retrieved June 14, 2005, from http://www.schoolnet.ca/aboriginal/issues/schools-e.html

Institute of Medicine. (2002). *Unequal treatment: What healthcare providers need to know about racial and ethnic disparities in health care.* Washington, DC: Institute of Medicine. Retrieved February 7, 2004, from http://www.iom.edu/report.asp?id=4475

Jezewski, M. A. (1995). Evolution of grounded theory: Conflict resolution through culture brokering. *Advances in Nursing Science, 17*(3), 14–30.

Kagawa-Singer, M., & Blackhall, L. J. (2001). Negotiating cross-cultural life issues at the end of life. *Journal of the American Medical Association, 23,* 2993–3001.

Kendall, J. K., & Hatton, D. (2002). Racism as a source of health disparity in families with attention deficit hyperactivity disorder. *Advances in Nursing Science, 25*(2), 22–39.

Kerr, M., Struthers, R., & Huynh, W. (2001). Workforce diversity. *American Association of Occupational Health Nursing Journal, 49*(1), 13–20.

King, T., & Wheeler, M. (2004). Inequality in health care: Unjust, inhumane, and unattended. *Annals of Internal Medicine, 141*(10), 815–817.

Kirmayer, L. J., & Minas, H. (2000). The future of cultural psychiatry: An international perspective. *Canadian Journal of Psychiatry, 45,* 438–446.

Kleinman, A., Eisenberg, L., & Good, B. (1978). Culture, illness, and care: Clinical lessons from anthropologic and cross cultural research. *Annals of Internal Medicine, 88,* 251–258.

Lavizzo-Mourney, R., & Mackenzie, E. (1996). Cultural competence: Essential measurements of quality for managed care organizations. *Annals of Internal Medicine, 124*(10), 919–921.

Leininger, M. (1991). The theory of culture care diversity and universality. In M. Leininger (Ed.), *Culture care diversity and universality: A theory of nursing* (pp. 5–72). New York: National League for Nursing.

Leininger, M. (1995). Transcultural nursing perspectives: Basic concepts, principles, and culture care incidents. In M. Leininger & M. R. McFarland (Eds.), *Transcultural nursing: Concepts, theories, research and practice* (2nd ed., pp. 57–92). New York: McGraw Hill.

Leininger, M. (2002a). Essential transcultural nursing care concepts, principles, examples, and policy statements. In M. Leininger & M. R. McFarland (Eds.), *Transcultural nursing: Concepts, theories, research and practice* (3rd ed., pp. 45–70). New York: McGraw Hill.

Leininger, M. (2002b). Theory of culture care and the ethnonursing research method. In M. Leininger & M. R. McFarland (Eds.), *Transcultural nursing: Concepts, theories, research and practice,* (3rd ed., pp. 71–98). New York: McGraw Hill.

Lock, M., & Bibeau, G. (1993). Healthy disputes: Some reflections on the practice of medical anthropology in Canada. *Health and Canadian Society,* *1*(1), 147–175.

Long, J., Chang, V., Ibrahim, S., & Asch, D. (2004). Update on health disparities literature. *Annals of Internal Medicine, 141*(10), 805–812.

Masi, R. (1988). Multiculturalism, medicine and health part I: Multicultural health care. *Canadian Family Physician, 34,* 2173–2178.

Meleis, A. (1999). Culturally competent care. *Journal of Transcultural Nursing, 10*(1), 12.

Mir, G., & Tovey, P. (2002). Cultural competency: Professional action and South Asian careers. *Journal of Management in Medicine, 16*(1), 7–19.

National Alliance for Hispanic Health. (2001). A primer for cultural proficiency. Washington: Estrella Press. Retrieved June 10, 2004, from http://www. hispanichealth.org/pdf/primer.pdf

O'Bryne, M. (2004). *A review of cross cultural training in mental health.* Montreal: McGill University Culture Consultation Service.

Ontario Ministry of Health. (1991). *Let's work together: Guidelines to promote cultural/ racial sensitivity and awareness in health are programs and services.* Toronto: Queen's Printer.

Popper, K. R. (1970). Normal science and its dangers. In I. Lakatos & A. Musgrave (Eds.), *Criticism and the growth of knowledge* (pp. 51–58). Cambridge, England: Cambridge University Press.

Registered Nurses Association of Ontario (2002a). *Racism.* Toronto: Author. Retrieved January 20, 2004, from http://www.rnao.org/html/pdf/policy_statement_racism.pdf

Registered Nurses Association of Ontario (2002b). *Nursing best practice guideline: Client-centred care.* Toronto: Author. Retrieved February 20, 2004, from http://www. rnao.org/bestpractices/pdf/BPG_cccare.pdfe

Rodriguez, B. (1999). *What is cultural competence?* Chicago: Family Resource Coalition.

Rootman, I., & Ronson, B. (2005). Literacy and health research. *Canadian Journal of Public Health, 96*(Suppl. 2), 62–77.

Rorie, J., Paine, L., & Barger, M. (1996). Cultural competence in primary care services. *Journal of Nurse–Midwifery, 41*(2), 92–100.

Rosenzweig, P. (1998). Managing the new global workforce: Fostering diversity, forging consistency. *European Management Journal, 16*(6), 644–652.

Rummens, J. A. (2004). Overlapping and intersecting identities. *Canadian Diversity, 3*(1), 5–9.

Smedley, B., Stith, A., & Nelson, A., (Eds.). (2002). *Unequal treatment: Confronting racial and ethnic disparities in health care.* Washington DC: National Academic Press.

Smith, L. S. (1998). Concept analysis: Cultural competence. *Journal of Cultural Diversity, 5*(1), 4–10.

Spitzer, D. (2005). Engendering health disparities. *Canadian Journal of Public Health*, *96*(Suppl. 2), 78–96.

Srivastava, R. (in press). Understanding clinical cultural competence. In J. A. Rummens & M. B. Beiser (Eds.), *Navigating diversity: Immigration, ethnicity and health*. Toronto: University of Toronto Press.

Statistics Canada. (2003). *Canada's ethnocultural portrait: The changing mosaic*. Ottawa: Ministry of Industry.

Sue, D. W. (2001). Multidimensional facets of cultural competence. *The Counseling Psychologist*, *29*(6), 790–821.

Thompson, D., (Ed.). (1998). *Oxford dictionary of current English*. New York: Oxford University Press.

Tripp-Reimer, T., Brink, P. J., & Saunders, J. M. (1984). Cultural assessment: Content and process. *Nursing Outlook*, *32*(2), 78–82.

Tripp-Reimer, T., Choi, E., Kelley, K., & Enslein, J. (2001). Cultural barriers to care: Inverting the problem. *Diabetes Spectrum*, *14*(1), 13–22.

Tsang, A. K. T., & George, U. (1998). Towards an integrated framework for cross cultural social work practice. *Canadian Social Work Review*, *15*(1), 73–93.

US Department of Health and Human Services. (2001). Mental health: Culture, race, and ethnicity—A supplement to mental health: A report of the surgeon general. Washington: Author. Retrieved February 10, 2004, from http://www.surgeongeneral.gov/library/mentalhealth/cre/

Villeneuve, M. J. (2002). Healthcare, race, and diversity: Time to act. *Hospital Quarterly* (Winter), 67–73.

Wenger, A. (1995). Cultural context, health and health care decision making. *Journal of Transcultural Nursing*, *7*(1), 3–14.

Wilson, A., Sanner, S., & McAllister, L. (2003). Building diverse relationships: Diversity white paper. Sigma Theta Tau International: Honor Society of Nursing. Retrieved December 18, 2004, from http://www.nursingsociety.org/about/Diversity_paper.pdf

Yagniza (2004). Cultural racism. Native American Holocaust Museum. Retrieved August 4, 2004, from http://nahm.org/cultural.html

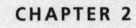

CHAPTER 2

Culture: Perspectives, Myths, and Misconceptions

RANI SRIVASTAVA

LEARNING OBJECTIVES

At the end of this chapter, the learner will be able to:
- Discuss the evolution of multicultural policy in Canada
- Describe the phases of multiculturalism
- Discuss three major perspectives on culture and diversity that have influenced healthcare literature and practice
- Identify the common myths and misconceptions associated with culture
- Recognize the paradoxical dilemmas associated with cultural competence

KEY TERMS

Assimilation	Ethno-specific
Bicultural staff	Explanatory model of illness
Cultural literacy	Multiculturalism
Cultural mosaic	Perspectives
Cultural relativism	Prejudice
Culture brokers	Stereotype
Equity	Strategy
Ethnic matching	

The purpose of this chapter is to provide an overview of the evolution of thought and knowledge concerning culture and diversity. Over the years, there have been different perspectives on how best to understand and apply cultural competence in healthcare practices. **Perspectives** can be thought of as conceptual landscapes or sets of ideas that form the overall picture on a given topic. To understand our current thinking about culture and diversity, it is important to have an understanding of the evolving social as well as the academic perspectives on the subject.

One way to examine the evolving social context of diversity is to look at government policies. For Canada, this means an examination of multiculturalism—

as it evolved in legislation and as it is experienced by Canadians. In this chapter, the legislative context is discussed separately from the conceptual perspectives for ease of understanding; in reality the two are interrelated.

Over the years, the academic discussions of culture also have undergone several evolutions. How we understand and view culture has been debated from varying, and at times conflicting, perspectives. Three main perspectives have emerged:

1. Cultural literacy or culturally specific approaches
2. Relational or intercultural approaches
3. Anti-racism and/or anti-oppression approaches

Although the academic perspectives highlighted in this chapter go beyond the national context, they are by no means all encompassing. Rather, they are drawn from the readily available healthcare literature thought to influence education and practice in Canada.

Multiculturalism: The Social and Legislative Context

Multiculturalism has been a part of Canadian society since the country's birth. The term refers to "a condition in which many cultures coexist in society and maintain their cultural differences" (*Webster's New Millennium Dictionary,* 2005). From the days of Confederation in 1867, English and French were accorded official constitutional status and a range of powers were assigned to the constituent member provinces. In the province of Quebec, where a large majority of residents were French speaking, these powers helped to protect and develop the French culture (Canadian Heritage, 2004).

Multiculturalism also refers to the public policy of managing cultural diversity in a multi-ethnic society in such a way that there is an emphasis on tolerance and respect for cultural diversity ("Multiculturalism," February 7, 2006). The origins of multiculturalism in Canada can be traced back to the Lester B. Pearson government's Royal Commission on Bilingualism and Biculturalism. The mid-1960s were a time of increasingly troubled relations between the French and English. Pearson appointed the royal commission to study and recommend solutions to these problems. At the same time, the immigration policy was undergoing change, and as a result, the cultures represented by new immigrants were changing. Although the royal commission was established to look at biculturalism and bilingualism, what it ended up hearing went beyond French and English relations. The result was a new model of citizenship based on public acceptance of difference and support of pluralism (existence of many cultures). Unlike the melting-pot model of the United States, which promoted **assimilation** (a process whereby a minority group gradually adopts the customs and attitudes of the dominant culture), Canada preferred the idea of a **cultural mosaic,** in which the various cultures were encouraged to preserve and celebrate their heritage. The term "cultural mosaic" refers to the multi-ethnic communities that form the fabric of Canadian society, where ethnicity is seen as a positive quality and not as a means of undermining Canadian identity (Centre for Canadian Studies, n.d.). The Canadian mosaic, however, was dominated by European heritage.

Esses and Gardner (1996) note that the multicultural policy was developed in response to three major forces in Canadian society. First, there were concerns expressed by ethnic minorities in response to the royal commission; second, an official policy on multiculturalism was an obvious next step in acknowledging acceptance of ethnic diversity after the liberalization of the immigration policy; and third, multiculturalism was set up as a national symbol for Canadians and fulfilled a need for a distinctive Canadian identity. Table 2-1 shows Canadian multicultural milestones with respect to official policy and legislation.

Phases of Multiculturalism

Multiculturalism was adopted as a national policy in Canada in 1971. Since that time, the policy has been said to evolve through several phases, each reflecting on and influencing the social climate of the time (Elliott, 1999).

Phase I: Cultural Preservation

The early 1970s have been described as the first phase of the multicultural policy—that of cultural preservation and reinforcement. When the policy was first established, it was developed to meet the needs of mainly European immigrant groups and their descendants (Esses & Gardner, 1996). It was implemented as support for cultural activities and for language and heritage education. Although the underlying notion that "everyone has a culture" was inherent in the definition of multiculturalism, in popular terms, culture was seen to belong to the minorities or to the various ethnic groups. During this time, ethnocultural groups, which previously might have struggled to preserve their cultural values and lifeways, were now able to celebrate them in public, through funding and legislative support. "It gave license to eat perogies in public, break open fortune cookies, or dance with kilts on . . . multiculturalism was viewed as letting ethnics play in their sandbox" (McClanagahan, 1995). With a focus on cultural celebrations, ethnocultural communities were able to affirm their religious and ethnic identities, and multiculturalism, for many Canadians, came to be viewed as the 4 Ds—dress, dance, dialect, and diet. Although the ethnocultural communities lived side by side, there was nothing that specifically encouraged interaction between them.

Phase II: Group Relations

The second phase of multiculturalism was evident by the late 1970s and was characterized by the shifting of focus from cultural celebrations to group relations (Elliott, 1999). Up to this point, multiculturalism had been important for the ethnocultural communities because it helped them affirm their identity and values. However, mainstream Canadian society's role in promoting multiculturalism was unclear. With the recognition that multiculturalism belonged to everyone, there was an increased call for cultural sensitivity, and those in the mainstream were encouraged to understand and respect the diverse cultural values.

Toward the late 1970s and early 1980s, Canadian immigration patterns began to experience a considerable shift. Previously, most of the immigrants had come

TABLE 2-1

Canadian Multicultural Milestones

1867:   Confederation
- English and French accorded official constitutional status

1960:   Passage of *Canadian Bill of Rights*
- Barred discrimination by federal agencies on the grounds of race, national origin, colour, religion, or sex

1962:   Changes to Canada's *Immigration Act*
- As a consequence, immigration became less European and the mix of source countries shifted to nations in southern Europe, Asia, and the West Indies

1969:   *Official Languages Act*
- Protected minority language rights

1971:   Canada adopted multiculturalism as an official policy
- Recognized the reality of cultural pluralism in Canada
- Acted to reverse the earlier attempt to assimilate
- Confirmed the rights of Aboriginal peoples and the status of two official languages
- Provided for programs and services to support ethnocultural associations and to help individuals overcome barriers to their full participation in Canadian society

1982:   *Canadian Charter of Rights and Freedoms*
- Multiculturalism now considered to be constitutional
- Equality rights without discrimination (in particular based on race, national or ethnic origin, colour, religion, sex, age, or mental or physical disability)
- Section 27 explicitly stated that this Charter shall be interpreted in a manner consistent with the preservation and enhancement of the multicultural heritage of Canadians; by virtue of this section of the Charter, Canada became a constitutional multicultural stage

1986:   *Employment Equity Act*
- Established to achieve equality in the workplace so that no person would be denied employment opportunities or benefits for reasons unrelated to ability
- Established the principle that employment equity means more than treating persons in the same way but also requires special measures and the accommodation of differences
- Identified four designated groups thought to experience disadvantage in employment: women, Aboriginal peoples, persons with disability, and persons in a visible minority (Human Resources and Skills Development Canada, 2001)

1988:   *Multiculturalism Act*
- Commits the government to assist communities and institutions in bringing about equal access and participation

1996:   Creation of the Canada Race Relations Foundation (CRRF)
- Established as one part of the 1988 Japanese Canadian Redress Agreement to combat all forms of racial discrimination in Canada, with special emphasis on systemic discrimination in education and employment

Modified from *Annual report on the operation of the Canadian Multicultural Act, 2002–2003*, Canadian Heritage, 2004: http://www.pch.gc.ca/progs/multi/reports/ann2002–2003/cont_e.cfm; *Multiculturalism in Canada*, by J.E. Goodrich, 2002, Canadian Studies at Mount Allison University: http://www.mta.ca/faculty/arts/canadian_studies/english/about/multi/index.htm.

from the United States or Western Europe. Now the majority of new immigrants were "visible minorities" coming from Asia, Africa, and the West Indies. As well, during this period there was a substantial increase in the number of immigrants admitted as refugees on humanitarian and compassionate grounds. As the ethnic mix of the country shifted, the multiculturalism policy was forced to deal with the concerns of the increasing numbers of visible minorities. Questions arose about how best to promote the cultural and economic integration of various groups, particularly in light of prejudice, discrimination, and differing values (McClanagahan, 1995).

The new and emerging communities were more concerned about equity and discrimination issues than about recognition and preservation of their heritage. The ethnocultural communities wanted equal access to jobs, housing, and education. Multiculturalism was required to move beyond support of cultural enrichment to elimination of racial prejudice and discrimination. As a result, the policy of multiculturalism expanded to include combating prejudice and discrimination and promoting full and equal participation in all aspects of society (Esses & Gardner, 1996). Race relations became part of the official agenda and subsequently became a main focus of the multicultural policy. With the passage of the *Canadian Charter of Rights and Freedoms* in 1982, multiculturalism was viewed as a constitutional right. The law protected equality, freedom from discrimination, and the importance of multicultural heritage (Canadian Heritage, 2004). While the law mandated equality, no clear policy or mandate emerged to stipulate that medical and social services should become ethnically sensitive institutions (Lock & Bibeau, 1993).

Phase III: Anti-Racism/Anti-Oppression

The late 1980s are characterized as the anti-racism and/or anti-oppression phase of multiculturalism. Although the multicultural policy had expanded to include race relations as a primary focus, many advocated for a specific anti-racism policy. Whereas multicultural policy focused on understanding and opening doors, anti-racism policy demanded a "level the playing field" approach through initiatives such as affirmative action and positive hiring (Elliott, 1999).

The *Multiculturalism Act* was passed in July 1988. Section 3 of the legislation declares that it is Canadian government policy to "recognize and promote understanding that multiculturalism reflects the cultural and racial diversity of Canadian society and acknowledges the freedom of all members of Canadian society to preserve, enhance, and share their cultural heritage" (Centre for Canadian Studies, n.d.). In 1996, the Canadian Race Relations Foundation was established to combat racism and all forms of racial discrimination in Canada, with a special emphasis on systemic discrimination in education and employment.

Phase IV: Integration

In the early twenty-first century, multiculturalism is said to be entering a new era that integrates the previous phases. The new focus includes cultural support and immigration adjustment, as well as human rights, anti-racism, and equity (Elliott, 1999). Much of the social perspective today is seen through the prism of increased globalization and shifting views on diversity. Canadian identity continues to be grounded in cultural pluralism, and the dialogue is once again shifting from anti-racism to identity, equity, and social justice. The multiculturalism program today therefore has three overall policy goals: identity, social justice, and civic participation. Specific objectives include fostering cross-cultural understanding, combating racism and discrimination, promoting shared citizenship, and making Canadian institutions more reflective of Canadian diversity (Canadian Heritage, 2004).

Academic Perspectives on Culture

The need for culturally sensitive and culturally appropriate health care has long been recognized in both Canadian society and the healthcare literature. The impact of cultural diversity on health care can be significant. Over the past four decades, the academic concept of culture has been profoundly transformed as the healthcare community has argued about the "correct" approach to understanding and addressing issues related to culture and diversity in health care. Over the years, the language of "difference," "diversity," "equity," and "intersectionality of multiple oppressions" has replaced the language of "culture," "multiculturalism," and "cultural pluralism." These perspectives can be broadly grouped into three major categories: cultural relativism or cultural literacy, relational or intercultural approaches, and the anti-racism/anti-oppression approaches. A fourth approach, an integrative social realist approach designed to examine health disparity, also is beginning to emerge. The perspectives, to some extent, parallel the legislative social context, and differ in their assumptions as well as suggested focus for cross-cultural learning and practice. Table 2-2 summarizes the first three approaches.

Cultural Literacy: The Traditional View

Early models of understanding culture reflected the anthropological perspective and focused on learning about the variations in values and beliefs regarding illness, health, and health care of different cultures or cultural literacy. The **cultural literacy** approach, also known as the culture-specific approach, reflects the principle of **cultural relativism,** meaning that behaviours of individuals should be understood and judged from the context of their own cultural systems (Baker, 1997). The emphasis is thus on healthcare providers becoming knowledgeable about the "cultures of their constituent patients and learning about their lifestyles and culturally determined health beliefs and behaviours" (Dreher & MacNaughton, 2002, p. 181).

In nursing, Madeleine Leininger—who links the concepts of culture and care—is widely recognized as a pioneer cultural literacy theorist. In Chapter 1, we discussed briefly that, through her Theory of Culture Care Diversity and Universality, she introduced the notion of transcultural nursing to the United States, Canada, and abroad as a legitimate and formal area of study and practice

TABLE 2-2

Approaches to Culture and Diversity

APPROACH	FOCUS OF APPROACH	LEARNING STRATEGY	FOCUS OF INTERVENTION	GOAL(S)
Cultural literacy	Individual level	Develop cultural sensitivity and awareness Become informed about cultural traditions, customs, and values in order to serve as an effective culture broker	Clients (individual or group)	Address cultural barriers by developing interventions that reflect/incorporate client cultural values (culturally congruent care)
Relational/ intercultural	Individual level	Develop self-awareness (be cautious of own ethnocentrism and response to difference Approach client from a position of not knowing and of learning from the other	Relationship between the client and the healthcare provider	Avoid cultural imposition Learn from clients about their needs and wishes and include those in the care provided
Anti-racism/ anti-oppression	Organizational or systemic level	Understand and challenge power and hierarchy inherent in all systems Gender, race, and class important categories of difference Challenge personal and institutional racist attitudes	Organizational systems and structures (policies and practices) Identify the various systemic factors that may be impacting on the client's expression and response to illness	Equity and access Social justice
Social realist/ integrative	Individual level and systemic level	Emphasize partnership and a sophisticated awareness of race and culture	System and client	Reduction of health disparities

From *Assessing the responsiveness of health care organizations to culturally diverse groups* (p. 260), by S. Bowen, 2004, Winnipeg: Department of Community Health Sciences, University of Manitoba.

focusing on "comparative human-care (caring) differences and similarities of the beliefs, values, patterned lifeways of cultures to provide culturally congruent, meaningful, and beneficial health care to people" (Leininger, 2002, pp. 5–6). The cultural literacy approach also has been referred to as the cross-cultural or multicultural approach. This approach is not unique to nursing but is also reflected in a broader range of clinical professions including psychology, psychiatry, and social work (Alaggia & Marziali, 2003; Sue, 2001).

From the perspective of traditional cultural literacy, culture is the central concept and the key to understanding differences. In this approach, cultural clashes are said to arise as a result of differences in values, beliefs, assumptions, and expectations of care. Therefore, healthcare providers are encouraged to acquire knowledge about different cultures and cultural patterns, which, in turn, will increase understanding and allow the client and the healthcare provider to work together effectively by accommodating or negotiating around expectations (Alaggia & Marziali, 2003; Leininger, 1991).

Inherent in the cultural literacy approach is the assumption that culture is "out there" to be discovered and that the cultural values related to health and illness are relatively homogeneous and unchanging (Alaggia & Marziali, 2003; Tsang & Bogo, 1997). This approach also minimizes the differences that may exist among members of a particular group. Although Leininger (1991) clearly articulated the concept of professional cultures and the need to understand the beliefs that the nurse or healthcare provider brings to the interaction, her focus was on discovering the healthcare values and patterns of expression related to the health and illness of specific cultural groups. Some critics came to view the cultural literacy path as a "cookbook" approach to health care, with values and beliefs as the identified ingredients. Depending on how culture was defined, there was inevitably an overemphasis on a singular aspect of culture (e.g., religion or ethnicity) without consideration of variations within the group or issues related to acculturation or generational differences. There was considerable concern that knowledge of cultural values would lead to increased stereotyping by healthcare providers (Dreher & MacNaughton, 2002; Duffy, 2001; Nance, 1995). A **stereotype** is when an individual or group is automatically designated to have certain characteristics without further exploration of what actually exists (Kendall, 2002).

As the cultural literacy approach developed, several other limitations became evident. The most obvious limitation is the practical challenge associated with learning about multiple cultures. In a multicultural society, a healthcare provider may encounter several ethnocultural groups in the course of a day. Thus, it would be impossible to expect him or her to learn about the multitude of cultures that he or she would come into contact with daily. The cultural literacy perspective also failed to acknowledge or address issues of discrimination, oppression, and racism (Duffy, 2001; Eisenbruch, 2001; Giest, 1994; Tsang & Bogo, 1997). Other limitations of the cultural literacy perspective included an inherent belief that culture was a "problem," that the "other" was inferior, and that the "norm" was what existed as the majority or status quo (Duffy, 2001; Tsang & Bogo, 1997).

Practically, within the healthcare system, the cultural literacy angle has been characterized as an "add on" approach to health care (Bowen, 2004), put into operation by placing the burden on the individual healthcare provider. The cultural literacy literature largely is targeted to individual healthcare providers, who are expected to add cultural knowledge to their repertoire by learning about the impact of culture on various aspects of health and health care and by learning about specific cultural values of their clients. The role of healthcare providers is to identify and respond to cultural needs and, in a sense, to act as **culture brokers** by striving to perceive the situation from the client's point of view, to compare it to their own, and to mediate between the two to achieve interventions that are mutually derived, satisfactory, and appropriate (DeSantis, 1994). While this approach recognizes the need for the healthcare provider to consciously examine his or her values so that they can be compared to that of the client (DeSantis, 1994; Leininger, 1991), the need for self-awareness is de-emphasized and the focus remains on the cultural "other." Over four decades, transcultural and multicultural scholars have conducted numerous studies on Western and non-Western cultures on a variety of issues related to health, illness, treatment, health care, and cure in a variety of clinical and non-clinical populations (Fernandez & Fernandez, 2005; Masi & Mensah, 1992; McFarland, 2002; Wilkins, 1993). Through research and case-study discussions, actual and potential differences in client and healthcare provider values were highlighted and the consequences of acknowledging and not acknowledging the cultural values and beliefs were discussed.

The need to provide health care that was culturally appropriate also led to the creation of **ethno-specific** (tailored to specific communities) services. Rather than serve a diverse client population, ethno-specific services fill an unmet need for one or more specific underserved population(s). Ethno-specific services can be part of mainstream healthcare organizations (e.g., counselling programs for gay, lesbian, transgendered, and transexual persons; or diabetes initiatives for the South Asian population) or function as agencies (e.g., a mental health agency to serve the Chinese-speaking population, or an Aboriginal health centre).

Ethno-specific agencies largely are found in urban centres where the community groups are significant in size and number. Many of these agencies have their roots in community support groups. Some of the issues that helped community support groups evolve from places to receive information and support into places to receive health care are as follows:

- Lack of culturally appropriate programming
- Non-availability of services in languages other than English
- Inaccessibility of services due to geography or timing

Typically, these ethno-specific agencies are small and use bicultural staff to meet the linguistic and cultural needs of their clients. **Bicultural staff** are individuals who are knowledgeable about the two cultures involved, have some legitimacy in both cultures, and can serve as culture brokers to bridge the cultural gap and negotiate across cultural misunderstandings.

While ethno-specific agencies serve to address a huge gap in services, they frequently operate parallel to the mainstream system and with many limitations in scope, capacity, and funding. Although there are examples of ethno-specific agencies that work together with the mainstream system (Baker, 2001), more often they exist as separate entities, with minimal interactions and without accounting for each other in their plans or activities (Siemiatycki, Rees, Ng, & Rahi, 2001). As clients move across these two solitudes, the risk of healthcare fragmentation grows. The bicultural healthcare workers also may risk heavy workloads and compromised job satisfaction as they attempt to negotiate across cultures and struggle to meet the expectations of multiple groups.

Designating ethno-specific services within mainstream organizations holds out the potential that the rest of the organization will be able to cater to such clients. However, ethno-specific services often are seen as creative initiatives by specific programs or departments, separate from the core functions of the organization. The ethno-specific service becomes the arm of the organization that addresses culture and diversity, often with a hidden underlying assumption that the mainstream system does not need to change.

Another challenge with ethno-specific models of health care is their limited scope. Ethno-specific services usually are targeted to the dominant ethnocultural groups and even then cannot meet all the healthcare needs of their community. Thus, often they focus on specific aspects of health (e.g., mental health) or specific subgroups (e.g., women or the elderly). Expectations of such services (on behalf of both the community and the healthcare provider) generally exceed capacity. Both the "offloading" of culturally diverse groups to ethno-specific healthcare providers and the limited scope of those groups can lead to fewer options for clients and a lack of skill development and change within the healthcare providers and the larger system (Bowen, 2004). The burden for addressing

CULTURAL COMPETENCE IN ACTION

Awareness of Difference
Try to think back to the first time you became aware of cultural differences and answer the following questions:
1. How did you recognize the difference? Perhaps it was when you travelled to a different country or became friends with someone from another background.
2. What was the difference?
3. Did it make you more aware of your own values?
4. Was the difference readily visible, and if so, did the visibility make it harder or easier for you to relate to the other person?

Now consider how you responded to the difference then, and how you might respond to the difference now. Did you have previous knowledge—or have you since acquired such knowledge—about the culture that helped you recognize or understand it? Did knowing about your own culture change the way you perceived certain behaviours or interactions? Did it change how you interacted with the other person?

We all have encounters with cultural differences every day. The extent to which we recognize the differences is important in our becoming aware of and learning from different cultures. The exposure to different cultures often lets us become aware of differences; however, it does not necessarily teach us how to work with the difference comfortably or effectively.

and negotiating cultural issues continues to rest in large part with individuals involved in direct care, who have little time, power, authority, or resources.

Health care organizations have made some attempts to strengthen their ability to respond to diversity. Apart from providing educational and policy support that addresses diversity, such initiatives largely have focused on offering interpreter services and increasing capacity by hiring multilingual staff.

Relational/Intercultural Approach: Postmodern View

Increasing recognition of the limitations associated with the cultural literacy approach gave rise to alternative perspectives. As with the multicultural policy, the academic literature also began to highlight the relational nature of cultural interactions. The contribution and criticism of the cultural literacy approach raised important questions about cultural differences. Should cultural differences between people be highlighted or minimized? As healthcare professionals continued to wrestle with how to apply the knowledge of a cultural group to an individual client without encountering the challenges of stereotyping, the emphasis shifted to meaning and communication. As the language shifted from "culture" to "difference," the healthcare professional's role and culture also gained increased recognition.

The relational approach is based on the belief that culture is individually and socially constructed, rather than a static entity to be discovered. The focus of this approach is on the structure and content of the clinical encounter between the healthcare provider and the client (Dreher & MacNaughton, 2002). This postmodern view highlighted the continually changing and evolving nature of cultures and challenged the healthcare provider's "culture knowledge." Rather than having superior knowledge or preconceived notions about the client, the healthcare provider is expected to approach the client from a position of not knowing, with a curiosity and desire to learn from him or her. As well, healthcare providers are advised to examine their own ethnocentrism to ensure that their own values do not become barriers to appropriate care (Herberg, 1993; Tsang & Bogo, 1997). The relational approach emphasizes development of shared meanings by recognizing and respecting differences between the healthcare provider and the client (Dean, 2001; Dreher & MacNaughton, 2002; Tsang & Bogo, 1997). In the cultural literacy approach, it is the healthcare provider's task to understand the cultural stranger; in the intercultural approach, the onus is on healthcare providers to consider themselves the stranger, recognize their own biases, and respect differences. Along the line, communication became the fundamental process through which cultural values were understood and acknowledged in the plan of care (Dreher & MacNaughton, 2002). Culture came to be viewed not as something that is possessed by individuals, but rather as a dynamic process of engagement that is subject to many influences (Nance, 1995).

At the Point of Care

Although the relational model focused on understanding the client's uniqueness, it has been criticized for imposing an additional burden on the client—that of "educating" the healthcare provider (Alaggia & Marziali, 2003). The inherent assumption is that the client and the healthcare provider have a reciprocal relationship and are able to mutually communicate and understand each other's perspectives. In reality, the assumption that all healthcare providers have the desire and the ability to be aware of their own biases is clearly false. Ethnocentrism on the part of the healthcare providers means that their espoused values are not always enacted (Lister, 1999).

Similarly, clients, especially when they are experiencing a health issue, are frequently unwilling or unable to express their needs and beliefs. The relationship with the healthcare providers also is culturally mediated. For example, among Cree and Ojibwa clients, there is an assumption that the relationship with the healer is one characterized by humility and a commitment to follow the healer's instructions, even if personal sacrifice is involved. As a result, Aboriginal clients may appear passive. However, the reticence of Aboriginal clients also may be due to "attitudes of resignation and alienation in biomedical settings, attitudes that are products of a colonial history" (Lock & Bibeau, 1993, p. 170). Even when beliefs are expressed by the client, they are subject to interpretation by the healthcare provider. Thus, without the contextual knowledge of the culture, the chances of misinterpreting clients' health issues increase significantly. A focus on individualizing problems further obscures the social context of illness to the detriment of the provision of good health care (Lock & Bibeau, 1993).

Three-Step Approach

Katon and Kleinman (1980) contend that socio-cultural factors exert a major influence on the construction of illness, and make a case for applying social science to medical practice. As such, illness is both a social and a biological phenomenon. The illness experience is recognized as being greater than the disease experience, and the biomedical model of health care is described as being considerably narrower than the bio-psycho-social approach. Katon and Kleinman propose a clinical method consisting of three main steps:
1. Determining the client's perception of illness
2. Determining the illness problems
3. Negotiating the care and treatment

Eliciting the client's perception of illness (i.e., Step 1 of Katon and Kleinman method) is also called determining the client's **explanatory model of illness**. The explanatory model of illness includes not just perceptions of the cause of illness, but also perceptions of the severity of illness, the expected treatment, and the prognosis. The explanatory model thus determines the meanings and expectations associated with the illness. The second step is to determine the additional problems that arise as a result of the illness experience (e.g., the experiential, family, economic, interpersonal, occupational, and daily life problems caused by the disease). The third step involves negotiation between the client's preferences for health care and the healthcare provider's recommendations. However, the authors point out that negotiations between healthcare providers and clients are based on unequal power relations and variables such as social class (Katon & Kleinman, 1980). Determining client preferences is a critical aspect of the negotiation process, as is the determination of who (client or key family member[s]) is regarded as the appropriate party to negotiate with. The authors caution, however, that although this broader sociocultural approach allows for consideration of a wider range of treatment options, most healthcare providers have their own preference regarding the therapeutic approach and thus run the risk of constructing symptoms in such a way as to justify their preferred intervention. The client's symptoms are made to fit the theory (Katon & Kleinman, 1980). While Katon and Kleinman's work is largely based in psychiatry, it has been widely adopted by other disciplines, including nursing, dentistry, and pharmacy (Bazaldua & Sias, 2004; College of Nurses of Ontario, 1999; DeSantis, 1994; Formicola Stavisky, & Lewy, 2003).

Katon and Kleinman's (1980) approach is similar to the intercultural approach in that, by focusing on the client's perspective and preferences, it relies on learning from the client rather than on preformed knowledge of cultures. However, the approach involves much more than simply listening to the client. Instead, it involves a complex awareness and understanding of socio-cultural issues and a concerted effort to elicit specific types of information from the client.

Anti-Racism/Anti-Oppression Approach: Socio-Political View

In the late 1980s and early 1990s, many authors began to emphasize that the real challenge facing healthcare clients and the wider society was not culture but the racialization or oppression that existed in society. The so-called different-ness of minority groups began to be recognized as the oppression of minority groups. Behaviour was seen to be influenced less by traditions and more by the way in which the group and individuals within the group were treated in the larger society. This is consistent with Katon and Kleinman's (1980) notion of the reciprocal relationship between the biological and the social course of illness, in which the client's general circumstances influence the severity and type of symptoms expressed, and that expression has a further impact on the client's circumstances (James & Prilleltensky, 2002). The anti-racism approach focuses less on the person and more on the dynamics of difference. The language of culture often is regarded as an excuse and coded logic for racism, and playing up cultural differences is seen as glossing over the client's self-identity or social reality.

The anti-racism approach acknowledges the following three key premises (Yee & Dumbrill, 2003):

1. Racism exists in society.
2. Conflict between racial minorities and dominant groups is due not to lack of contact or to cultural misunderstanding between groups, but rather to power differentials between the dominant group and ethno-racial minorities.
3. One's social, political, and economic relationships are racially structured.

Anti-racism has been described as an action-oriented strategy for institutional change that challenges existing power structures and addresses racism and other interlocking systems of oppression, and is therefore regarded as an effective alternative to multiculturalism (Tsang & George, 1998).

Within the anti-racism perspective, the definition of culture expanded beyond ethnic boundaries and started to highlight the influence of "non-ethnic" variables such as race, class, gender, sexual orientation, and physical ability. The terms "multicultural" and "transcultural" were replaced by terms such as "ethno-racial" and "diversity." Multicultural communities were referred to first as ethno-racial communities, and then as diverse communities, and ultimately the idea of culture got lost in the language of power, inequity, and difference (Srivastava & Leininger, 2002).

The anti-racism perspective clearly highlighted that the concept of power had been missing from the cultural perspective. As well, the newer perspective began to question White power and privilege and its rationale for dominance. From an anti-racism perspective, the "barrier" was not culture or even race; rather, it was the dominance of "Whiteness." The perspective shifted from promoting cultural diversity toward challenging the power and privilege associated with dominance, all of which was synonymous with "Whiteness" (Yee & Dumbrill, 2003).

Although the anti-racism perspective has made a major contribution to the cultural perspectives, it also has several limitations. Anti-racism is aimed primarily at a systemic or organizational level, and it advocates changing the system itself rather than altering what the system does or how it functions. Thus, it has been extremely difficult to gain acceptance for anti-racism among some of the key players in the system, who, one could argue, are largely of members of the dominant group (Yee & Dumbrill, 2003). Anti-racism also has been challenged for its focus on race and its view of cultural difference as simply a source of division and weakness in the struggle against racism (George & Tsang, 1999). Anti-racism has been criticized for lacking sufficient theoretical grounding; instead, the anti-oppression approach is proposed as the base upon which one moves toward the awareness of self, of social inequalities, and of difference among all people (George, 2004). As the perspective of "difference" gained popularity, the variables of race, class, and gender in particular became major categories for understanding difference. However, it can be argued that these concepts are inherently about power relations, inequality, and the way humans relate socially, not about difference itself. In other words, we need to regard "gender," "race," and "class" as terms associated with social difference and not as basic categories of difference (Bottero & Irwin, 2003).

Healthcare providers have found it difficult to apply the anti-racism approach in clinical practice. Even when we can best understand the health issues by placing them in the broader context of racism and can recognize the need for systemic change, it is unclear exactly how the healthcare provider should act to make a difference for a particular client. Although healthcare providers may be aware of the differences in values, beliefs, and expectations, and may be concerned about potential miscommunication, misdiagnosis, and inappropriate care, the anti-racism approach has provided little guidance for translating such awareness into practice.

As is evident from the above discussion, the perspectives on diversity have themselves evolved over time, with each perspective highlighting particular aspects of culture and diversity, and each making a contribution toward an increasingly sophisticated understanding of culture and its role in illness, health, and health care.

The current perspective of the twenty-first century calls for models of integration. Recent models value cultural difference; advocate for insight and awareness into our own values, behaviours, and prejudicial beliefs; and understand the individual problem within such broader issues as racism, oppression, inequity, discrimination, and exclusion (Alaggia & Marziali, 2003; Burchum, 2002; Cortis, 2003; Tsang & George, 1998). In New Zealand, Maori nurse leaders developed the concept of cultural safety to provide a critical lens through which to examine the healthcare interactions between the country's indigenous Maori people and the primary White, European-descendant healthcare providers. Cultural safety extends the cultural focus of understanding health beliefs and practices of different groups to include an examination of power inequities, individual and systemic discrimination, and the unequal power relations in health care (Papps & Ramsden, 1996). Anderson and colleagues (2003) argue for a "rewriting" of this concept to include the social context of illness for all clients and as a way to examine how the social pegging of the client and the healthcare provider affect care (Anderson et al., 2003).

For too long, healthcare providers have struggled to find the "right" language and approach to effectively address issues of culture and diversity in health care. The evolutionary perspectives have led to a more sophisticated understanding of cultural issues as well as the dynamics associated with the broader social environment. There also is an increased call to examine health outcomes, not just approaches to healthcare. The concepts of health disparity and inequity are prominent in the current perspective and development of multi-level cultural competence is seen as a key strategy to address these disparities.

Misconceptions and Myths

The various perspectives on culture and diversity have resulted in a greater understanding of the issues as well as increased confusion and conflict. As a result, a number of cultural myths and misconceptions have arisen that must be examined and challenged in order to develop cultural competence (Masi, 1996). Many of the myths presented in this section were initially identified and discussed by Masi (1996).

Myth #1: The Myth of Equality

This myth refers to the view that fairness means equal treatment for all. It is characteristic of what Williams (2001) describes as the "meritocratist" perspective on diversity, which values hard work, self-reliance, and individualism. Proponents of this perspective cite success stories throughout history in which individuals of all ethnic, racial, and gender backgrounds have achieved goals and outcomes based on their hard work and merit; they argue that if some can succeed, so can all (Williams, 2001). However, this view reflects a lack of awareness, or insensitivity, to systemic barriers and institutional racism. Further, it places the responsibility for success solely on the individual without acknowledging systemic inequities, and may, in fact, lead to unconscious bias and prejudice against individuals and groups who are unable to achieve the desired outcomes with respect to health and illness.

It is widely recognized that while all people may be created equal, they are not created the same. Therefore, the concept of equality must be differentiated from the concept of equity. **Equity** refers to equality with respect to opportunity, access, and outcome and the notion of giving each person her or his due. Achieving equity often requires differential treatment of individuals in order to achieve the same results. In order to provide appropriate and equitable care, healthcare providers have to be aware of differences between groups and biases that may be inherent in the healthcare processes. According to the Canadian Human Rights Commission (McLachlin, 2003), "true equality means a respect for people's different needs" (p. 3).

Myth #2: The Myth of Sameness

This myth suggests that clients receive the best care from healthcare providers of their own background. Attempts to match clients and healthcare providers of the same ethnic background is referred to as **ethnic matching** and is based on the assumption that cultural differences between client and healthcare provider can lead to miscommunication, misdiagnosis, and inappropriate care. Therefore, it follows that if we decreased or eliminated the "difference" between healthcare provider and client, we also would substantially decrease the possibility of miscommunication. This is particularly true if healthcare providers and clients can be matched on the basis of language because language differences are one of the most pervasive issues encountered in cross-cultural health care. The approach is supported by proponents of the anti-racism approach, as well as by healthcare administrators who argue that the dominant culture lacks or has limited sensitivity to the life experiences of clients from so-called minority cultural groups (Bowen, 2004).

Masi (1996) refers to this myth as the fallacy of "like should treat like" (p. 150). There are at least three questions that must be asked when assessing this fallacy:

1. How do we determine that "like" really is "like"?
2. Do the clients prefer someone who is from a "like" culture or someone from a different culture?
3. What is the impact of this myth on the healthcare provider?

The assumption that someone who shares the client's ethnicity and language will provide more effective healthcare needs to be challenged. The visible similarity may only be skin deep and many other factors may influence similarity and the provision of care. The presence of bicultural workers does not always ensure a cultural fit, nor does it address the underlying issues of racism and discrimination. Further, since the capacity to deal with a specific culture depends on particular individuals, it is transient—as people leave, the ability to provide culturally specific health care is drastically reduced, leading to ongoing challenges in the continuity and sustainability of care.

Research evidence on ethnic matching is mixed. There is some evidence that it leads not only to improved communication but also to enhanced trust and confidence, appropriate use (e.g., decreased visits to the emergency room and crisis services, and increased follow-up in outpatient programs), and improved satisfaction (Bowen, 2004; Chin & Humikowski, 2002; Gray & Stodared, 1997; Snowden, Hu, & Jerrell, 1995; Ziguras, Klimidis, Lewis, & Stuart, 2003); however, the processes that lead to the success are unclear. Variables such as gender, class, education, and occupation (i.e., factors associated with social difference) can outweigh shared cultural origins, and thus it is the similarity in values that is more critical than race or ethnicity (Masi, 1996).

Increasing workforce diversity is commonly identified as a way that organizations can become culturally responsive; however, the view that this is *the* answer also is a misconception. Ensuring that healthcare providers are from diverse ethnic communities does not in itself address issues of good health care. All healthcare providers, regardless of their personal background, need to develop the necessary competence to provide health care in a multicultural society.

The myth of sameness also denies client preferences and needs. There are many instances where clients will prefer *not* to seek a provider with the same culture. The reasons most frequently cited for this are confidentiality, social distance, and perceived (or actual) cultural bias on the part of the provider. Cultural communities often are small and close knit, and clients sometimes express concerns about the potential for breaches in confidentiality when they can expect to encounter their healthcare providers in social situations. In addition, if particular conditions, diseases, or treatment are considered culturally unacceptable, clients may shy away from seeking a healthcare provider from that culture. A woman seeking an abortion, for example, may be hesitant about going to a physician affiliated with an orthodox Roman Catholic Church (Masi, 1996).

The myth of sameness presents other challenges. Not only can ethnic matching go against the client's best interests, but it is frequently contrary to the healthcare provider's best interests. Even when the "like" is in fact "like," we have to be aware of the dynamics and expectations that may be created for the clients. Clients frequently have different expectations of heathcare providers who share their own ethnocultural heritage than they do of other healthcare providers. Clients may believe that the similarity will translate into increased understanding and an ability to provide something extra or different than routine care. Such expectations can lead to challenges for the healthcare provider in maintaining professional boundaries. The expectation that certain healthcare providers work primarily with members of their own communities also can be limiting and affect professional career and growth opportunities for the healthcare providers (Masi, 1996). US research also indicates that although minority clients are more likely to seek and receive health care from minority physicians, there may be financial and other disadvantages to using the non-White physicians (Moy & Bartman, 1996). While targeted use of staff resources can be helpful, particularly in the short term, the long-term goal should focus on increasing the capacity of the individual healthcare providers and the system to deal with clients from non-dominant cultures.

CULTURAL CONSIDERATIONS IN CARE

A Special Bond with the Client

Ms. Singh, a 23-year-old East Indian woman, was referred to the nephrology program for chronic renal failure. She needed dialysis until a kidney transplant became available.

The nephrology team consisted of a physician (of British background), a social worker (a White female Canadian), and a clinical nurse specialist (CNS) of East Indian origin. The client's first language was Punjabi, but she was able to communicate in English. The CNS was fluent in Hindi and had some familiarity with Punjabi, and the client had sufficient familiarity with Hindi to be able to communicate with the CNS in a mixture of Hindi and Punjabi; subsequently, the two developed a special bond.

Ms. Singh started to regard the CNS as a big sister, which she even stated on more than one occasion. As a result, the client started to disclose personal information regarding her marriage and family, but insisted that this information not be shared with other members of the healthcare team. The social worker was involved in Ms. Singh's health care with respect to assisting with financial support and making arrangements for dialysis supplies. The client did not share the marital and family concerns with the social worker as she did not feel comfortable talking about her personal affairs with strangers and also because she feared that issues would be taken out of the cultural context and create difficulties for her family members.

Friction occurred within the team. The social worker became frustrated and felt that she was being underutilized by the client and that the CNS was undermining her role. Subsequently, the client received a transplant and was unwilling to let go of the CNS, and continued to direct questions and concerns toward the CNS instead of the transplantation team. Ms. Singh would frequently leave messages for the CNS that led to delays in the overall response to client issues, which interfered with the communication and relationship with the transplantation team. The CNS also felt torn: on the one hand, she wanted to provide continuity in care and support for the client, but on the other, the relationship was creating difficulties.

1. Discuss this scenario from the perspective of the client, the CNS, and the other team members.
2. Identify strategies that could best make use of the diversity within the team and prevent some of the difficulties encountered.

Myth #3: Cultural Differences Are a Problem

Within health care, issues of culture and diversity have largely been viewed from a negative standpoint, with a focus on cultural differences and the resulting problems. Culture is frequently regarded as a barrier to be overcome. It is true that differences in cultural values may, at times, lead to conflict, but it is important to remember that values and beliefs play significant positive roles in people's lives. The view of culture as a barrier or a problem can limit the healthcare provider's ability to understand the positive aspects of beliefs and values, particularly when they are different from those of the healthcare provider.

Seeing culture as a barrier often leads to a response of avoidance. Consider what most people do when they encounter a barrier: they tend to go around it or over it with the hopes of getting to the other side as quickly and efficiently as possible. When culture is regarded as a barrier to be overcome, the healthcare provider is likely to focus on ways of getting the client to accept predetermined goals or solutions. However, experience shows that people will ultimately choose what they think is right for them. While a healthcare provider may be successful in minimizing the influence of cultural values and beliefs in the short term, the cultural issues are likely to resurface.

It would be more effective to recognize that the barriers do not result from the clients' cultures but rather from the values and beliefs inherent in the biomedical culture, and from insufficient professional training as well as barriers in the healthcare system (Tripp-Reimer, Choi, Kelley, & Enslein, 2001). An alternative concept is to view culture not as problem to be overcome but as a leverage point—a point that can affect the outcome significantly if energy is focused on it. Focusing on cultural consideration in health care can be a powerful tool in providing health care that is relevant and meaningful for the client, and in turn will lead to more positive outcomes in the actual health of clients.

Myth #4: Everything Must Be Acceptable

Many healthcare providers struggle with the boundaries of what is acceptable when it comes to cultural issues. There is a perception that if something is a "cultural value," it must be accepted (Masi, 1996). This is simply not true. Respect must not be confused with acceptance. Health care must be provided within the parameters of legal and professional boundaries, and behaviours have to be interpreted within the context of the legal system. Clients need to be informed about unacceptable behaviour and its consequences. However, wherever

---

CULTURAL CONSIDERATIONS IN CARE

Exorcism as Part of the Plan of Care
Within the mental health setting, clients and families may have concepts of illness that are vastly different from the physicians'.

In eliciting one particular client and family's explanatory model of illness, it became apparent that the client and family believed that supernatural forces were behind the illness, and they wished to have an exorcism performed by a spiritual leader. Although the psychiatrist did not believe in exorcism or subscribe to this explanatory model, he understood the family's need for such an intervention and negotiated with them to have the treatment performed outside the hospital. By doing so, he was able to maintain a trusting relationship with the family and to continue to provide care from the biomedical perspective.

The message here is that respect does not equal acceptance or endorsement; rather, it means respecting client choices even when they are not understood or sanctioned by the healthcare provider.

possible, this needs to be done in ways that continue to acknowledge respect and with a view toward maintaining the healthcare provider–client relationship for future interactions (College of Nurses of Ontario, 1999). Masi (1996) uses the example of child abuse to illustrate this misconception. Child abuse, clearly, is unacceptable in our society. However, what constitutes child abuse may vary with different individuals. Cultural practices such as "scratching the wind"—where bruises are caused by cupping and scratches are created by running a coin on the skin for the purpose of relieving fever or illness—may not be considered to be child abuse in some cultures (Masi, 1996). Of course, healthcare providers must not overlook suspected abuse, but they also need to understand the cultural context in which such practices may not be malevolent in intent.

Other behaviours, such as substance abuse or partner violence in immigrant communities, need to be understood in the context of the unique vulnerabilities of the population in question but should not be confused with acceptable cultural practice.

Myth #5: Generalizations Are Unacceptable

Many professionals claim that generalizations about any cultural group are inappropriate (Masi, 1996). The cultural literacy approach is criticized chiefly on the basis that generalizations are not appropriate because they ignore variations within a cultural group and therefore stereotype individuals. The term "culture" refers to shared values, beliefs, norms, and patterns. Shared values do not preclude individual differences. Generalizations are necessary to understand groups, but they should not be imposed upon individuals within the groups. It is important to differentiate between generalizations and stereotypes. Generalizations are a necessary beginning point, indicating trends and patterns that require additional information as to their appropriateness and applicability to specific individuals and situations; stereotypes are an "end point" in which complexities are not explored and assumptions are imposed (Kendall, 2002, p. 22). Generalizations often are useful in helping healthcare providers begin a conversation with some understanding of common traits that may be relatively consistent within and across populations. Stereotypes close conversations and knowledge development.

There are many compelling reasons why healthcare professionals need to be careful about generalizations. However, the need for caution must not be confused with inappropriateness. Learning about the needs of cardiac clients does not mean stereotyping all cardiac clients to have exactly the same needs and does not preclude individualized care. Healthcare providers do not impose the knowledge or the predetermined intervention on the client without validating need and appropriateness. Similarly, learning about communities based on shared characteristics other than illness or diagnosis need not be considered problematic.

Myth #6: Familiarity Equals Competence

For many Canadians, living in a diverse society has made us complacent and over-confident about our understanding of diversity. Frequently, healthcare providers will state that they are comfortable with diversity since a multicultural clientele is a regular feature of their practice, and yet they are unable to describe the impact that diversity has on their practice, especially with respect to how they engage with the client and the subsequent health care and treatment that is offered (Srivastava, 2004). Familiarity with difference paradoxically makes the difference invisible. Similarly, international exposure through travel may be helpful but is not on a par with the systematic development of cultural knowledge and understanding. Cultural competence requires a desire and a commitment to learn both about and from the cultures to which one is exposed locally, nationally, and internationally.

Cultural Paradoxes

The varied perspectives, myths, and misconceptions about culture clearly reveal that cultural issues are a dynamic, complex, and often paradoxical phenomenon. Within a group, they are both universal and diverse. The paradoxical nature of cultural issues can be understood through the principles of complexity thinking—a way of thinking that simultaneously seeks to distinguish (but not separate) and to connect. "To understand complexity is to know how to accept ambiguity, contradiction, the inaccuracy of concepts and the phenomenon and to accept the unexplainable" (Browaeys & Baets, 2003, p. 336).

The following three key aspects of complexity thinking can be used to help understand cultural competence:

1. The dialogic principle
2. The principle of recursivity
3. The hologrammic perspective

The term "dialogic" means that two logics can exist together without the dual nature being lost in the unit. The dialogic principle allows for contradictory notions to exist together. Culture is about groups in a system as well as about individuals, where the individual is simultaneously part of and separate from the group. The principle of recursivity means that causes simultaneously are effects. "Individuals create the society which in turn creates the individuals [and] this is a recursive process" (Browaeys & Baets, 2003, p. 336). Culture is about differences and the differences in turn have an impact on cultural ways of being. Individuals create culture through their interactions; at the same time, culture influences the interactions that occur. In the hologrammic principle, parts and wholes co-exist simultaneously. It is similar to the dialogic principle in that the parts are present in the whole; the difference is that the whole also is reflected in the parts. This principle "goes beyond reductionism, that only sees the parts, and holism, that only sees the whole. Holons or whole/parts are entities that are both wholes and parts of ever greater wholes" (Browaeys & Baets, 2003, p. 336). Similarly, individuals are whole entities but also are part of a cultural group and carry the culture as a whole around with them.

Another characteristic of complexity thinking is that it suggests a strategy or an approach instead of a specific program of knowledge. **Strategy** means a "guide in the uncertainty" (Browaeys & Baets, 2003, p. 339), and is based on the particular circumstance or objective. Strategy is not a predetermined method that is applicable in all situations; rather, it allows healthcare providers to move forward with an approach that can be modified as the situation unfolds. Viewing culture and cultural competence through the prism of complexity means that the development of cultural competence is an approach or a strategy, not a program full of specific content and information.

The Culture Care Framework described in the next chapter is presented as an approach to developing cultural competence. It is a strategy that can be applied by healthcare providers to develop their understanding of cultures and to apply the principles of cultural competence in their clinical encounters. There are no universal methods that work in all circumstances or across all cultures. The framework will guide the healthcare provider in exploring the uncertain world of cultures and assisting in navigating the complexities to allow new discoveries of what is possible.

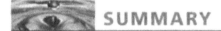 ## SUMMARY

This chapter has presented an evolution of thinking on culture and diversity. In addition to discussing the multicultural policy in Canada, it examined three major perspectives on culture and health care with respect to their strengths, limitations, and contributions to current thinking on cultural competence. These perspectives are: (1) The traditional approach of cultural literacy. It has helped us to recognize that there are different world views and ways of being that are critical to the client's health experience. The approach has highlighted the need to negotiate care based on the clients' values, and recognized that the values of the healthcare provider may be different. (2) The relational/intercultural perspective. It holds that cultures need to be understood in context, and has helped to alert healthcare providers to potential miscommunication, inaccurate diagnosis, and ineffective care. (3) The anti-racism/anti-oppression perspective. This has helped identify the need to look at power, the inherent barriers within the healthcare system, and the impact of multiple factors and oppressions on the expression and experience of illness and health.

Common myths and misconceptions that can become hindrances to developing cultural competence also were discussed. The chapter ended with a discussion of the principles of complexity thinking that illustrated the paradoxes of cultural issues and the need to develop an approach to cultural competence that provides a strategy or guide instead of a program of knowledge.

REFERENCES

Alaggia, R., & Marziali, E. (2003). Social work with Canadians of Italian background: Applying cultural concepts to bicultural and intergenerational issues in clinical practice. In A. Al-Krenaw & J. R. Graham (Eds.), *Multicultural social work in Canada* (pp. 150–173). Don Mills: Oxford University Press.

American Heritage Dictionaries (2000). *The American heritage dictionary of the English language* (4th ed.). Boston: Houghton Mifflin Company.

Anderson, J., Perry, J., Blue, C., Brown, A., Henderson, A., Basu Khan, K., Reimer Kikham, S., Lynam, J., Semeniuk, P., & Smye V. (2003). Rewriting cultural safety within the postcolonial and postnational feminist project: Towards new epistemologies of healing. *Advances in Nursing Science, 26*(3), 196–214.

Baker, C. (1997). Cultural relativism and cultural diversity: Implications for nursing practice. *Advances in Nursing Science, 20*(1), 3–11.

Baker, C. (2001). *Service provision by representative institutions and identity.* Halifax: Department of Canadian Heritage.

Bazaldua, O., & Sias, J. (2004). Cultural competence: A pharmacy perspective. *Journal of Pharmacy Practice, 17*(3), 160–166.

Bottero, W., & Irwin, S. (2003). Locating difference, class, race, and gender, and the shaping of social inequalities. *The Sociological Review, 51*(4), 463–483.

Bowen, S. (2004). *Assessing the responsiveness of health care organizations to culturally diverse groups.* Winnipeg: Department of Community Health Sciences. University of Manitoba.

Browaeys, M., & Baets, W. (2003). Cultural complexity: A new epistemological perspective. *The Learning Organization, 10*(6), 332–339.

Browne, A. J., & Smye, V. (2002). A post-colonial analysis of health care discourses addressing Aboriginal women. *Nurse Researcher, 9*(3), 28–41.

Burchum, J. L. (2002). Cultural competence: An evolutionary perspective. *Nursing Forum, 37*(4), 5–11.

Canadian Heritage. (2004). Annual report on the operation of the *Canadian Multicultural Act*, 2002–2003. Retrieved June 14, 2004, from http://www.pch.gc.ca/progs/multi/reports/ann2002–2003/cont_e.cfm

Centre for Canadian Studies. (n.d.). *Multiculturalism in Canada.* Sackville, NB: Mount Allison University, Centre for Canadian Studies. Retrieved February 21, 2004, from http://www.mta.ca/faculty/arts/canadian_studies/english/about/multi/

Chin, M. H., & Humikowski, C. A. (2002). When is risk stratification by race or ethnicity justified in medical care? *Academic Medicine, 77*(3), 202–208.

College of Nurses of Ontario. (1999). *Guidelines for providing culturally sensitive care.* Toronto, Author.

Cortis, J. D. (2003). Culture, values and racism: Application to nursing. *International Nursing Review, 50*, 55–64.

Dean, R. (2001). The myth of cross-cultural competence. *Families in Society, 82*(6), 623–630.

DeSantis, L. (1994). Making anthropology clinically relevant to nursing care. *Journal of Advanced Nursing, 20*(4), 707–715.

Dreher, M., & MacNaughton, N. (2002). Cultural competence in nursing: Foundation or fallacy. *Nursing Outlook, 50*(5), 181–186.

Duffy, M. E. (2001). A critique of cultural education in nursing. *Journal of Advanced Nursing, 36*(4), 487–495.

Eisenbruch, M. (2001). National review of nursing education: Multicultural nursing education, Sydney: University of New South Wales, Higher Education Division. Retrieved June 10, 2004, from http://www.dest.gov.au/archive/highered/nursing/pubs/multi_cultural/1.htm

Elliott, G. (1999). *Cross cultural awareness in an aging society: Effective strategies for communication and caring.* Hamilton, ON: McMaster University, Office of Gerontological Studies.

Esses, V., & Gardner, R. C. (1996). Multiculturalism in Canada: Context and current status. *Canadian Journal of Behavioural Science, 28*(3), 145–154.

Fernandez, V., & Fernandez, K. (2005). *Transcultural nursing: Basic concepts and case studies.* Retrieved July 7, 2005, from http://www.culturediversity.org

Formicola, A., Stavisky, J., & Lewy, R. (2003). Cultural competence: Dentistry and medicine learning from one another. *Journal of Dental Education, 67*(8), 869–875.

George, U. (2004). *Diversity and equity in professional education.* Presentation made to Faculty of Nursing Symposium. Perspectives on diversity and equity in professional education. (January 21, 2004). Toronto: University of Toronto.

George, U., & Tsang, A. K. T. (1999). Towards an inclusive paradigm in social work: The diversity framework. *The Indian Journal of Social Work, 60*(1), 57–68.

Giest, P. (1994). Negotiating cultural understanding in health care communication. In R. Porter, & L. Samovar (Eds.), *Intercultural Communication: A Reader.* (pp. 311–319). Belmont, CA: Wadsworth.

Gray, B., & Stodared, J. (1997). Patient–physician pairing: Does racial and ethnic congruity influence selection of a regular physician? *Journal of Community Health, 22*(4), 247–259.

Herberg, D. C. (1993). *Frameworks for cultural and racial diversity.* Toronto: Canadian Scholars' Press.

Human Resources and Skills Development Canada. (2001). *Employment Equity Act review: A report to the Standing Committee on Human Resources Development and the Status of Persons with Disabilities, Ottawa.* Retrieved December 31, 2005, from http://www.hrsdc.gc.ca/en/lp/lo/lswe/we/review/report/main.shtml#2

James, S., & Prilleltensky, I. (2002). Cultural diversity and mental health: Towards integrative practice. *Clinical Psychology Review, 22,* 1133–1154.

Katon, W., & Kleinman, A. (1980). Doctor–patient negotiation and other social science strategies in patient care. In L. Eisenberg & S. Klimidis (Eds.), *The Relevance of Social Science for Medicine.* (pp. 253–279). Boston: D. Reidel Publishing.

Kendall, J. K. (2002). Racism as a source of health disparity in families with attention deficit hyperactivity disorder. *Advances in Nursing Science, 25*(2), 22–39.

Leininger, M. (1991). The theory of culture care diversity and universality. In M. Leininger (Ed.), *Culture care diversity and universality: A theory of nursing* (pp. 5–72). New York: National League for Nursing.

Leininger, M. (2002). Transcultural nursing and globalization of health care. In M. Leininger & M. R. McFarland (Eds.), *Transcultural nursing: Concepts, theories, research and practice* (3rd ed., pp. 3–43). New York: McGraw Hill.

Lister, P. (1999). A taxonomy for developing cultural competence. *Nursing Education Today, 19,* 313–318.

Lock, M., & Bibeau, G. (1993). Healthy disputes: Some reflections on the practice of medical anthropology in Canada. *Health and Canadian Society/Santé et Sociétée Canadienne, 1*(1): 147–175.

Masi, R. (1996). Inclusion: How can a health system respond to diversity. In A. S. Zieberth (Ed.), *Pinched: A management guide to the Canadian health care archipelago* (pp.147–157). Nepean, ON: Pinched Press.

Masi, R., & Mensah, L. (Eds.). (1992). *Health and cultures: Exploring the relationships.* Oakville, ON: Mosaic Press.

McClanagahan, L. (1995). *Diversity: Corporate Canada from an international perspective.* Simon Fraser University at Harbour Centre: Centre for International Communication. Retrieved February 8, 2005, from http://www.cic.sfu.ca/forum/NeilMcDonaldSummary.html

McFarland, M. R. (2002). Selected research findings from the culture care theory. In M. Leininger & M. R. McFarland (Eds.), *Transcultural nursing: Concepts, theories, research and practice* (3rd ed., pp. 99–116). New York: McGraw Hill.

McLachlin, B. (Ed.). (2003). A place for all: A guide to creating an inclusive workplace. (Cat. No. HR21-55/2001). Ottawa: Minister of Public Works and Government Services. Canadian Human Rights Commission.

Moy, E., & Bartman, B. (1996). Physician race and care of medically indigent patients. *Journal of the American Medical Association, 273*(19): 1515–1520.

"Mutliculturalism" (February 7, 2006). *Wikipedia, The Free Encyclopedia.* Retrieved February 8, 2006, from http://en.wikipedia.org/wiki/Multiculturalism

Nance, T. (1995). Intercultural communication: Finding common ground. *Journal of Obstetric, Gynecologic, and Neonatal Nursing, 24*(3): 249–255.

Papps, E., & Ramsden, I. (1996). Cultural safety in nursing: The New Zealand experience. *International Journal of Quality Health Care, 8*(5): 491–497.

Siemiatycki, M., Rees, T., Ng, R., & Rahi, K. (2001). *Integrating community diversity in Toronto: On whose terms?* Toronto: CERIS.

Snowden, L., Hu, T., & Jerrell, J. M. (1995). Emergency care avoidance: Ethnic matching and participation in minority-serving programs. *Community Mental Health Journal, 31*(5): 463–467.

Srivastava, R. (2004). *Influence of organizational factors on clinical cultural competence.* Toronto: University of Toronto, Institute of Medical Sciences.

Srivastava, R., & Leininger, M. (2002). Canadian transcultural nursing: Trends and issues. In M. Leininger & M. R. McFarland (Eds.), *Transcultural nursing: Concepts, theories, research and practice* (3rd ed., pp. 493–502). New York: McGraw-Hill.

Sue, D. W. (2001). Multidimensional facets of cultural competence. *The Counseling Psychologist, 29*(6): 790–821.

Tripp-Reimer, T., Choi, E., Kelley, L., & Enslein, J. (2001). Cultural barriers to care: Inverting the problem. *Diabetes Spectrum, 14*(1): 13–22.

Tsang, A. K. T., & Bogo, M. (1997). Engaging with clients cross culturally: Towards developing a research based practice. *Journal of Multicultural Social Work, 6*(3–4): 73–91.

Tsang, A. K. T., & George, U. (1998). Towards an integrated framework for cross cultural social work practice. *Canadian Social Work Review, 15*(1): 73–93.

Webster's New Millennium Dictionary of English, Preview Edition (2005). Longbeach, CA: Lexico Publishing Group, LLC.

Wilkins, H. (1993). Transcultural nursing: A selective review of the literature, 1985–1991. *Journal of Advanced Nursing, 18*: 602–612.

Williams, M. (2001). *The 10 lenses: Your guide to living and working in a multicultural world.* Sterling, VA: Capital Books.

Yee, J. Y., & Dumbrill, G. C. (2003). Whiteout: Looking for race in Canadian social work practice. In A. Al-Krenaw & J. R. Graham (Eds.), *Multicultural social work in Canada* (pp. 98–121). Toronto: Oxford University.

Ziguras, S., Klimidis, S., Lewis, J., & Stuart, G. (2003). Ethnic matching of clients and clinicians and use of mental health services by ethnic minority clients. *Psychiatric Services, 54*, 535–541.

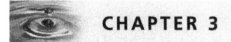

CHAPTER 3

Culture Care Framework I: Overview and Cultural Sensitivity

RANI SRIVASTAVA

LEARNING OBJECTIVES

At the end of this chapter, the learner will be able to:

- Describe the assumptions and main features of the Culture Care Framework
- Discuss cultural sensitivity, cultural knowledge, and cultural resources and how they work together to foster cultural competence
- Apply the framework to facilitate personal development of cultural sensitivity
- Discuss the factors that influence the cultural dynamics of a healthcare provider–client relationship
- Discuss the barriers and building blocks to equity and how they can be purposefully applied to promote cultural competence in clinical care

KEY TERMS

Cultural knowledge	Legacies
Cultural resources	Meritocracy
Cultural sensitivity	Power
Culturally congruent care	Privilege
Culture care	Self-reflexivity
Equity	Specific cultural knowledge
Generic cultural knowledge	Trust
Identity	World view
Layers	

This chapter begins with an examination of the Culture Care Framework, including a discussion of its development, salient features, and applicability in practice. The chapter focuses largely on the first element of the framework: cultural sensitivity. This is a critical part of the foundation of cultural competence and often is the aspect that is hardest to understand. Chapter 4 will provide further discussion of the cultural knowledge and resources aspects of the framework, as well as strategies to bridge the gap across cultures.

The aim of the Culture Care Framework is to make culture visible and to give healthcare providers a way of understanding and working with cultural complexities and cultural influences on health and health care. As noted throughout the discussion, the framework is based on, and uses, many of the core concepts in Madeleine Leininger's Theory of Culture Care Diversity and Universality (Leininger 1995). However, the framework is a more integrative and practical approach, reflecting the issues of power as well as cultural patterns. Figure 3-1 presents the core principle underlying the framework.

The Culture Care Framework was first developed by Rani Srivastava (1996). It has evolved out of her attempts to apply and teach cultural understanding in clinical situations as well as from ongoing discussions with nurses (from a variety of clinical settings), physicians, social workers, dieticians, and volunteers. Healthcare providers practising in a diverse, multicultural society are acutely aware of the need to provide care that is consistent with a client's cultural values, but they continue to face the challenge, often on a daily basis, of how to apply this understanding in practice. Leininger (1995) defined **culture care** as "subjectively and objectively learned and transmitted values, beliefs, and patterned lifeways that assist, support, facilitate, or enable another individual or group to maintain well-being and health, to improve the human condition and lifeway, or to deal

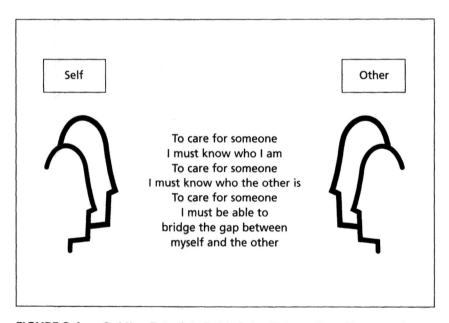

FIGURE 3-1 ▪ **Guiding Principle Behind the Culture Care Framework**
From "The cultural context of caring," by J. Anderson, 1987, *Canadian Critical Care Nursing Journal, 4*(4), 7–13.

with illness, handicaps, and death" (p. 105). Simply put, the term "culture care" reflects the goal of integrating the issues of culture into all aspects of health care. Table 3-1 highlights the main features of the Culture Care Framework.

Overview of the Framework

Culture care can be described as an approach to health care that stresses understanding and interacting in a manner that respects and integrates the values, beliefs, and expectations of others. In order for clinical practice to reflect cultural competence, healthcare providers need to learn to do the following:

- Be aware of the care processes that may be affected by culture
- Be able to ascertain client values and preferences
- Recognize the gaps that may exist between client values and healthcare provider values
- Work with clients to bridge the gaps that may exist between client values and needs, healthcare provider values and needs, and the care that is provided

The complexities of culture can make this an overwhelming task; however, the framework offers an approach that allows for these issues to be addressed in clinical care.

Assumptions Behind the Culture Care Framework

Set out below are the assumptions behind the culture care framework:

- Culture influences every aspect of our lives, yet rarely intrudes into conscious thought (Leininger, 1990).
- Culture is both individual and shared. Culture is universal in the human experience, yet each local, regional, or individual manifestation of it is unique (Leininger, 1990). In other words, while individuals may share characteristics, values, and beliefs with others, the degree to which the characteristics are shared can vary greatly.
- Individuals may belong to many cultures.
- We all approach a situation from our own individual and cultural bias.
- Cultural differences are not about right or wrong—just differences.
- Self-awareness is the first and most critical step for developing cultural competence.

TABLE 3-1

Salient Features of the Culture Care Framework

- Integrates patterns and power perspectives of cultural diversity
- Focuses on self-awareness
- Provides a way of "knowing the other"
- Suggests strategies for bridging the gap between self and other
- Recognizes the interactions between the individual and his or her context
- Provides a way of moving beyond understanding and awareness to application

▪ Responses to situations are shaped by beliefs as well as circumstances. That is, some responses are similar regardless of circumstances, while others are largely determined by circumstances. Most often, responses reflect a combination of the two.

▪ Responses to differences are automatic, frequently negative, often unconscious, and influence the dynamics of all interactions.

Goal(s) for Integrating Culture into Health Care

One of the difficulties associated with translating cultural awareness into practice is uncertainty about the exact goal. Ridley, Baker, and Hill (2001) note that, despite the vast amount of literature available, most healthcare providers cannot verify that their clinical practices actually demonstrate cultural competence. In a study of clinical cultural competence, Srivastava (2004) interviewed healthcare providers and asked what cultural competence looks like in practice. The need for integrating client values was readily acknowledged, but healthcare providers (nurses, doctors, social workers, and occupational therapists) had difficulty expressing how these values were elicited and, more important, how they were integrated into care. Healthcare providers also had difficulty identifying how they knew they had been successful in demonstrating cultural competence (Srivastava, 2004).

In the Culture Care Framework, the goal of care is identified as **culturally congruent care**. The notion of congruence is important because it suggests a "fit" between two or more parties. Leininger (1995) defines culturally congruent care as "acts or decisions that are tailor made to fit with individual, group, or institutional cultural values, beliefs, and lifeways in order to provide or support meaningful, beneficial, and satisfying health care or well-being services" (p. 106). Although Leininger's definition is comprehensive, it can seem overwhelming to healthcare providers in a fast-paced healthcare environment. The Culture Care Framework offers a simpler interpretation, defining culturally congruent care as care that incorporates key values and beliefs of the client in a given situation. Healthcare providers are not expected to be familiar with all aspects of a client's culture; rather, the intent is to identify the most important client and healthcare provider values that may be affecting the situation at hand. The goal of congruence serves as a reminder for healthcare providers to ensure that client and healthcare provider values have been made explicit and that the plan of care reflects client goals—not only the goals established by the clinical team. Healthcare providers can use this criterion to audit their own practice for cultural competence. There are different approaches that can be taken to elicit client values and goals and to achieve congruence; these will be further discussed in the next chapter on bridging the gap across cultures.

Structural Elements of the Framework

An overview of the Culture Care Framework appears in Figure 3-2. Essentially, the framework consists of three broad elements: cultural sensitivity, cultural knowledge, and cultural resources. The framework contends that all three elements are needed to provide culturally congruent care and that true cultural competence requires development in each of the three areas.

Cultural sensitivity refers to awareness, understanding, and attitude toward culture, and places the focus on the self. **Cultural knowledge** identifies that cultural competence is more than just an attitude and is, in fact, knowledge-based care. Cultural knowledge has two components: **generic cultural knowledge** or fundamental knowledge that can be applied across cultural and clinical populations, and **specific cultural knowledge** that is focused on specific clinical or cultural populations. The third element, **cultural resources,** recognizes that what happens in a particular clinical interaction depends not only on the competence of the healthcare provider but also on the resources available in the healthcare environment.

Finally, the framework is action-oriented and uses Leininger's (1995) modes of decision making as the basic approaches for bridging the gap across cultures. In order for cultural competence to be truly put into practice, it is necessary to go beyond merely understanding culture. Healthcare providers need models that will guide them on what to do differently within specific instances of their work to be more culturally competent (Ridley et al., 2001). Leininger's (1995) modes of decision making offer that guidance.

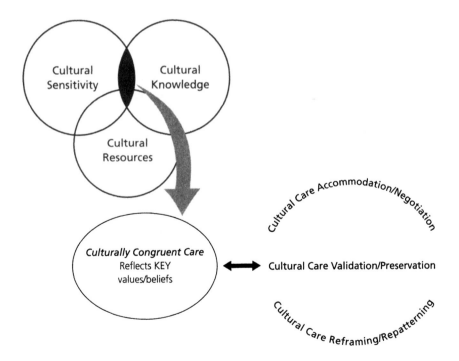

FIGURE 3-2 ▪ **Overview of the Culture Care Framework**
For a complete discussion of the terms accommodation/negotiation, validation/preservation, and reframing/repatterning, please refer to Chapter 4.

Cultural Sensitivity

The concept of cultural sensitivity is broad and includes the notion of cultural awareness. Cultural awareness has been described as "the deliberate cognitive process in which healthcare providers become appreciative and sensitive to the values, beliefs, lifeways, practices, and problem solving strategies of clients' cultures" (Camphina-Bacote, 1999, p. 204). Cultural sensitivity, as depicted in the Culture Care Framework, is neither an inherent personality trait nor a simple matter of focus; rather, it is a complex set of perceptions about culture, oneself, and the dynamics associated with issues of difference (see Figure 3-3). Although cultural awareness can be considered as "knowing that," sensitivity requires a greater degree of proficiency and includes "knowing how." The concepts of "knowing that" and "knowing how" have been discussed by authors such as Patricia Benner (1984) in the context of nursing skill development from novice to expert. "Knowing that" is described as theoretical knowledge acquired through systematically examining a phenomenon; "knowing how" is considered to be practical knowledge and the skills acquired through experience and practice.

Cultural sensitivity requires developing insight as follows:

- Understanding the concept of culture
- Understanding our own culture, including values, biases, and prejudices
- Understanding the dynamics of difference and relationships

Understanding Culture

As discussed in Chapter 1, culture is a difficult concept to grasp. The definitions are complex and ambiguous at the same time and essentially describe culture as something that applies to any group of people whose members share values and ways of thinking and acting that differ from those of people outside the group. A simple description of culture is reflected by the letters C.U.L.T.U.R.E. (see "Definition of Culture" box).

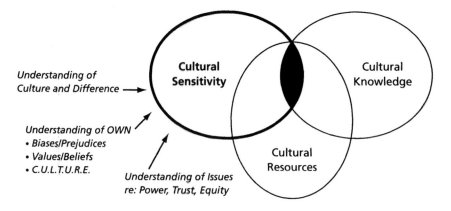

FIGURE 3-3 ▪ **Cultural Sensitivity**

DEFINITION OF CULTURE

Culture is...
    Commonly
    Understood
    Learned
    Traditions and
    Unconscious
    Rules of
    Engagement

Culture is something *commonly understood* by those who share it—it is the common world view, values, and beliefs that are clear to those who are a part of the cultural group, but foreign to others. A **world view** is the "way in which an individual or group looks out on and understands their world about them as a value, stance, picture, or perspective about life or the world" (Leininger, 2002, p. 83). In other words, it is the way in which we perceive, interpret, and relate to the world around us.

Culture is *learned* from birth, through language acquisition and socialization. Individuals are not born with culture; they are born into a culture. Similarly, healthcare providers are socialized into professional cultures as they learn about and take on the norms, values, and expectations of the profession. Culture also is about *traditions* and rituals—what is done, when is it done (or not done), and how it is done. Different groups have different ways of doing things.

Culture is not only commonly understood, but it is *unconscious* and automatic. It reflects a norm based on underlying values and assumptions about the world: values and beliefs that are taken for granted and rarely examined or enacted consciously. Often, it is only when we are confronted with difference that traditions and rituals are recognizable for what they are and what they represent.

Last, cultural values determine the *rules of engagement* with the situations and events in our lives, including illness and health care. Cultural values serve several key functions:

- Provide a basis for attitudes, beliefs, and behaviours
- Serve as a reference point for determining our individual identity
- Influence perception of and reaction to people, events, and situations
- Determine acceptable and unacceptable behaviour

Culture provides the map for interacting with the events and circumstances in our lives. How we communicate, verbally and non-verbally, and how we make decisions, define the boundaries of the private and public, and determine what is respectful and what is rude are all processes that are culturally bound. Culture influences how we interact and engage with others on a routine basis as well as under particular circumstances.

Characteristics of Culture

Culture has a number of distinguishing features. Culture is:

- *Learned*—not innate. We experience culture from infancy and learn to internalize the patterns of behaviour around us. What we learn is not static or timeless; rather, it evolves and changes based on events and experiences.
- *Adaptive*—based on history and context. Culture is an adaptation to specific activities related to environmental and technological factors.
- *Dynamic*—not static. Culture is not genetically inherited, fixed, or static. Although culture represents strength and stability and is the foundation for how we exist in the world, it also changes in response to new situations and pressures.
- *Invisible*—is experienced, not seen. Although culture is recognizable through symbols such as language, rituals, dress, and celebrations, culture itself is not visible.
- *Shared*—in varying degrees. Although values, beliefs, and patterns of behaviour are shared by members of a cultural group, individual differences continue to exist and everyone is ultimately unique.
- *Selective*—differentiates between insiders and outsiders. Culture defines the boundaries of which behaviours are desired, acceptable, or unacceptable. Culture influences the perception of, and the response to, situations and issues.

Culture as Identity

By definition, culture refers to shared identities because of the shared values, beliefs, norms, and other characteristics involved. The extent to which particular cultural traits are shared varies across individuals within a culture, so that, although culture is shared, no two people within a culture are identical. It is therefore challenging to understand the individual within the context of a shared culture. To understand the individual's culture we have to understand the concept of identity.

The term **identity** has its roots in the French word *identité* and the Latin adjective *idem*, meaning "the same," and is essentially a comparative concept that emphasizes a degree of sameness that individuals reveal with regard to a particular characteristic (Rummens, 2003). There are many types of identities, each reflecting a different set of criteria that may be used to differentiate among individuals or to reinforce commonalities (sameness). Almost on a daily basis, all of us negotiate and navigate multiple identities, including, for example, parent, student, doctor, immigrant, or member of visible minority. Three features should be noted regarding identity:

1. Different identities are prominent under different circumstances.
2. Intersections of identities can significantly influence experience (e.g., a healthcare provider who belongs to a visible minority group may experience a situation differently than another healthcare provider or another member of a visible minority who is not a healthcare provider).
3. Identities are often ascribed by others and may have different meanings for those people than for the individuals being appraised or labelled. For

example, a first-generation immigrant woman from India may be described by others as an immigrant woman, a woman of colour, and an Indo-Canadian, South Asian, or East Indian; however, the woman may have come to Canada as a child and not identify with the label "immigrant woman" or feel comfortable being referred to as South Asian rather than East Indian.

In reality, we each comprise multiple identities that may be based on religion, ethnicity, race, sexual orientation, socio-economic status, professional status, developmental stage of life, and so on. Each individual thus shares a sense of "sameness" and belonging with multiple groups and is therefore simultaneously a part of multiple cultures. Identity is shaped by heritage as well as by experiences. A word of caution here: identity should not be considered a blueprint for culture. Social labels of identity neither dictate nor predict particular ways of thinking; they simply point to possible interpretations and experiences that may influence the way of thinking (Wear, 2003).

Culture serves a dual function, with the integrative values and beliefs giving an individual the following:

■ A sense of identity
■ The rules of engagement with the surrounding world

Culture is about shared ways or patterns of understanding and expression. Understanding a client's culture therefore requires an understanding of the concept of culture in general and also understanding the client's identity, which in turn may provide information on the client's interpretation of, and ways of interacting with, a given situation. Figure 3-4 presents a visual image of culture as being composed of multiple dimensions of identities.

How does one begin to understand an individual's culture? The Culture Care Framework recognizes that multiple identities exist within the individual. The

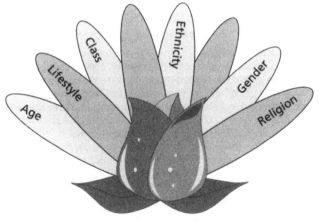

CULTURE

FIGURE 3-4 ■ **Conceptualization of Culture as Multi-Dimensional Identities**

different petals in Figure 3-4 reflect the different identities that contribute to the individual's overall unique identity. The framework recognizes that the different identities may be more important or less important at different times and in different ways. The challenge for the healthcare provider is to identify the potential identities that could be affecting a situation at any given time. Only then is it possible to begin to understand the cultures that really are influencing the interaction. Cultural sensitivity is not about understanding one culture but rather identifying and understanding the impact of various identities on a given interaction. The question to ask ourselves is how the various dimensions of age, gender, race, ethnicity, and sexual orientation, among others, have an impact on the current situation. Are there some dimensions that take on a greater significance in the current health context than others? Sometimes challenges arise from the combination of identities; it therefore becomes essential to consider not just which identity or identities are most important, but also the potential impact of the combination.

Understanding Your Own Values, Biases, and Prejudices

Self-awareness is a critical component of cultural competence. Cultural dynamics are part of all interactions, whether or not they are recognized. Although it may not be possible to remove personal biases, it is by recognizing their own cultural values and biases that healthcare providers can learn about or remove unintentional influences (Camphina-Bacote, 1999).

It is important for healthcare providers to understand not only what they value, but also what they dislike, fear, or are otherwise biased against. Everyone has biases and prejudices. One way for healthcare providers to check their own biases is to ask themselves: "Why do I believe or think what I do in this situation? Would someone else looking at this situation come to the same conclusion, or

---

CULTURAL COMPETENCE IN ACTION

Understanding My Culture
How would you describe your cultural identity? What groups are you like? Consider gender, age, professional role, family status, immigration status, sexual orientation, race, ethnicity, acculturation, and so on.

If you were to discuss your answers in a group, are there some identities that you would be comfortable talking about and others that you would not be comfortable talking about? Why might they be?

If you discuss your answers with others, you are likely to find that different identities are important to different people. Individuals may identify aspects of identity (e.g., immigration status) that others may not have even considered to be important.

Pick one or two identities and discuss some of the characteristics associated with it/them. During the discussion, you are likely to discover that different people have differing beliefs about particular identities.

CULTURAL COMPETENCE IN ACTION

The Changing and Unchanging Nature of Values
Identify two values that your parents (or elders) taught you when you were growing up. Consider values like independence, co-operation, duty, desire, obedience, individuality, allegiance to family, and questioning or challenging the status quo.

From the above list, identify two values that you would like to teach your children (or your niece or nephew, or young people in general). Are the values the same as the ones that were taught to you? Are they different? Can you identify the reasons for any differences? Does the gender of the child or person influence your answer?

This exercise highlights that while values and preferences may remain the same across generations, they can also change over time based on circumstances and life experiences. Gender role expectations can also influence value preferences.

could they come up with a different interpretation?" The answers can be illuminating and may reveal implicit assumptions that are influencing the perception of the situation.

Our perception of the world is influenced by our own history—our values, beliefs, and what we have learned and experienced. Williams (2001) notes that these perceptions are based on both legacies and layers. **Legacies** are powerful historical events experienced by our ancestors, family, and community of origin that continue to have ripple effects in our lives today. Examples of legacies include colonization, slavery, capture and redistribution of land, and the civil rights movement. Even though these events may have happened decades ago, the impact was so powerful that the influence extends across time and generations. Everyone brings these legacies into his or her interactions daily.

Layers are the various dimensions of our identity and life experiences that shape perception. As suggested earlier, they can include race, ethnicity, gender, age, marital status, education level, socio-economic level, religion, sexual orientation, profession, political affiliation, and leisure activities. Layers and legacies are dynamically intertwined, and they contribute to our ideas and beliefs about a variety of issues, such as those related to culture, diversity, and health. For healthcare providers, it is critical to consider all the layers of identity as well as the legacies that lead to assumptions and biases on the part of everyone involved. Awareness of the various perspectives is important for two reasons:

1. On a personal level, healthcare providers' understanding of their own preferences helps to identify the biases and ideologies that influence their interactions.
2. On a team level, it is critical to recognize that team members do not all have the same beliefs. Variations in perceptions and perspectives can lead to inconsistencies and ineffectiveness in the health care provided.

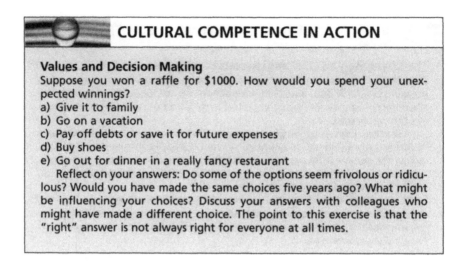

CULTURAL COMPETENCE IN ACTION

Values and Decision Making
Suppose you won a raffle for $1000. How would you spend your unexpected winnings?
a) Give it to family
b) Go on a vacation
c) Pay off debts or save it for future expenses
d) Buy shoes
e) Go out for dinner in a really fancy restaurant
 Reflect on your answers: Do some of the options seem frivolous or ridiculous? Would you have made the same choices five years ago? What might be influencing your choices? Discuss your answers with colleagues who might have made a different choice. The point to this exercise is that the "right" answer is not always right for everyone at all times.

As discussed in Chapter 2, a common misconception surrounding cultural competence is that we must accept everything. This is simply not true. Respecting the choices of others does not mean endorsing those choices or the values involved. Nor does it mean forsaking our own values. Everyone has preferences, and embracing cultural diversity does not diminish our own values. In fact, self-awareness and personal insight can strengthen appreciation for our own culture as well as develop respect for other cultures. Cultural clashes often are less about differing values than about how the differences are treated. Consider the difference between having discriminatory tastes and being discriminatory: the first is generally regarded positively and often is a desired trait, whereas the second is usually regarded in a negative light and deemed unacceptable. The difference is in the impact of the choices. Having discriminatory tastes usually is associated with being selective and having high expectations or standards. The impact largely is on oneself. However, being discriminatory has an impact on others; it is an imposition of personal choices on others, is associated with exclusion, and has an adverse impact on the ability of others to participate fully in their environment. Healthcare providers must be aware of their personal and professional cultures in order to avoid being discriminatory or imposing their views and values on clients both consciously and unconsciously.

Understanding our culture goes beyond being clear about our own values and beliefs. It also is critical to understand the legacies and layers involved, and issues of power and privilege associated with social position.

Privilege can be described as unearned resources (Shore, 2003) and is a difficult concept to make visible. In a study of Canadian medical students exposed to a new course aimed at fostering ethnocultural and gender sensitivity in physicians, Beagan (2003) notes that "very few students were able to identify the advantages, or privileges enjoyed by students from the dominant social groups" (p. 611). The majority of students viewed "class" purely as an issue of money, with only a few students identifying the more subtle signs of class, such as privilege and the advan-

CULTURAL CONSIDERATIONS IN CARE

Dialysis Training—With a Thoughtful Twist

North American society places a high value on independence. Often, treatments are geared toward helping individuals gain as much as independence as possible. Consider what happens when we encounter an individual who attaches a different significance to independence.

In many cultures, the elderly value independence differently from the North American norm. Instead, there is an expectation of being cared for in one's old age by members of one's family. An example of this occurred in a home dialysis program that was teaching clients how to maintain themselves on continuous ambulatory peritoneal dialysis. One of the biggest advantages of this therapy over other types of dialysis is that it allows clients to do the dialysis themselves and thus be completely independent. However, the staff soon realized that many of the elderly clients, particularly those from Eastern backgrounds, were relying on their spouses or children to actually do the procedure. This was of concern since the spouses and children had not received the training on how to do the procedure safely.

Initially, the team's response was to emphasize the need for the client to do the procedure and express disapproval when this was not being done. Some clients continued to rely on other family members for the procedure. As the team took time to reflect on what was happening, team members understood the issue differently and they built greater flexibility into the program to allow for training not just the client but also the key family member(s) who might be doing the procedure. The concern for client safety was addressed, along with the family's need to care for its ill family member.

tages held by people from upper-class or upper-middle-class backgrounds (Beagan, 2003). This study and others emphasize the need to shift away from a passive acquisition of information about particular groups or populations, toward an approach that encourages self-awareness and self-reflexivity. **Self-reflexivity** refers to processes of critical self-examination aimed at challenging a neutral stance and instead focusing on our own reality and the assumptions on which it is based. Accepting the notion of privilege means giving up the notion of **meritocracy** (a belief that individual success is based on merit, hard work, ability, and accomplishment). This can be particularly difficult for a society that values individual success, freedom, opportunity, and equality.

Understanding the Dynamics of Difference

As human beings, we are conditioned to respond to the unusual and unfamiliar with vigilance and suspicion. Reactions to differences generally are automatic, often subconscious, and are based on inherent cultural assumptions. Fear and lack of familiarity or experience with something are the most common barriers to providing culturally sensitive care (College of Nurses of Ontario, 1999). Fear often involves the fear of losing something, such as control, power, values, or traditions.

In clinical situations, this may be a fear about losing control over the care delivery process or losing personal status as the expert healthcare provider; familiarity with procedures and other team members may decrease fear but does not necessarily promote understanding. Such responses influence the dynamics of all relationships.

Identifying and understanding the dynamics of difference is the first step to managing the dynamics in ways that minimize the negative and optimize the positive opportunities associated with cultural diversity. It is important for healthcare professionals to understand the dynamics of difference at multiple levels. Healthcare providers need to understand how marginalization in society can lead to increased health risks for both clients and communities (Meleis, 1999). It is equally important for healthcare providers to recognize the dynamics of difference within the healthcare provider–client relationship itself that can lead to client values and choices being ignored or excluded in the health care provided.

Consider the following quotation by Ralph Waldo Emerson: "Who you are speaks so loudly, I can't hear what you're saying." Several interpretations are possible, including the following:

- ◾ Actions speak louder than words.
- ◾ What you do determines who you are.
- ◾ Often our beliefs (stereotypes) about people determine our judgements regarding their ability and credibility; it is not necessarily about words or actions but rather about the interpretation or meaning ascribed to the words or actions by others.

Cultural sensitivity requires that healthcare providers become aware of their own assumptions and avoid labelling and judging people, but it also requires that they become aware of the assumptions that others may have or make about them. When healthcare providers know how they might come across to others in particular situations, they can better understand and manage the dynamics proactively, and thus avoid—or at least minimize—misinterpretations or unintentional influences. For example, when we are aware that some clients may say "yes" simply to show respect for the healthcare provider's authority, we can manage the potential impact of authority by using other questions to elicit client views.

Many factors influence the dynamics of an interaction. The Culture Care Framework focuses on three—trust, equity, and power—which are all important in healthcare interactions and affect healthcare provider–client relationships where an issue of difference is involved.

Trust

Trust is an everyday concept with an implied meaning. It is fundamental to all helping relationships and influences what clients disclose, as well as when and to whom (Clair, Beatty, & MacLean, 2005). In a healthcare environment, client trust is based on expectations that the healthcare provider will be knowledgeable, will take responsibility for the care that is needed, and will make the client's welfare a high priority (Hupcey, Penrod, Morse, & Mitcham, 2001).

Many healthcare providers feel that their professional status automatically makes them deserving of trust. This assumption may be wrong. The healthcare

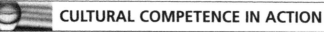

CULTURAL COMPETENCE IN ACTION

Managing Others' Perceptions
Evelyn is a nurse of Asian background. She has become aware that individuals with her background often do not differentiate between the gendered pronouns "he" and "she" in the way that lifelong English speakers do. The pronoun difference led to communication difficulties with colleagues when she talked about her clients during rounds, as well as difficulties with families when she inadvertently used the wrong gendered pronoun (e.g., referring to the daughter as "he").

Since Evelyn became aware of how her culture can have an adverse impact on the effectiveness of her communication, she has developed two strategies to minimize any negative impact:

1. She tries to avoid pronoun problems by referring to clients by name (or by relationship, such as "your mother") when speaking to families.
2. She has acknowledged this difficulty with her colleagues and asked them to let her know if they are not certain whom she is talking about (previously, colleagues were reluctant to appear rude).

***

Saira is a health educator who is passionate about her work, and articulate and animated in her discussions. However, she has recognized that her passion can be misinterpreted as anger by some and may be intimidating to others. Her "loudness" can be a barrier that prevents others from hearing the message she intends to convey. This was becoming a challenge in her personal life as well because her partner's "cultural expectations" require women to be soft-spoken.

Saira now manages this potential for miscommunication by monitoring two areas of behaviour:

1. Her own behaviour
2. Other people's response to her

Previously, when she saw someone withdrawing from her, she assumed they did not understand or were uninterested; thus, her natural response was to become more animated. Now she takes more cues from others and tries a softer style of engagement. She also recognizes that although she has explained to her partner that her "loudness" is passion, not anger, cultural reactions often are unconscious and hard to change; the couple therefore worked out a system whereby he can give her feedback without it interfering with the communication. Now, when Saira and her partner have a passionate, animated discussion that becomes "too loud" for him, he simply reminds her that they are in the same room and next to each other. The loudness is addressed in a non-threatening way so that they can each hear what the other is truly saying. Saira also has been able to apply this understanding to her clinical work by explaining to her clients that she can get really passionate and asking them to let her know when that passion starts to interfere with the clarity of the message, and also by being more aware of her clients' verbal and non-verbal responses.

system expects clients to disclose a great deal of information, some of which the client may not feel is relevant, at least during the initial visit. Clients may have difficulty trusting an unfamiliar system that they cannot interact with effectively and that does not seem to understand them. The trust is in danger of further erosion if there has been any talk in their community about a lack of respect, miscommunication, or misdiagnosis.

Healthcare providers need to remember that trust is likely to be fragile at the beginning of a relationship (College of Nurses of Ontario, 1999) and that clients' trust can increase or decrease based on their interactions with healthcare professionals and the healthcare system (Clair et al., 2005). Although trust often takes time to develop, the impact of first impressions cannot be underestimated. Experience with non-English-speaking clients indicates that these clients, in particular, tend to determine trustworthiness of the provider very early in the interaction, through perceptions of non-verbal cues and nuances (Browne, 1997; Leininger, 1995). Therefore, it is important to ensure that sufficient time and effort is spent early in the relationship to gain (or confirm) a client's trust, instead of taking the trust for granted. Key steps in building trust may include acknowledging the client's potential mistrust of the healthcare system, while building a personal commitment to learning the client's perspective and developing a relationship that is respectful and non-judgemental (Betancourt, 2004).

Equity

Equity is a difficult concept to define. Many countries have only one word to cover both equity and equality (Almond, 2002), but the two concepts are not the same (also see Chapter 2). Equality is rooted in the concept of equal opportunity, a cherished value within North American society, and focuses on equality in the process. By contrast, **equity** focuses on equality of outcomes. In other words, equity means that people with unequal need require different or differential treatment to achieve identical results (Almond, 2002; Sue, 2001). All inequities, whether based on gender, race, social status, age, professional status, or geography, are sustained by social norms that make dominant groups privileged and exclude or exploit subordinate groups. Thus, equity becomes something that challenges the norms and looks for ways to balance or counter exclusion or exploitation.

Within health care, there is ample evidence that "equal" or same treatment for all results in health disparity or inequitable health outcomes for some (Institute of Medicine, 2002; Spitzer, 2005). To ensure equal access to health care for all individuals, we have to examine the barriers to equity. For example, offering care only on weekdays between 9 A.M. and 5 P.M. threatens potential clients' access to care if they cannot afford to take time off from regular work.

In the early 1990s, the Ontario anti-racism secretariat produced a document that identified five barriers to equity which, when understood and put to good use, can turn into the building blocks for equity (Ontario Ministry of Citizenship, 1995). These building blocks masquerading as barriers are as follows:

1. Information
2. Connections
3. Experience and expertise
4. Resources
5. Decision making

The building blocks also can be considered as elements or sources of power.

Power

Power is a complex concept. The therapeutic relationship, by its very nature, is one of unequal power. The following factors ensure that the healthcare provider has more power than the client (College of Nurses of Ontario, 1999):

- The authority within the healthcare system that comes with the position
- Specialized knowledge
- The ability to influence and access other healthcare providers and other parts of the system
- Access to privileged information

Healthcare providers are expected to use their power appropriately. They are expected to make certain that a client's vulnerable position is not taken advantage of, and at the same time to use their power and privilege to enhance the relationship with the client to help the client achieve health equity. When the healthcare provider understands the power dynamics involved in health interactions and social processes, he or she can use the building-block elements to purposefully balance the power.

INFORMATION. Most of us would agree that information is power. It is important that, in their day-to-day work, healthcare providers consider not only issues involving access to information (e.g., language and literacy) but also the kind of information that people access, from where (i.e., sources of information or knowledge), and the kind of information that is considered legitimate or relevant (e.g., teaching nutrition using the typical Canadian diet may not be helpful to someone who recently moved here from Jamaica and eats different foods).

The information barrier can be turned into a building block when its influence is recognized and purposefully used to improve the following:

- Accessibility (e.g., when information is conveyed in the client's language and appropriate literacy level, maybe even communicated through ethnic media)
- Credibility (i.e., the information comes from a credible or trusted source, such as community leaders and healers)
- Relevance (i.e., the information uses and builds on concepts that are familiar and important to the client)

CONNECTIONS. A great deal of communication happens informally through networks. Groups that are excluded from dominant networks are at risk for missing information or opportunities. Connections can be critical to gaining access to information and resources, and for developing credibility. Connections also serve to reinforce thoughts and can thus help to reinforce the status quo or particular ideas or perspectives. Healthcare providers must consider the connections that a client has and the potential influences of those connections. For example, a client whose community stigmatizes mental illness may experience difficulty seeking and accepting help, as well as integrating back into society. Recognizing the strengths and limitations of connections also helps us identify perspectives that may be missing from our day-to-day interactions. For example, clients unfamiliar with a particular treatment option may find comfort in connecting with members of their own community who have had experience with this type of treatment.

Healthcare providers also need to reflect on their own connections. Discussing situations with like-minded individuals will probably result in a high degree of agreement. However, seeking out individuals who could have a different perspective is likely to result in a broader range of interpretations and possibilities. Purposeful development and use of connections can broaden the world view of both the healthcare provider and the client. Healthcare providers who seek out information about a particular community and cultural influences on care are more likely than others to achieve the following:

▪ Enhance their own assessment skills
▪ Be able to provide care to a more diverse population
▪ Develop credibility within the community

EXPERIENCE/EXPERTISE. In any health interaction, it is critical to recognize what expertise is being valued and what may be discarded by the client, the healthcare provider, or both. For example, healthcare providers may ask about a client's experience with a particular medication but may not think about posing similar questions about herbal or other non-pharmacological agents. Client stories often remain unheard because healthcare providers are looking only for particular information and the client's other perceptions or beliefs are not considered valid or legitimate. Clients may place greater value on whether or not a healthcare provider seems trustworthy, and less on professional credentials.

CULTURAL CONSIDERATIONS IN CARE

Rigid Formats Can Trigger Challenging Encounters

Seeking information in particular ways occurs in a variety of settings. Consider the situation of a new immigrant going into a fast-food restaurant. The traditional first question here is, "Eat in or take out?" Being unfamiliar with this phraseology and more focused on what food to choose, the individual may not answer the question and instead launch straight into giving the order (hamburger with fries, and so on).

Some cashiers won't mind if the eat-in or take-out question is not answered until later, but others won't be able to move to the next step until the first question has been answered. Imagine a cashier continuing to repeat the question, often in an increasingly loud tone, and the customer becoming increasingly frustrated at not understanding and/or not being understood. Meanwhile, the lineup becomes longer and other customers begin to form judgements about the individual. The simple act of ordering a meal has become a challenging cultural encounter.

In health care, we also have rules and specific sequences—sometimes rigid—in which we ask questions to gain a good history and assessment. Clients, however, may have a different sequence in which they want to convey what is important to them. For example, healthcare providers often expect to ask questions and receive information about health history in chronological order. A client who does not provide information in that way runs the risk of being labelled a poor historian, losing credibility with the health team, and being unlikely to have his or her concerns heard or addressed adequately.

CULTURAL CONSIDERATIONS IN CARE

Keeping Written Records Doesn't Thrill Everyone
Mainstream North American society relies heavily on data and trends as noted by graphs. For self-care management, clients are often asked to maintain a diary or record of their symptoms or response to treatment (e.g., documenting blood pressure, blood sugar, fluid intake, or temperature). However, people vary as to their preference and value for written documentation. There is a real possibility that clients will come for follow-up appointments with incomplete records or, worse, with records that have been completed to please the healthcare provider.

DECISION MAKING. Both the process and outcomes of decision making are a reflection of underlying values. To achieve equity, is it important to reflect on how decisions are made? Who has input and who is actually at the table when various options are being considered? The role of consultations in the ultimate decision also needs to be clear. Is the consultation or input being sought simply to inform someone else's decision, or is it expected that the input will be reflected in the final outcome? It also is important to consider the decision maker and the basis on which decisions are made. Often, the context significantly influences people's ability to participate effectively in decision making. A client who does not speak English and cannot access an interpreter is unable to participate effectively in decisions regarding health care. Similarly, if a client cannot relate to the treatment being proposed, the cultural barrier remains, even if an interpreter is used to address the linguistic barrier. Clients also may wish to consult others before decisions are made, and while some consultations may be recognized and supported by the healthcare setting (e.g., consultations with immediate family), others may not (e.g., consultations with extended family, community healers, or elders).

The consequences of decisions also need to be considered from a multidimensional perspective. For example, consider the situation of a client who chooses not to take medications during a period of fasting. What decision is being made here: to honour the fast or to disregard the medication? What are the consequences of this decision on the client's physical and spiritual health, and on the client's relationship with the healthcare team, particularly if some members of the team perceive the refusal to take medications as "non-compliance"?

RESOURCES. Resources are fundamental to achieving equity. We need to consider the manner in which we allocate and provide access to resources. For example, if interpreter services are available to healthcare providers but no clear mechanism exists to inform clients that they can request or arrange for an interpreter, access is still compromised.

Frequently, healthcare providers feel that if a client seeks help through an emergency room or walk-in clinic, he or she is clearly indicating willing acceptance of any treatment offered. This assumption is erroneous. The client may not know in advance what type of treatment to expect and/or may be unfamiliar with the treatment that is offered. Even if clients know that a medical approach is

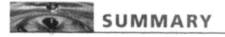

CULTURAL COMPETENCE IN ACTION

Clients May Be Experts Too

Gcina visited her family physician with her daughter, Thoka, and provided a history in the following manner: "For the past four days, my daughter has had a low-grade fever during the day and it spikes in the evening." At this point the doctor interrupted and asked Gcina if she had measured the temperature with a thermometer and recorded it on paper to see the trend she was describing. Gcina's response was "no." The doctor responded by saying, "So you can tell temperature by touch, can you?" Gcina was embarrassed and perceived this as a dismissive response. She did not know how to respond further and said little throughout the rest of the interaction.

Consider this situation from the physician's point of view: Is the physician's expectation of the temperature record appropriate and legitimate? How might Gcina have contributed to this expectation? Does it make a difference to know that Gcina is a nurse and has considerable experience in the pediatric setting?

How could the physician handle such an interaction differently to both benefit from a mother's expert knowledge of her child and meet his need for specific data on which to base a diagnosis and intervention?

different from what they are used to, they simply may not know what else to do or may not have access to any other resources, so they access what they can, likely with a combination of fear, trepidation, and hope.

SUMMARY

The cultural sensitivity element of the Culture Care Framework focuses largely on awareness and understanding of self and the dynamics of difference within the healthcare provider–client relationship. Cultural sensitivity is about learning "who I am." The various exercises and reflections presented in this section are intended to foster critical self-reflection. Students and healthcare providers can continue to develop their own cultural sensitivity through ongoing reflection and dialogue with themselves and with others.

The Culture Care Framework describes cultural sensitivity with respect to awareness and understanding—not only about our own values and reactions to difference but also about how we may be perceived by others. The framework also describes the dynamics of difference created by systemic barriers to equity. Culturally sensitive healthcare providers have both theoretical knowledge ("knowing that") and practical knowledge ("knowing how"). They value diversity in all individuals, understand the dynamics of difference, and are able to use their knowledge and understanding to turn barriers into building blocks.

Although cultural sensitivity is a critical part of cultural competence, it is only one element. As noted in this chapter, the other two elements are cultural knowledge and cultural resources. Chapter 4 discusses these other elements and examines how the healthcare provider can apply cultural knowledge in a way that focuses on the client's needs and integrates cultural needs and values into care.

REFERENCES

Almond, P. (2002). An analysis of the concept of equity and its application to health visiting. *Journal of Advanced Nursing, 37*(6), 598–606.

Anderson, J. (1987). The cultural context of caring. *Canadian Critical Care Nursing Journal, 4*(4), 7–13.

Arnold, R., Burke, B., James, C., D'Arcy, M., & Thomas, B. (1991). *Educating for a change.* Toronto, ON: Between the Lines and Doris Marshall Institute for Education and Action.

Beagan, B. (2003). Teaching social and cultural awareness to medical students: It's all very nice to talk about it in theory, but ultimately it makes no difference. *Academic Medicine, 78*(6), 605–614.

Benner, P. (1984). *From novice to expert.* Menlo Park, CA: Addison Wesley.

Betancourt, J. (2004). Cultural competence—Marginal or mainstream movement. *New England Journal of Medicine, 351*(10), 953–955.

Browne, A. (1997). A concept analysis of respect applying the hybrid model in cross-cultural settings. *Western Journal of Nursing Research, 19*(6), 762–781.

Camphina-Bacote, J. (1999). A model and instrument for addressing cultural competence in health care. *Journal of Nursing Education, 38*(5), 203–207.

Clair, J., Beatty, J. E., & MacLean, T. L. (2005). Out of sight but not out of mind: Managing invisible social identities in the workplace. *Academy of Management Review, 30*(1), 78–95.

College of Nurses of Ontario. (1999). Guidelines for providing culturally sensitive care. Toronto: Author.

Hupcey, J. E, Penrod, J., Morse, J. M., & Mitcham, C. (2001). An exploration and advancement of the concept of trust. *Journal of Advanced Nursing, 36*(2), 282–293.

Institute of Medicine. (2002). *Unequal treatment: What healthcare providers need to know about racial and ethnic disparities in health care.* Washington, DC: Author.

Leininger, M. (1990). The significance of cultural concepts in nursing. *Journal of Transcultural Nursing, 2*(1), 52–59.

Leininger, M. (1995). Overview of Leininger's culture care theory. In M. Leininger & M. R. McFarland (Eds.), *Transcultural nursing: Concepts, theories, research and practice* (2nd ed., pp. 93–114). New York: McGraw Hill.

Leininger, M. (2002). Theory of culture care and the ethnonursing research method. In M. Leininger & M. R. McFarland (Eds.), *Transcultural nursing: Concepts, theories, research and practice* (3rd ed., pp. 71–98). New York: McGraw Hill.

Meleis, A. (1999). Culturally competent care. *Journal of Transcultural Nursing, 10*(1), 12.

Ontario Ministry of Citizenship. (1995). *Building blocks to equity.* Toronto: Author.

Ridley, C. R., Baker, D. M., & Hill, C. L. (2001). Critical issues concerning cultural competence. *The Counseling Psychologist, 29*(6), 822–833.

Rummens, J. A. (2003). Conceptualising identity and diversity: Overlaps, intersections, and processes. *Canadian Ethnic Studies 35*(3), 10–25.

Shore, S. (2003). What's whiteness got to do with it? *Literacies,* (Fall), 19–28.

Spitzer, D. (2005). Engendering health disparities. *Canadian Journal of Public Health, 96*(Suppl. 2), 78–96.

Srivastava (1996). Culture care framework: An approach to integrating culture into practice. Unpublished report for Access and Equity Initiative, Toronto: Wellesley Hospital.

Srivastava, R. (2004). Influence of organizational factors on clinical cultural competence. Unpublished report Toronto: University of Toronto, Institute of Medical Sciences.

Sue, S. (2001). Ethnic and racial issues: Why can't we all just get along? Dateline UC Davis. Retrieved July 30, 2005, from http://www-dateline.ucdavis.edu/100501/DL_ stansueconvo.html

Wear, D. (2003). Insurgent multiculturalism: Rethinking how and why we teach culture in medical education. *Academic Medicine 78*, 549–554.

Williams, M. (2001). *The 10 lenses: Your guide to living & working in a multicultural world.* Sterling, VA: Capital Books.

CHAPTER 4

Culture Care Framework II: Cultural Knowledge, Resources, and Bridging the Gap

RANI SRIVASTAVA

LEARNING OBJECTIVES

At the end of this chapter, the learner will be able to:
- Describe cultural knowledge and cultural resources
- Examine the two dimensions of cultural knowledge
- Describe care processes that are shaped by culture
- Discuss strategies to bridge the gap across cultures
- Apply the strategies of cultural care validation, accommodation, and reframing to clinical situations

KEY TERMS

Cultural care
  accommodation/negotiation
Cultural care reframing/
  repatterning
Cultural care validation/
  preservation
Cultural knowledge

Cultural resources
Explanatory model of illness
Generic cultural knowledge
Holding knowledge
Specific cultural knowledge

This chapter continues the discussion of the Culture Care Framework that began in Chapter 3 with both an overview and an examination of one framework element, cultural sensitivity. Chapter 4 examines the elements of cultural knowledge and cultural resources, and describes ways to apply sensitivity, knowledge, and resources in clinical practice in order to work effectively across cultures.

Cultural Knowledge

Cultural knowledge is widely recognized as a critical element of cultural competence, but exactly what makes up the base of that knowledge is murky. What, for example, do we mean by "knowledge"? The term can be defined as "familiarity, awareness, or understanding gained through experience or study" (American Heritage Dictionaries, 2000). Frequently, when healthcare providers hold particular viewpoints, these are perceived as the culmination of what has been learned through professional education and socialization and built upon by clinical experience. Conversely, when it comes to clients and other cultures, we often talk about cultural beliefs. A belief is defined as a mental acceptance of, and conviction in, the truth, actuality, or validity of something (American Heritage Dictionaries, 2000). The implication is that the knowledge that healthcare providers possess is superior to the beliefs that clients hold. It is important for healthcare providers to closely examine their own sources of knowledge and to accept client cultural knowledge as legitimate, even when it is not part of the healthcare providers' own world view (Taylor, 2003).

Cultural knowledge in the healthcare setting is said to involve a number of factors:

- Understanding world views across populations
- Obtaining information about specific physical, biological, and physiological variations among ethnic groups
- Obtaining information about local and national demographics
- Understanding inequalities in general health
- Understanding linguistic and communication issues
- Understanding group healthcare practices and epidemiology
- Being familiar with cultural representations of illness and healthcare services (Betancourt, Green, & Carrillo, 2002; Campinha-Bacote, 1999; Cortis, 2003; Leininger, 1995; Office of Minority Health Resource Center, 2001; Purnell, 2000)

The vast variety and quantity of cultural information can be overwhelming. The Culture Care Framework provides a streamlined approach that allows healthcare providers to focus on two broad areas of cultural knowledge:

1. **Generic cultural knowledge**—basic knowledge about cultures that applies across a wide variety of cultural groups
2. **Specific cultural knowledge**—knowledge that focuses on the specific cultural groups one serves, including the important cultural issues associated with such groups

Examples of generic cultural knowledge include an understanding of cross-cultural communication, care processes that are shaped by culture, and cultural issues related to families. Examples of specific cultural knowledge could involve focusing on the values and beliefs of specific cultural groups such as the Aboriginal population or the Chinese community, or the health issues faced by particular populations such as immigrant women. The generic and specific areas work hand in hand because a strong grasp of generic cultural knowledge serves to alert the healthcare provider as to what kind of information to seek in specific clinical situations. Both types of knowledge are necessary for the development of cultural competence in a multicultural society (see Figure 4-1).

Generic Cultural Knowledge

Cultural generalities should not be used to obscure individual differences, but the generalities are helpful in recognizing and understanding cultural patterns. Consider the saying by Thomas Khun, "You don't see something until you have the right metaphor to perceive it" (Gleick, 1987, p. 262). Cultural knowledge is about understanding a variety of world views so that we can expand our own repertoire of metaphors. Pattern recognition is easier when the pattern is familiar and meaningful. Leininger (1995) refers to this understanding of cultural patterns as **holding knowledge**—knowledge of cultural patterns that is held by the healthcare provider and used to reflect on ideas and experiences and not to make stereotypical judgements. Healthcare providers have always studied facets of particular groups (e.g., psychosocial concerns of cardiac clients) and patterns (e.g., stages of grieving), without the expectation that all clients who fall into the general group (e.g., cardiac patients and those experiencing grief) will exhibit identical behaviours; instead, this knowledge is "held" by providers and used in care selectively, when it is relevant. Similarly, cultural knowledge is knowledge of particular groups that needs to be used selectively to better understand and manage the clinical encounter.

Different authors have identified different domains of culture as important for healthcare providers to understand (Bonder, Martin, & Miracle, 2002; Leininger, 1995; Purnell, 2000). The concepts and processes identified in Table 4-1 are based on key concepts from the literature as well as feedback from healthcare providers and should be regarded as essential knowledge for starting to build a foundation for clinical competence.

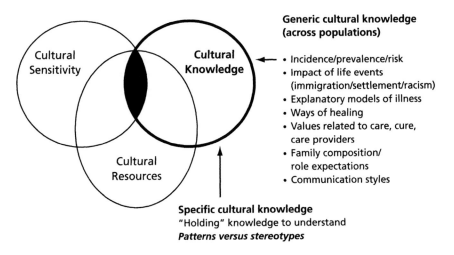

FIGURE 4-1 ▪ **Cultural Knowledge**

TABLE 4-1

Healthcare Processes Shaped by Culture

Communication
Biology, physiology, incidence, and prevalence
Pharmacology
Time orientation
Personal space (public/private; what is disclosed)
Views toward care, cure, and caregivers
Models of illness and systems of healing
Self-care/independence
Role of family in decision making and caregiving
Rituals/customs related to treatment including diet and prayer

Understanding how culture shapes the processes noted in Table 4-1 can be described as generic cultural knowledge. Such cultural knowledge (i.e., for understanding a variety of healthcare processes from communication through rituals or customs like diet and prayer) is applicable across clinical populations and healthcare settings. The knowledge required to understand cultural variations in biology, physiology, incidence, prevalence, and pharmacology varies considerably depending on the clinical setting; however, it is important for all healthcare providers to have a basic understanding that these processes are susceptible to cultural variations.

The discussion below offers a brief explanation of how cross-cultural variations may affect these processes. (We look at the issue in more depth in Sections II and III of the book.)

Communication

Effective communication is critical for good clinical care. Culture and diversity affect many aspects of communication, the most obvious being language, whether verbal or non-verbal, including eye contact, hand gestures, facial expressions, and tone of voice. Communication has an impact on not only what is said but also on how it is said, to whom it is said, and what remains unsaid. Cross-cultural communication skills are fundamental to cultural competence because without effective communication, every phase of the clinical encounter can be compromised—from establishing the therapeutic relationship to making an assessment and following through with interventions. Cross-cultural communication issues and working effectively with interpreters are discussed in greater depth in Chapters 5 and 6.

Biology/Physiology/Pharmacology

In recent years, healthcare providers have begun to acknowledge gender differences in the expression of illness and the response to pharmaceutical agents. Racial and ethnic differences also exist regarding the incidence and prevalence of illness, as well as in response to many medications, including psychotropic drugs and calcium channel blockers (Campinha-Bacote, 1995; Goldbloom, 2003). Two categories of factors influence the responses to drugs in ethnic or racial groups:

1. Genetic factors (e.g., inherent metabolic differences and specific enzyme deficiencies) may influence a drug's action by altering its absorption and excretion rate, leading to toxicity in smaller dosages.
2. Environmental factors (e.g., diet, including herbal remedies) also could have significant effects on drug metabolism (Campinha-Bacote, 2000).

Healthcare providers need to be aware of differences in the incidence, prevalence, and risk factors associated with illness and medication for different ethnocultural groups, and should explore the reasons for the differences. Caution must be exercised to avoid labelling people indiscriminately; rather, the key is to assess for potential differences across population groups. For example, African Americans are one of the populations that have been noted to have comparatively high frequencies of diagnosis of psychosis and fewer diagnoses of depression (Campinha-Bacote, 2000). Does this mean that the group actually has a higher incidence of psychosis, or does it mean that many African Americans' presentation of illness is such that it is interpreted as psychosis, or that psychosis is more culturally acceptable than depression? Similar issues often are raised for South Asian populations who frequently express mental health issues through somatic complaints. Being aware of the incidence of illness is helpful, but healthcare providers also need to understand the complex factors that may underlie the etiology. For example, it is well known that diabetes is a major health concern for Aboriginal peoples around the world. In Canada, the prevalence of non-insulin-dependent diabetes mellitus (NIDDM) in First Nations, Inuit, and Métis peoples is between three and five times the national average, with rates being higher among women and those living on reserves (Adelson, 2005). The basis for this disproportion may include genetics, but factors such as changing diets, poverty, limited work options, social stressors, cultural variations of foodstuffs, and access to resources may also be significant (Adelson, 2005).

Biological variations across ethnocultural groups are based on several factors, such as the following:

▪ Skin pigmentation
▪ Bone density
▪ Skin disorders
▪ Pathophysiology of some illnesses

It is important for healthcare providers to understand how to assess for conditions such as cyanosis, inflammation, jaundice, and petechiae in clients who are dark skinned. The usual assessment skills of visual inspection for colour may need to be augmented. For example, when assessing for inflammation in dark-skinned clients, health providers should palpate the skin for warmth, edema, tightness, or induration. Similarly, to assess for cyanosis in dark-skinned clients, healthcare providers need to observe the oral mucosa or conjunctiva, and jaundice is assessed by observing for yellow discoloration in the palms of the hands, the soles of the feet, and the sclera of the eyes (Purnell, 2000). Purnell further notes that African Americans have higher bone density and longer bones than European Americans, Asians, and Hispanics, and that genetically this population is more prone to retaining sodium, which contributes to the high incidence of hypertension among African Americans (Purnell, 2000). However, like the basis of NIDDM in the Aboriginal population, the basis for the high incidence of hypertension is not racial or cultural traits but rather a complex set of biological and social factors.

Time Orientation

Healthcare agencies frequently note that they experience challenging variations in client punctuality for appointments and in the value that clients place on time generally. Healthcare systems, particularly hospitals, are highly dependent on appointments and schedules, with little flexibility to accommodate people who appear at non-scheduled times. However, although mainstream North American society is highly oriented toward the 24-hour clock and punctuality is a cherished value, other cultures often value time differently. In some cultures, schedules are perceived as guidelines rather than strict rules, and being late—especially when there is a good reason—is not considered inappropriate. That said, healthcare professionals also must consider that a host of reasons may cause clients to be tardy about appointment times, including the following:

- Value placed on time may differ from the healthcare system norm
- Issues related to accessibility
- Issues related to work
- Inability to find childcare
- Client needs time to find friend or family member to accompany him or her
- Religious days or inauspicious (unfavourable or unlucky) days
- Transportation difficulties

Rather than simply giving an appointment time, it is important to take a few minutes to verify that the time is suitable, offering alternatives if it is not, and providing the information necessary to change the appointment if needed. Other helpful steps include anticipating potential challenges and assisting clients with planning and accessing the necessary support systems and resources.

Time orientation also can affect a client's medication habits, particularly with respect to the interval between doses. Healthcare providers can teach clients the optimum times for taking medicine, ask when exactly they see themselves being able to take it, explain how much latitude exists in the schedule, and discuss issues involving skipped doses (e.g., fasting). Despite the explanations and coaching, however, some clients may still have difficulty with issues of time management or following instructions that are dictated by the clock. These difficulties need to be understood in the context of the client's life and should not be attributed to the "naughtiness" of the client (Adelson, 2005).

Personal Space

The amount of personal space we are comfortable with varies across cultures; the same is true for what we consider to be private and what activities we are comfortable with in the presence of others. Many healthcare processes require close physical contact and/or discussions of an intimate nature; thus, personal boundaries can be particularly significant with respect to client disclosure and co-operation with activities. Issues concerning personal space and gender often surface during activities involving physical assessment and personal care. Healthcare providers need to use sensitivity and to talk with clients to find approaches that best fit the clients' healthcare needs and personal preferences. Cultural rules for personal and intimate activities can vary greatly across cultures. For example, individuals may feel uncomfortable undressing in front of others, including people of their own gender, yet be totally comfortable sharing a bed with same-gender family members. In many cultures, it is normal for infants and children to share a bed with their parents or other relatives every night. This is in sharp contrast with North American society, where parents and children have separate sleeping quarters, only intimate partners share a bed night after night, and some degree of nudity in front of members of the same gender is not regarded as inappropriate in a locker room.

Care/Cure/Caregivers

Cultural norms influence our personal preferences regarding who provides care and what kind of care or treatment is involved. Consulting professional caregivers is commonplace in some cultures; relying only on one's family or community is the norm in others. Clients may also have different expectations about the type of care or treatment they expect to receive. Different treatments may have different goals, including the following:

- Strengthening the body's capacity to fight illness
- Maintaining the balance among physical, spiritual, and emotional health
- Addressing the symptoms of illness
- Addressing the root cause of the illness

Consider common treatments for a cold: while some people prefer hot liquids (e.g., tea or chicken soup), others advocate citrus juices (usually served cold in North America), and still others seek out medications to either boost their immune system or control the symptoms related to the cold.

When it comes to the caregivers themselves, Canadian and American healthcare systems are based on a team approach, with different members of the team having different roles, often with clear boundaries in terms of who does what. Many cultures, however, are used to a single caregiver, who may be a spiritual healer, medical doctor, or trusted elder. Clients may therefore be unfamiliar with the kinds of roles that comprise a team, or their perceptions of specific roles may be at odds with the reality they now face. In many cultures, for example, nurses are regarded as the doctors, or as families' handmaidens; social workers are sometimes seen as representatives of the state rather than as advocates for clients. It is critical

---

CULTURAL COMPETENCE IN ACTION

Opposite Practices Have a Common Thread
In your childhood days, how did your family react when a child had a fever—put on additional layers of clothing, or take layers off? How was the practice explained?

The two responses may seem completely opposite, yet ultimately they serve a similar purpose. The stated purpose behind adding layers is to encourage the body to break into a sweat, which cools the body as it evaporates. Advocates of taking layers off are also trying to promote body cooling through heat loss. Interestingly, the practice that is most familiar is also likely to feel more comfortable physically and emotionally.

that healthcare providers not assume that the client knows what they do, and they should take the time to discuss their role in a way that is relevant to the client.

Systems of Health Care and Models of Illness

An **explanatory model of illness** is the way a client conceptualizes a sickness episode (Patcher, 1994). Explanatory models are influenced by cultural concepts, beliefs, and values (see Chapter 2). Beliefs about etiology, or origin of illness, are likely to influence the type of care or therapy needed. If an invasion (e.g., by bacteria) is viewed as the cause of an illness, the approach is to attack and conquer (through mechanical or chemical means); if an illness is seen as penance or punishment, it is tolerated and accepted.

The biomedical system of health care (also called allopathy) is frequently referred to in North America as the conventional treatment; however, it is only one of several scientifically based systems of healing. Systems of healing that are based on philosophical and scientific approaches including the following:

- Homeopathy
- Traditional Chinese medicine
- Aboriginal medicine
- Ayurveda
- Allopathy

Although it is impossible for a healthcare provider to have expertise in all the healing systems, it is important to be aware of some of the major ones and to have respect for the foundations they are built on and the therapies they entail. (This is discussed in greater detail in Chapter 8.) It is important to recognize that individuals may make use of more than one source of care during a single episode of illness. While seeking care from biomedical healthcare providers, clients may simultaneously be consulting traditional healers and using herbal remedies and other complementary therapies.

Role of the Family in Care

The roles of various family members in healthcare decisions and interventions also are influenced by cultures. Understanding how to work effectively with families across cultures is a key aspect of generic cultural knowledge and will be discussed in greater depth in Chapter 7. The brief discussion here is meant simply to introduce the issue.

Self-Care/Independence

North American society in general focuses strongly on the individual and on individuals' abilities to maintain or achieve independence and be able to take care of themselves. In many cultures, the concept of being sick means dependence and being taken care of, and taking care of others is part of the family role. Some elders, in particular, expect to be taken care of and see it as the children's duty to take care of them. Parents often view "doing for" as an expression of love and support; others—particularly healthcare providers—may interpret the same behaviour as fostering dependence. Conflict can occur when there are discrepan-

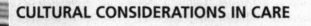

CULTURAL CONSIDERATIONS IN CARE

Different Dynamics in Decision Making

In mainstream North America, the focus generally is on the individual, with the family seen as a contextual support (or a burden, in some instances). Decisions are based on a client's rights and best interests. In many other cultures, the value is on the collective and decisions are made on the basis of the family's best interests.

Differences also exist regarding who is considered the decision maker. In some instances, the grandparent, eldest brother, or eldest son may be the critical decision maker. Therefore, it is important to understand the decision-making patterns and roles within the family system. Gendered and relational role expectations also exist regarding caregiving: daughters-in-law or sons may be the key caregivers in one culture, whereas in other cultures it is the daughter, or else the caregiving responsibilities are shared equally among the children.

Healthcare providers are in a pivotal position to influence assumptions and decisions that are made by a family, but only after the family's values and reasons are understood.

cies between family members and between the family and healthcare providers. It is important that healthcare providers determine and explain the reasons behind the desired behaviours and strive to maintain a balance between clients' achieving independence and feeling that they are being cared for.

Specific Cultural Knowledge

In keeping with the Culture Care Framework's two-step approach to developing cultural knowledge, the preceding discussion focused on core issues that health providers need to be able to recognize and study. The other step in the framework is to develop more in-depth knowledge about populations and issues specific to one's practice. The two steps are intertwined: knowledge of specific cultures and issues allows us to reflect on generic processes, and understanding generic processes provides a context in which we can recognize the specific. Being able to recognize the two types of cultural knowledge also promotes a critical-thinking approach. Healthcare providers always need to assess situations to identify the extent to which the issues involved can be categorized as (1) unique to the individual, (2) reflective of the broader culture or cultures, and (3) reflective of cultural processes in general.

Specific cultural knowledge can be described various ways. Populations may be defined by the following characteristics:

- Clinical specialty (e.g., mental health)
- Cultural group based on ethnic identity (e.g., the Asian community)
- Developmental stage (e.g., end of life)
- Location where health care is accessed (e.g., hospital or community)

Each population has issues that are of particular importance for healthcare providers to understand. Section III of this book offers a range of population-specific examples.

Cultural knowledge begins to address the second half of the guiding principle behind the Culture Care Framework, "To care for someone I must know who the other is," which was presented in Chapter 3 (see Figure 3-1). Both generic and specific cultural knowledge can help us know the other, but only with respect to whom the other *might* be. A critical step of knowing the other is to apply this cultural knowledge to individual assessments (see "Bridging the Gap," later in this chapter).

Cultural Resources

Cultural resources are the third element in the Culture Care Framework. Understanding and developing such resources is a critical part of the journey to cultural competence because, as has been stressed, the healthcare provider is not expected to have all the answers and needs to develop a way to acquire the knowledge and skills and to access the resources that will provide appropriate and effective interventions. As we learned in Chapter 1, the initial call for cultural competence was directed toward individual healthcare providers; however, now it is widely recognized that excellence in care results from competence among healthcare providers as well as from practice environments that support the cultural competence philosophy (College of Nurses of Ontario, 1999). Cultural resources need to be developed at the individual level as well as the broader organizational and systemic level (see Figure 4-2).

Individual-Level Resources

Individual healthcare providers can develop cultural competence in several ways:
- By seeking information
- By reflecting on experiences
- By developing diverse connections

Relevant experiences and connections are essential to developing the confidence and competence necessary to provide good care across populations. The first requirement is a genuine desire to learn *from* the other, not just *about* the other— in other words, to engage in cultural networking. Like other personal networks, cultural networks develop over time. Seeking out opportunities to interact with people (including colleagues) from different cultural communities is a good beginning; it is important, though, to go beyond dance, dialect, dress, and diet to engage with people and learn about different world views and approaches to health, illness, caring, and healing. This requires taking the risk of being unwelcome and not being offended or discouraged should that occur. Being able to examine the reasons and processes behind a lack of welcome provides a unique learning opportunity.

Learning a second language is another way of strengthening an individual's capacity to connect with diverse groups. Films, books, and other media also are rich sources of cultural knowledge. Healthcare professionals can access a variety of informational resources that are made available on the Internet through various associations and interest groups (see Table 4-2 on page 87). Resources related to

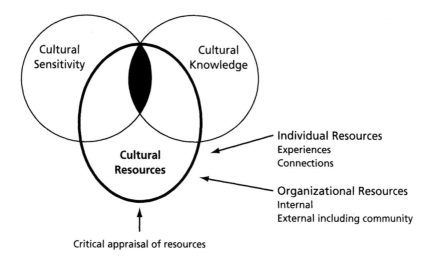

FIGURE 4-2 ■ **Cultural Resources**

specific issues and populations are identified where necessary at the ends of later chapters.

Organizational-Level Resources

Even though resources that are developed by individuals (such as personal contacts) can be invaluable, over-reliance on those resources can be counterproductive. Imagine a healthcare system in which referrals to other agencies, communities, or specialty services cannot take place until individual team members have initiated searches for the services involved or for the specialists needed to make the referrals. Not only would this lead to client delays in accessing services, it would lead to duplication of effort and inappropriate referrals, which in turn would further compromise the efficiency and effectiveness of health care. Cultural resources need to be considered in a similar light.

Organizational resources may be both internal and external to the organization. Internal resources include policies and guidelines that create an expectation for cultural competence in clinical care. Internal organizational resources also include support from a diverse workforce, as well as interpreter services, multifaith religious and spiritual care, and services that offer complementary therapies. Although is it important to have the resources, it is equally important to consider how to make good use of them. Having a diverse workforce may increase an organization's potential capacity to meet the needs of a diverse population, for example, but it also increases the potential for conflict. Without recognizing this potential, and without introducing effective processes to manage the conflict, an organization may have a diverse workforce that remains an untapped resource. Healthcare providers need to be able to tap into this expertise and develop an environment that encourages learning from others. As discussed in Chapter 1, developing team-level cultural competence is important, but that can occur only when individuals within the team make the commitment and provide leadership and support for each other. Clients and families also can be excellent resources for healthcare providers to learn from, provided that the healthcare provider recognizes and values the experience and expertise they offer.

External organizational resources may include services noted above (e.g., interpreter services or religious support) and a variety of partnerships (e.g., with community leaders and groups, non-mainstream healthcare agencies, and alternative therapy providers). Strategies to develop such partnerships are similar to strategies for developing personal networks. It is important to identify the potential resources that are in the community—particularly individuals and groups who may not be connected to the healthcare agency—and to explore opportunities to get them into the organization, for example, through community forums and community advisory groups. Offering to share organizational expertise and resources with community groups is another way to begin an alliance.

When we work with resources such as culture-specific services, one issue that often arises is the balance between referring to a service and seeking advice from a service. As discussed in Chapter 1, ethno-specific services have limited capacity, and mainstream agencies need to develop greater responsiveness. It is critical that healthcare providers view such services as learning resources to help develop their own abilities as well as a resource that clients can use to receive care.

Critical Appraisal and Use of Resources

Having access to resources is essential for the provision of culturally appropriate care; however, healthcare providers also need to use critical-thinking skills to assess how applicable the resource is. In the technologically enriched twenty-first century, with a variety of Internet search engines at our disposal, the challenge is not in finding information but in assessing the quality, adequacy, and applicability of information. When we use a cultural resource, no matter what the form— printed, electronic, human, or experiential—we need to practise ongoing individualized assessment. A single experience with a culture tells us only about that encounter; the experience may or may not be typical of, or similar to, other experiences with that culture. A single individual from a culture can be a valuable informant, but no individual represents all aspects of a culture. Culture is about possible patterns, not universal truths. Resources can help us recognize patterns, interpret information, or generate hypotheses, but ultimately the interpretation needs to be validated with the client and refined for the specific situation.

The list of useful Web sites provided in Table 4-2 should in no way be considered exhaustive. New information is constantly being generated, and readers are encouraged to develop their own lists of information sources based on areas of interest and focus.

Thus far, the discussion of the Culture Care Framework has been limited to the three elements of sensitivity, knowledge, and resources. Ultimately, however, success lies in translating awareness into practice, which is the topic of the second part of the Culture Care Framework discussion.

TABLE 4-2

Selected Web Sites as Cultural Resources

Canadian Sites

www.cprn.org/en/diversity.cfm
Developed by the Canadian Policy Research Network (CPRN), Diversity Gateway presents information on diversity issues from a Canadian perspective. CPRN's mission is to create knowledge and lead public debate on social and economic issues important to the well-being of Canadians. The site provides historical and statistical information, and information on the meaning of pluralism and citizenship. There is a particular focus on youth and the future.

www.culture.ca
An initiative of the federal Department of Heritage, Culture.ca aims to engage Canadians in cultural life, to educate and entertain Web surfers with the stories of many peoples, and to provide access to the best of Canadian culture online.

www.settlement.org
Developed by Citizenship and Immigration Canada and the Province of Ontario, Settlement.org provides information to and for newcomers to Ontario and those who work with them.

www.cp-pc.ca/english/index.htm
This URL is the gateway to cultural profiles for more than 100 countries. The profiles have been developed by Citizenship and Immigration Canada, in association with the AMNI Centre, at the Faculty of Social Work, University of Toronto. Each cultural profile provides an overview of life and customs in the featured country. Information about health care and communication also is included. Although each profile provides insight into some customs, it does not cover all facets of life, and the customs described may not apply in equal measure to all newcomers from the profiled country.

www.ag.gov.bc.ca/sam/index.htm
The Settlement and Multiculturalism Division of British Columbia's Ministry of Attorney General focuses on settlement and adaptation as well as anti-racism and multiculturalism programs. The site offers information for newcomers as well as information about community resources within the area.

www.ceris.metropolis.net
The Joint Centre of Excellence for Research on Immigration and Settlement, Toronto (CERIS), is a consortium of Toronto-area universities and community partners. It is one of four such research centres across Canada. The Metropolis Project provides resources, including information for research and policy on migration, diversity, and changing cities. The Web site includes access to a virtual library and newsletters.

International Sites

http://depts.washington.edu/pfes/cultureclues.html
Culture Clues™ are tip sheets for clinicians, designed to increase awareness about concepts and preferences of clients from the diverse cultures served by the University of Washington Medical Center. Prepared by a cultural anthropologist, this Web site provides health-related information on specific cultures. Topics covered include communication, family and gender issues, pain, end-of-life considerations, pregnancy and childbirth, and health-related practices.

continued

TABLE 4-2 *continued*

http://iccnetwork.org/cancerfacts/
Prepared by the Intercultural Cancer Council (ICC), this Web site contains brief
(one- to two-page) descriptions of cancer issues for various cultures. Each
section includes an extensive reference list. The ICC promotes policies, programs,
partnerships, and research to eliminate disparities surrounding cancer among
racial and ethnic minorities and medically underserved populations in the
United States and its associated territories.

www.omhrc.gov/clas
Produced for the US Department of Health and Human Services's Office of Minority
Health, this Web site provides information regarding the national standards for
Culturally and Linguistically Appropriate Services (CLAS) in health care. These
standards were developed with input from a national advisory committee of
policymakers, healthcare providers, and researchers. Each standard is accompanied
by commentary that addresses the proposed guideline's relationship to existing
laws and standards, and offers recommendations for implementation.

http://bphc.hrsa.gov/quality/default.htm
This Web site, prepared by the US Department of Health and Human Services's
Bureau of Primary Health Care, provides a link to *The Provider's Guide to Quality
& Culture*, a new Web resource to help healthcare professionals provide good-
quality culturally and linguistically appropriate services to multicultural populations. Content includes information on health disparities, client–healthcare
provider interactions, cultural groups, and culturally competent organizations.

www.diversityrx.org
Supported by several institutions—the US National Conference of State
Legislatures (NCSL), Resources for Cross Cultural Health Care (RCCHC), and the
Henry J. Kaiser Family Foundation of Menlo Park, CA—Diversity Rx is a US-based
clearing house of information on how to meet the language and cultural needs
of minorities, immigrants, refugees, and other diverse populations seeking
health care. Sections provide information on models, (US) policy, expert
opinions, and annual conference highlights.

www.health.qld.gov.au/multicultural/default.asp
Developed by Queensland Health, Australia, this Web site provides guides and
policies to support the provision of culturally sensitive health care in hospitals
and community health services. There are cultural profiles on specific
communities and information for health providers on issues such as language,
understanding hospital systems, admission, diagnostic investigations, birthing
practices, and gender and modesty.

www.ethnicityonline.net/default.htm
This UK Web site aims to provide a resource for the multidisciplinary,
multicultural healthcare community that will help people's understanding of,
and involvement in, cross-cultural issues affecting the giving or receiving of
health care. The Web site provides information about several ethnic groups;
cultural issues that might arise in everyday healthcare situations; and links to
groups where further help, support, and advice can be found.

www.rcn.org.uk/resources/transcultural/
This UK Web site presents a series of learning modules by a variety of authors.
The materials have been piloted across several institutions in the UK. Topics
include practice areas such as child health, adult health, and learning disability,
as well as broader topics such as the politics of diversity, race-equality
management, and epidemiology of diversity.

Bridging the Gap

The Culture Care Framework identifies the need to go beyond knowing oneself and the other and to overcome any cultural rift separating the health provider and the client. Although specific theoretical principles exist regarding how to bridge the gap (e.g., respect and negotiation), practical interpretations and behavioural guidelines are not as clear. The Culture Care Framework draws on works by Arthur Kleinman (Kleinman, Eisenberg, & Good, 1978) and Madeleine Leininger (Leininger, 1995) to provide practical and concrete strategies to bridge the gap.

The first step in the process is to understand the similarities and differences between the client's and the healthcare provider's interpretation of the situation. Leininger's Theory of Culture Care Diversity and Universality explicitly recognizes the interactions between clients' generic folk-care (emic) practices and healthcare providers' care-cure (etic) practices (Leininger, 1995). Leininger notes that it is important to obtain a client's emic knowledge before reflecting on etic or healthcare-provider knowledge in order to "discover" care meanings and avoid imposing the values of the healthcare provider (Leininger, 1995). Although this can seem like an unrealistic expectation for clinical interactions, understanding client perspectives and preferences is a fundamental tenet of all client-centred or client-focused care approaches. Simply put, being client-centred means that it is important to elicit the client's perspective and priorities in every clinical encounter.

Kleinman et al. (1978) refer to the understanding of client perspectives as understanding client "agendas" and offer a framework for drawing out clients' explanatory models of illness and care through a series of eight questions that can be readily incorporated into various assessment approaches. The College of Nurses of Ontario (1999) guidelines expanded the initial list to include four questions that address not just perceptions of the illness but also aspects of treatment preferences. The dozen questions are presented in Table 4-3.

The questions in Table 4-3 are useful and adaptable. They are open ended, and they begin with the current issue and expand outward to what else may be

TABLE 4-3

Understanding the Client's Explanatory Models of Illness and Care

1. What do you call the problem?
2. What do you think has caused the problem?
3. Why do you think it started when it did?
4. What do you think the sickness does to you? How does it work?
5. How severe is the sickness? Will it have a short or long course?
6. What are the major problems or difficulties that the sickness has caused in your life?
7. What have you done for this problem up to now?
8. What kind of treatment do you think you should receive?
9. What are the most important results you hope to achieve from this treatment?
10. What do you fear most about the sickness?
11. What do you fear most about the treatment?
12. Who else should be consulted or involved in your (or your family member's) care?

significant. This contrasts with many cultural-assessment tools, which begin with an exploration of background factors and then ask the healthcare provider to determine what is relevant. The open-ended nature of the questions reinforces the need to value client expertise in the interaction.

The questions are a tool and serve as a guide; healthcare providers should assess the situation to determine exactly when and what to ask clients, modifying the words and tone as needed to fit the setting and the relationship. A useful strategy is to listen to the words that the client uses and to reflect them in the questions. For example, the client may refer to his or her problem as a problem, illness, sickness, or condition; the healthcare providers can use the same word as a way of acknowledging the client's expertise and building mutual understanding. The order of questioning is not critical and not all the information needs to be collected during the first interaction. Sometimes it is useful to depersonalize the questions. In some circumstances, clients may be reluctant to disclose their own beliefs but may be more willing to share beliefs held by the community in general or some individuals within the community. In such circumstances, questions can be phrased so to ask how the problem would be treated in the family or community, or what the client thinks others fear about the illness or treatment. Similarly, when working in pediatric settings, the questions can be modified to elicit both a parent's and a child's point of view (Goldbloom, 2003). Using the list of questions with different family members can alert the healthcare provider to conflicting viewpoints within the family, which in turn may influence acceptance of the suggested interventions.

Exploring the client's explanatory model of illness is a useful way to generate a comprehensive list of issues and can help the healthcare provider identify key values that may be influencing the healthcare encounter and should be included in the plan of care.

Modes of Action and Decision

Madeleine Leininger's "three modes of nursing action and decision" serve as guidelines for general healthcare interventions based on the care values identified by the client. The chosen mode(s) needs to fit the client's world views as well as incorporate provider expertise that may benefit the client. The modes of action identified in the Culture Care Framework are based on Leininger's (1995) work and comprise **cultural care validation/preservation**, **cultural care accommodation/ negotiation**; and **cultural care reframing/repatterning** (see Figure 4-3).

Cultural Care Validation/Preservation

Cultural care "preservation" refers to actions and decisions that help clients retain their meaningful care values and lifeways (Leininger, 1995). This approach means making efforts to integrate a client's preferences into the plan of care when these preferences are important to the client's physical, spiritual, or emotional health. The Culture Care Framework uses the additional term "validation" to emphasize the need for client values to be recognized as legitimate preferences

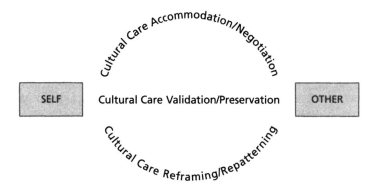

FIGURE 4-3 ▪ **Strategies to Bridge the Gap**

and not just idiosyncratic beliefs. Cultural care validation/preservation is most appropriate when the client's preference poses no risk of harming the client or others (College of Nurses of Ontario, 1999).

It should be noted that acknowledging and supporting others in preserving their values, traditions, or practices does not mean that the healthcare provider has to agree with or endorse those practices. Cultural care validation/preservation encourages healthcare providers to find the values and practices that are important to the client and, where possible, work with these values and practices as a foundation for mutual goal-setting. In a discussion of how acquired immune deficiency syndrome (AIDS) should be explained within different cultural communities, Lechky (1997) highlights the importance of recognizing and working with cultural values and norms. Cultural validation/preservation occurs when healthcare providers present information in ways and places that are acceptable and valued in the client's culture. For example, for communities where sexual behaviour is considered a private topic, it is important to respect cultural norms and use materials without graphic drawings of body parts or physical contact (Lechky, 1997).

Despite the fact that acknowledging client preferences is a foundation for good practice, healthcare providers generally under-use cultural care validation/ preservation strategies when the values in question are not problematic and remain invisible. However, acknowledging or validating care values that are important for clients to preserve can have extremely positive effects with respect to the relationship. It also signals to the client that the healthcare provider has an understanding of and respect for cultures, which increases the likelihood of subsequent disclosure on issues that may be more personal or controversial.

Cultural Care Accommodation/Negotiation

The term "accommodation" means to make suitable or adapt. It can, however, also imply doing a favour or obliging someone. It is important to recognize that cultural care accommodation is not about obliging; rather, it is about assisting clients and healthcare providers in adapting their ways to include courses of

CULTURAL COMPETENCE IN ACTION

Religious Insight Goes a Long Way
An 18-year-old client arrived in the emergency room after a motor vehicle accident. From the admission sheet, the nurse noted that the client's stated religion was Islam. During the nutritional assessment, the nurse sought out the client's food preferences and also asked him whether he was fasting during Ramadan and how that might impact on the care he could receive while in hospital.

The client reacted with considerable surprise that not only was the nurse aware of the Islamic tradition of fasting during Ramadan, a special month of the year when keeping fasts is obligatory for most Muslims, but, more important, was willing to consider how this practice could be incorporated into the care schedule. This initial question enhanced the trust within the nurse–client relationship and allowed the client to be more comfortable in discussing his nutritional as well as spiritual needs.

action that may have been previously unfamiliar or inaccessible to the client. Leininger (1995) defines cultural care accommodation/negotiation as provider actions or decisions that help people of one culture adapt to or negotiate with others for meaningful and beneficial healthcare outcomes. In this mode of action, the healthcare provider is encouraged to explore ways to accommodate client choice by minimizing risks and finding ways to overcome barriers (College of Nurses of Ontario, 1999). Common examples of accommodation include using interpreters to ensure that the clients are able to participate in their care; allowing different/multiple family members to visit and/or participate in care; and scheduling procedures and tests around times of prayer or significant visits.

Like validation, the act of negotiation itself can be very useful to decrease the power imbalance in the healthcare provider–client relationship by signalling to the client that his or her perspectives and wishes are important. The first step in clinical negotiation is to develop trust in the therapeutic relationship (Katon & Kleinman, 1980). Negotiation implies a balancing of competing priorities and occurs when there are differences between the client's and the healthcare provider's preferences and the healthcare provider feels strongly that his or her medical interventions are essential to the client's care. This means first making those preferences and priorities explicit by eliciting the client's explanatory model of illness. If the healthcare provider doesn't understand the client's explanatory model, negotiation can occur in a parallel universe, with the healthcare provider focusing on one problem and the client focusing on other illness-related issues. For negotiation to be successful, it needs to be supported by education (Katon & Kleinman, 1980) so that the choices that are made are informed. Negotiation often occurs around therapies such as medications that the client may be reluctant to accept because of a preference for herbal or other kinds of treatments. It is important that healthcare providers both learn about and provide information on the various therapies under consideration. In this instance, it may be possible to negotiate with the client to take the medication and the complementary treatment, as long as the two treatments are not incompatible (College of Nurses of Ontario, 1999).

When considering the mode of cultural care accommodation/negotiation, healthcare providers should avoid seeing the strategies as "either/or" and should explore the "this and . . ." approach instead. A useful question to ask is, "What would it take to _____?"; the blank can be filled with whatever the client's values are demanding. The answer may, in turn, generate another "What would it take" question. Consider the example of a Middle Eastern family requesting that their father not be cared for by female nurses. If one uses the "What would it take" question, the first answer would obviously be a male nurse. However, if there were no male nurses scheduled on that shift, accommodation in the short term would not be possible. It then becomes important to negotiate with the family what care needs to be performed and who can perform it. The question then may become, "What would it take to provide the care in a culturally acceptable manner?" In some instances, male family members may be willing to take on some responsibility while female nurses carry out other medical interventions. Other answers for "What would it take" questions could be to request a male nurse in the form of a temporary member of staff. However, that may not be possible due to either budgetary limitations (in this

---

CULTURAL COMPETENCE IN ACTION

Family Visits
Mrs. Porkapolos is an elderly Greek woman who often has many family members visiting her, even though signs are posted that clearly restrict the number of visitors per client. The family often becomes very loud and disturbs the other client in the room. Nursing staff are unsure how to deal with this situation.

Some staff members allow the extra visitors in order to accommodate the client's cultural needs. They recognize that close family in this culture includes members of the extended family and that the role of family is significant in care. Other healthcare providers, however, are concerned about the needs of the other client and the disruption that the family causes. The inconsistency leads to frustration for both the family and the hospital staff.

How would you handle this situation? Several strategies can be tried. The most important thing is to have a consistent plan of care so that individual healthcare providers are not required to make decisions independently or arbitrarily. Recognizing and involving the family is critical but can be done in ways that avoid allowing multiple visitors. Staff can acknowledge the value of family support while raising their own concerns and limitations. Potential solutions can include assisting Mrs. Porkapolos to the lounge area when she can have visitors, to minimize their impact on the other client; encouraging the family to take turns and maintain a stronger presence rather than all coming at once; and determining whether one or two family members could serve as spokespersons and co-ordinators of the family activities.

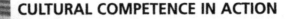

CULTURAL COMPETENCE IN ACTION

Arranging an Exorcism
Chachkes and Christ cite the following example in their discussion on cross-cultural issues in client education:

> A 12-year-old Hispanic boy was hospitalized because of the acute onset of auditory hallucinations. The boy's grandmother, his legal guardian, refused to give the physician permission to medicate the boy. She insisted he was possessed, and the devil needed to be exorcised. The grandmother was a respected *Bruja* in her community who could do the exorcism. A negotiated agreement was reached: the grandmother could do the exorcism in the hospital, following which she would sign the medication consent. She understood her grandson's reluctance to take medication, so she offered to bless the medication tray in a ritual he could witness. The outcome was very positive and replaced the previous impasse between family and healthcare staff. Even a North American solution, such as a court order to override the grandmother's objections, would not have assured the essential medication compliance.

From "Cross cultural issues in patient education," by E. Chachkes and G. Christ, 1996, *Patient Education and Counselling, 27*, 13–21.

instance, the family may be willing to bear the cost of private duty nurses if the hospital agrees) or lack of availability (all nurses who are qualified are female). Even if the request is not accommodated successfully, the family is likely to be more accepting of the limitation when they believe that genuine attempts have been made to accommodate them; the healthcare providers and family would then work together to determine the appropriate actions given the circumstances. Sometimes "What would it take" is a policy that needs to be changed or a resource that needs to be developed. Raising the issue becomes the first step in addressing it, and although the change may not occur in time to be beneficial to the client who instigated the question, it may benefit other clients in the future.

Cultural Care Reframing/Repatterning

Cultural care repatterning helps clients to reorder, change, or modify their life-ways to discover new possibilities and ways of achieving health goals (College of Nurses of Ontario, 1999; Leininger, 1995). Leininger called this mode repatterning/restructuring. The mode of action is about reframing preconceived ideas to discover new meanings and new patterns, hence the term reframing. Reframing is about seeing something differently; repatterning is about changing our patterns to do things differently. Cultural care reframing/repatterning must be differentiated from cultural imposition, in which the healthcare provider's viewpoint is assumed to be somehow superior and efforts are made to convince the client to accept the viewpoint.

Reframing offers the client alternative ways of understanding behaviour and discovering new patterns and meanings if the client chooses to try it. For example, Western society is heavily focused on the individual and the value of taking care of oneself. As noted previously, in many other cultures, the comparable value is to care for others; in these cultures, putting oneself first is not considered a priority and may even be regarded as selfish behaviour, especially by the women. Women of Eastern cultures often are unwilling to seek health care for complaints perceived to be minor or engage in exercise programs focused toward improving their own health and well-being. Healthcare providers working with this context must acknowledge the value of taking care of others but offer the alternative explanation that being healthy is a prerequisite to being able to take care of others. An analogy of airline safety practices can be used to illustrate the point. In the safety instructions on all flights, passengers are advised that if oxygen masks become necessary, adults should put on their masks before assisting children or others needing assistance.

The mode of cultural care reframing and repatterning is not limited to clients; it can apply equally to healthcare providers. In many cultures, for example—including both the Navajo people in the United States and the Dene people in Canada—speaking explicitly about terminal illness and death is said to hasten death. As a result, families may request that news of this nature not be communicated directly to the client (Ellerby, McKenzie, McKay, Gariepy, & Kaufert, 2000). Some healthcare providers may regard compliance with such a request as withholding the truth, and they may feel obligated to disregard family wishes and tell the client the information. However, others may consider that going against the family wishes would constitute imposing the truth. Recognizing the different ways of framing a situation may allow both parties to consider a third option, that of offering the truth and "allowing the person to define the level and explicitness of the information they require to interpret care options" (Ellerby et al., 2000, p. 847).

Another example at a broader healthcare system level is the recognition of practices such as therapeutic touch. A couple of decades ago, this practice may have been considered an unscientific ritual with little place in Western health care; today it is recognized in many jurisdictions as a valuable and legitimate therapy and has been integrated into many hospitals and professions. The reframing/repatterning mode is based on the need for continually challenging old assumptions and creating new possibilities that lead to more options for clients, healthcare providers, and the healthcare system.

The above discussion on modes of action and decision offers a practical approach to addressing gaps that cultural differences may have created. The modes we have discussed can serve as the bridge over the cultural divide. It is important to recognize that there are no clear answers or strategies that work in all circumstances. Instead, multiple strategies will need to be used simultaneously to validate, accommodate, and reframe the values and meanings that underlie behaviour. Successful interactions will result in positive learning experiences for both the client and the healthcare provider.

CULTURAL COMPETENCE IN ACTION

When Male Partners Do the Talking

Nancy is a nurse who works in the women's outpatient program in a hospital that serves a large number of refugees and recent immigrants to Canada. In her practice, Nancy frequently encounters situations in which the male partner accompanies the woman to her appointment, answers the questions on her behalf, and essentially does not allow the woman to interact directly with the healthcare providers.

Nancy has found this extremely frustrating. Although she recognizes that many cultures have different gender roles and behaviours, she feels that because the women are now in Canada, the healthcare providers needs to help empower them to claim equal status. Nancy is also concerned from a practice perspective. She is aware of the increased potential for domestic violence in immigrant communities that has been associated with the stress of migration, underemployment, and changing family roles, and she finds it difficult to assess for this risk without an opportunity to interact with the woman alone.

In a discussion about cultural competence, Nancy realizes that much of her reaction has been influenced by her own feminist background and her beliefs related to gender roles and the associated history of women's rights in society. However, she still finds this situation extremely challenging to deal with.

What advice would you give Nancy in working through this situation? Would you agree that the male partner's behaviour is oppressive and its influence needs to be minimized? Would any other explanations account for the male partner's behaviour?

In your discussion, imagine the following scenario: you have travelled to a strange country with someone you care for very much (e.g., spouse, child, sibling, or parent). Your significant other becomes ill and needs health care; however, the language as well as the healthcare system is unfamiliar. When seeking health care, would you accompany your significant other? Are there circumstances under which you might speak for them (bearing in mind that many native-born Canadians do that when they think their significant others will not be clear or complete about their symptoms)? How would you react if you felt that people were trying very hard to separate you from your significant other?

This scenario illustrates that what may be labelled as oppressive behaviour could in fact be an expression of caring. Nancy's attempts to ignore or distance the male partner are likely to have the opposite impact by increasing distrust. The alternative explanation does not mean that the first hypothesis was incorrect, but it does caution against premature judgement and suggests the need for additional data. Nancy's desire to empower women (or at least to set the tone) on their initial visits is reflective of her priority and not necessarily that of her client. If, however, Nancy is successful in developing a relationship with both the woman and the male partner, the woman is likely to feel safer and in subsequent interactions may share any concerns she has related to her partner and/or domestic stress and abuse.

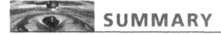

SUMMARY

This chapter has presented two of the three elements of the Culture Care Framework: cultural knowledge and cultural resources. It is important for healthcare providers to develop generic cultural knowledge that applies across populations and also knowledge that is focused on specific cultures or clinical populations. Cultural resources need to be developed at the individual as well as the organizational level. These two elements, together with cultural sensitivity (which was discussed in Chapter 3), are critical for the development and application of clinical cultural competence.

The three elements allow healthcare providers to understand themselves and others; however, identifying a cultural gap does not automatically mean we know how to bridge it. The framework therefore includes strategies for determining key client values and priorities and for addressing differences that may exist between the client's and the healthcare provider's explanatory models of illness and treatment. Although the need for negotiation and accommodation is widely recognized, the framework also includes the strategies of validation and reframing. Both validation and reframing are critical supports for the negotiation process.

The Culture Care Framework can thus be summarized as a framework that recognizes three key elements that are necessary to develop cultural competence: cultural sensitivity, cultural knowledge, and cultural resources. All three elements are needed to assist healthcare providers in identifying key cultural values that affect the clinical encounter. The key cultural values can then be incorporated into health care by actions aimed at validation, negotiation, and reframing to help ensure that the care is culturally suitable.

REFERENCES

Adelson, N. (2005). The embodiment of inequity. *Canadian Journal of Public Health*, *96*(Suppl. 2), 45–61.

American Heritage Dictionaries. (2000). *The American Heritage Dictionary of the English Language* (4th ed.). Boston: Houghton Mifflin.

Betancourt, J., Green, A. R., & Carrillo, J. E. (2002). *Cultural competence in health care: Emerging frameworks and practical approaches.* New York: The Commonwealth Fund.

Bonder, B., Martin, L., & Miracle, A. (2002). *Culture in clinical care.* Thorofare, NJ: Slack.

Campinha-Bacote, J. (1995). The quest for cultural competence in nursing care. *Nursing Forum*, *30*(4), 19–25.

Campinha-Bacote, J. (1999). A model and instrument for addressing cultural competence in health care. *Journal of Nursing Education, 38*(5), 203–207.

Campinha-Bacote, J. (2000). A review of ethnic psycho-pharmacology: A neglected area of cultural competence in psychiatric and mental health nursing. In J. Campinha-Bacote (Ed.), *Readings and resources in transcultural health care and mental health*, (12th ed., pp. 127–35). Cincinnati, OH: Josepha Campinha-Bacote.

Chachkes, E., & Christ, G. (1996). Cross cultural issues in patient education. *Patient Education and Counseling, 27,* 13–21.

College of Nurses of Ontario (1999). *Guidelines for providing culturally sensitive care.* Toronto, Author.

Cortis, J. (2003). Managing society's difference and diversity. *Nursing Standard, 18*(14–16), 33–39.

Ellerby, J., McKenzie, J., McKay, S., Gariepy, G., & Kaufert, J. M. (2000). Bioethics for clinicians: Aboriginal cultures. *Canadian Medical Association Journal, 163*(7), 845–850.

Gleick, J. (1987). *Chaos: Making a new science.* New York: Viking.

Goldbloom, R. B. (2003). *Skills for culturally sensitive pediatric care.* Philadelphia: Saunders.

Katon, W., & Kleinman, A. (1980). Doctor–patient negotiation and other social science strategies in patient care. In L. Eisenberg & S. Klimidis (Eds.), *The relevance of social science for medicine* (pp. 253–279). Boston: D. Reidel Publishing.

Kleinman, A., Eisenberg, L., & Good, B. (1978). Culture, illness, and care: Clinical lessons from anthropologic and cross cultural research. *Annals of Internal Medicine, 88,* 251–258.

Lechky, O. (1997). Multiculturalism and AIDS. *Canadian Medical Association Journal, 156,* 1446–1448.

Leininger, M. (1995). *Overview of Leininger's theory of culture care.* In M. Leininger (Ed.), *Transcultural nursing: Concepts, theories, research and practice* (2nd ed., pp. 93–114). New York: John Wiley & Sons.

Office of Minority Health Resource Center. (2001). Assuring cultural competence in health care: Recommendations for national standards and an outcomes focused research agenda. Retrieved May 19, 2004, from http://www.omhrc.gov/CLAS/

Patcher, L. (1994). Culture and clinical care: Folk illness beliefs and behaviors and their implications for health care delivery. *Journal of the American Medical Association, 271*(9), 690–694.

Purnell, L. (2000). A description of the Purnell model for cultural competence. *Journal of Transcultural Nursing, 11*(1), 40–46.

Taylor, J. (2003). Confronting 'culture' in medicine's 'culture of no culture'. *Academic Medicine, 78*(6), 555–559.

SECTION II

Universally Applicable Cultural Knowledge

This section presents four chapters that systematically examine communication, interpretation, family, illness beliefs, and ways of healing. The issues and strategies discussed are considered to be generic cultural knowledge (a fundamental requirement for cultural competence), regardless of the specific cultural or clinical population that a healthcare provider may work with. References to specific cultural groups appear throughout the chapters for illustrative purposes only, and readers are reminded to remain alert to individual variations when dealing with clients in order to avoid stereotyping. It is also important for readers to constantly remain self-aware regarding the issues presented in each discussion.

Chapter 5 begins with a discussion of communication issues that arise between the professional healthcare culture and that of the client, regardless of ethnic and cultural similarity or dissimilarity. Providing health care for any client presents challenges, which become more complex when the cultural dimensions of race, ethnicity, language, and religion are added into the equation.

Chapter 6 focuses specifically on communication that involves limited English language proficiency and/or working with interpreters. Since interpreters are an essential part of clinical care, healthcare providers must be well versed in how best to collaborate with them. This chapter therefore offers practical strategies and tips for strengthening three-way communication.

Chapter 7 presents an overview of the main cultural issues involved in caring for diverse families. Just as no two families are alike, unique combinations of issues and strategies apply to individual families. The chapter presents a number of the key issues related to family roles and rules that are influenced by cultural leanings toward individualism or collectivism and that, in turn, influence the general use of health services and the acceptance of specific forms of care.

Chapter 8 provides an overview of health and illness models and discusses such traditional forms of healing as Aboriginal medicine, traditional Chinese medicine, Ayurveda, and homeopathy. It is important to remember that what one person views as "alternative" or "complementary" is, in fact, the familiar and traditional approach for others. Readers are strongly encouraged to consult other sources to build on the foundation of knowledge about the healing paradigm that this chapter aims to provide.

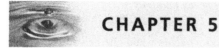

CHAPTER 5

Cross-Cultural Communication

RANI SRIVASTAVA

Special thanks to Angela McNabb for her contribution to this chapter.

LEARNING OBJECTIVES

At the end of this chapter, the learner will be able to:

- Identify the influence of culture on verbal and non-verbal communication
- Distinguish between high-context and low-context communication styles and identify strategies to work with each of them
- Identify the impact of power and authority on communication styles
- Acquire practical skills for enhancing communication with clients who have limited English proficiency
- Describe the characteristics of effective conversations
- Differentiate between inquiring and dismissive responses

KEY TERMS

Bi-directional conversations	Idioms
Collectivism	Individualism
Decoding	Inquiring responses
Encoding	Low-context communication
Face	Monochronic time (M-time)
High-context communication	Polychronic time (P-time)

Communication is the main tool that healthcare providers use to supply health-care services. Successful communication is a two-way street, and the healthcare setting demands considerable communication skills on the part of both the healthcare provider and the client. Complex issues must be mutually understood; subsequent decisions about treatment concern issues of great importance that affect all facets of life and are frequently emotionally charged (McJannett, Butow, Tattersall, & Thompson, 2003).

At its most basic level, communication occurs when one person (the sender or encoder) sends a message to another person (the receiver or decoder) (Munoz & Luckmann, 2005). **Encoding** refers to the processes we use to put thoughts, emotions, feelings, or attitudes into forms that others can recognize; **decoding** is the process of perceiving and interpreting the incoming messages. Culture affects both the encoding and decoding of messages. Because communication is an ongoing, dynamic process, encoding and decoding happen together and influence each other. What is decoded (i.e., understood) influences what is encoded (i.e., sent in response) and vice versa (Gudykunst & Young, 1992). It is important to remember that while messages can be transmitted from one person to another, meanings cannot.

Communication and cultural competence go hand in hand. Healthcare providers who want to develop cultural competence need to understand cross-cultural communication patterns and work out ways to strengthen their own communication skills. If we develop cultural sensitivity (one of the elements of the Culture Care Framework discussed in Chapters 3 and 4), we by implication recognize that the communication patterns we are familiar with may not apply; cultural sensitivity, however, does not help create new ones. Knowledge is necessary to recognize and develop new patterns.

This chapter begins with a brief discussion of the vital role that communication plays in health care. As we examine the influence of culture on communication, we discuss the various ways that cultures can differ. Language issues—including those associated with limited proficiency in the dominant language—also are presented. For the purposes of this chapter, the dominant language is assumed to be English. The chapter ends with a discussion about effective conversations and strategies to foster communication.

Communication and Health Care

Communication is important in all healthcare services. It has been associated with client satisfaction with health care as well as healthcare outcomes (Cruz & Pincus, 2002; Suraez-Almazor, 2004; Thorne, Harris, Mahoney, Con, & McGuiness, 2004). Communication is critical to processes of establishing trust (Baker, 2001; Pope, 2004), informed consent (Barnes, Davis, Moran, Portillo, & Koenig, 1998), decision making (Degner et al., 1997), and self-management of chronic illnesses (Hussein & Partridge, 2002; Rogers, Kennedy, Nelson, Robinson, 2005; Thorne et al., 2004). The authors Roter, Hall, and Aoki (2002) note that even when English-speaking clients speak with English-speaking physicians, they often have difficulty understanding what was said and feeling empowered enough to ask for clarification (Pope, 2004).

As noted by Suarez-Almazor (2004), the medical or healthcare interview involves three essential functions:

1. Information gathering
2. Relationship building
3. Client education

In reality, however, much time is spent on information gathering and information giving (versus client education).

Research indicates that communication in a healthcare context is more likely to centre around the healthcare provider than the client (Kaufert, Putsch, & Lavallee, 1999; Rogers et al., 2005; Suraez-Almazor, 2004). Healthcare provider–centred approaches reflect a view that the healthcare provider is the expert, and are characterized by the healthcare provider dominating the conversation, asking closed-ended questions, and interrupting or dismissing client questions, opinions, or contexts (Suraez-Almazor, 2004). In this type of interaction, the healthcare provider's perspective determines the meaning, and client self-management may be defined as medical compliance only, with the healthcare provider dismissing the client's efforts to explore alternatives (Rogers et al., 2005). In contrast, client-centred approaches are characterized by being attentive to client interpretations of symptoms; discussing lifestyle and treatment choices in an open, non-judgemental way; and understanding client views, information needs, and concerns (Suraez-Almazor, 2004; Thorne et al., 2004).

In a healthcare encounter, a number of factors can have a negative impact on the client's ability to understand what is being communicated. Clinical experience shows that these include the following:

▪ The client is under physical stress and experiencing at least some degree of emotional distress.
▪ The healthcare provider uses technical language or professional jargon.
▪ The client typically has little time with the doctor and the encounter is frequently rushed.
▪ The healthcare provider fails to grasp the situation from the client's point of view.

Healthcare literature involving cancer clients indicates not only that clients have a variety of preferences when it comes to decision making, but also that discrepancies exist between what clients prefer and what they experience. Significant discrepancies have been noted between women clients' preferred versus actual roles in decision making; factors cited as hindering the women's involvement in the process include insufficient information and pressure to make decisions quickly (Degner et al., 1997). Thus, it is clearly evident that communication in the healthcare context is a complex phenomenon with multiple, ongoing challenges.

Communication and Culture

Communication in the healthcare system poses challenges for all individuals, but the challenges can have particularly grave consequences and seem insurmountable when there are cultural differences and language barriers between clients and healthcare providers. Cultural dissimilarity has been identified as a leading cause of ineffective communication between two ethnic groups (King, 2000). Conversely, communication has been identified as the main barrier to providing culturally sensitive care (Coffman, 2004).

Ineffective communication across cultures goes beyond undermining the healthcare provider–client relationship; it also leads to the following:

▪ Neglect
▪ Misdiagnosis
▪ An inability to obtain genuine informed consent

- An inadequate healthcare teaching
- Dissatisfaction with care
- An inability on the client's part to access and follow through with health-care services and treatments
(Baker, 2001; Barnes et al., 1998; Chachkes & Christ, 1996; Coffman, 2004; Hussein & Partridge, 2002; McPhee, 2002; Mir & Tovey, 2002; Robb & Douglas, 2004; Rogers et al., 2005).

Although language is the most obvious and frequently cited challenge to cross-cultural communication (Coffman, 2004), it is important to remember that communication is a multi-dimensional concept and involves much more than the spoken word. Among the major reasons for difficulties in cross-cultural communication is the fact that persons from different cultures have different understandings and expectations of the interaction process, and different styles of communication (Korac-Kakabadse, Kouzmin, Korac-Kakabadse, & Savery, 2001).

Differences in Communication Style

Communication takes place at varying levels of awareness. A large number of interactions occur at very low levels of awareness—these are things we do automatically without a great deal of conscious thought. Although we vary our communication approaches based on the situation, patterns tend to surface unless we make a deliberate attempt to act differently.

Communication Context: High versus Low

The influence of culture on communication goes beyond the language spoken and includes communication styles and/or patterns (DuPraw & Axner, 1997; Gudykunst & Young, 1992; Korac-Kakabadse et al., 2001). Anthropologist Edward Hall developed a theoretical model of cultural variability (i.e., ways in which cultures differ) based on the concepts of information processing, time orientation, and the interaction patterns used by particular cultures (Korac-Kakabadse et al., 2001). Hall notes that context (i.e., the relevant circumstances) is critical to understanding the meaning of information. Based on observations that people from different cultures do not all use the same information-processing systems for the information they take in, Hall proposed a continuum of low- and high-context-oriented styles of communication. The two styles differ as follows:

1. **Low-context communication**: the assumption is that the listener knows very little and must be told practically everything. The message is in the spoken word.
2. **High-context communication**: the listener is already contextualized (i.e. knows all the relevant circumstances) and therefore has the necessary background information to understand the concerns and key messages (Korac-Kakabadse et al., 2001). The message is not as much in the spoken word as it is embedded in the context.

An example of high-context communication is the everyday conversation between partners (life or professional) who share so much history that they understand each other without having to say very much. Teaching–learning situations, in which every detail is made explicit, provide an example of low-context communication; teachers start out by defining what will be reviewed, then they review the content, and in concluding they repeat key points. Although there are no cultures at the extreme ends of the continuum, the Scandinavian nations and countries such as Canada, the United States, and Germany tend to fall toward the lower-context end (Gudykunst & Young, 1992). However, within Canada there are several groups—including people with Asian backgrounds and Aboriginal peoples—who are more likely to exhibit high-context communication. Healthcare providers need to be aware of these patterns and to take a conscious approach to communication that includes a greater emphasis on listening and noting responses in body language as well as speech (Ellerby, McKenzie, McKay, Gariépy, & Kaufert, 2000). Table 5-1 presents characteristics of high- and low-context cultures.

In general, high-context cultures tend to be more concerned with the overall emotional quality of the interaction than with the meaning of particular words and sentences. How something is said and what is not said are just as important as what is said. Courtesy often takes precedence over truthfulness, and members of high-context cultures tend to have moderate or suppressed expression of negative or confrontational messages (Gudykunst & Young, 1992). People in this group are more likely to give an agreeable and pleasant answer to a question if the factual answer is seen to be embarrassing or unpleasant. Expressions of agreement such as "Yes" can range in meaning from "I understand what you are saying," with no agreement or commitment to follow through, to "I agree" and will follow through. This can be particularly challenging in health care, where mutual goal-setting and

TABLE 5-1

Characteristics of High- and Low-Context Communication

HIGH-CONTEXT COMMUNICATION	LOW-CONTEXT COMMUNICATION
■ Most of the message is in the physical context or internalized in the person, and less is explicit	■ Most of the information is made explicit in the language used
■ More emphasis on what is left unspoken; more likely to "read into" the interactions	■ Information often is repeated for emphasis to ensure there is no misunderstanding (if it is relevant and important, it must be stated; if it is not stated, it is not relevant)
■ Less reliance on verbal communication—the obvious does not need to be stated	■ The responsibility for communication clearly lies with the speaker; it is better to over-communicate and be clear than to leave things unsaid
■ More responsibility on the listener— to hear, to interpret, and then to act	■ Silence and pauses are often misunderstood as signs of agreement or a lack of interest
■ More need for silence; longer pauses (to reflect, understand the context, and process the message)	

a negotiated plan of care are important elements of the services provided. Subsequent lack of follow-through often is viewed as breach of contract and leads to frustration and labels of non-compliance.

A high-context orientation in communication also is highly related to how the members of a culture use silence and time (Korac-Kakabadse et al., 2001). Views of time can vary from linear or **monochronic time (M-time)** to circular or **polychronic time (P-time)** (Goleman, 2003). M-time cultures, such as Canada and the United States, emphasize schedules, appointments, and promptness. People on P-time (such as Middle Eastern, Latin American, Asian, and Aboriginal cultures) are more apt to do several things at once and value involvement with others over schedules and appointments. As a result, P-timers may come to appointments late or change schedules frequently, much to the frustration of their M-time colleagues or healthcare providers (Olson, 2004). High-context cultures also make use of silence more than low-context cultures. It is critical that health-care providers recognize the valuable role silence plays in high-context communication by promoting reflection, and that they not interrupt the silence with questions or comments.

Emotional Expression

Adding emotion and intonation to words is a common way of adding meaning to the spoken sentence. However, it is important that the receiver receives the meaning that is intended by the sender. Cultural variations influence the meaning behind emotional expression. For example, generally in the West, raised voices are considered to be a sign of tension or aggression; however, in some Black, Jewish, and Italian cultures, the increase in volume is a sign of exciting conversations among friends. The correct interpretation is critical to determining the appropriate response (alarm or pleasure) and subsequent action (DuPraw & Axner, 1997). Similarly, people who speak quietly or slowly may do so because they are using a second language or because of cultural norms of respect and reflection, and not because they are inarticulate or lack confidence in their thoughts. Clients and family members who exhibit such behaviours are at risk of being misunderstood as uninterested and passive. The lack of self-importance or humility on a client's part should not be confused with indifference (Chachkes & Christ, 1996).

Differences in tone and emotion also can be expressed by words that indicate formality or informality. Many cultures equate the formal form of address (e.g., Dr., Mr., Mrs., Ms.) with respect; others see informality as a sign of closeness and friendship.

Non-Verbal Communication

People all over the world use their hands, heads, and other body parts to communicate expressively. Sixty percent of all communication is non-verbal (Imai, 1996). The non-verbal aspects of communication are said to convey stronger messages than the verbal, often reinforcing or contradicting the verbal response. For instance, when a manager indicates verbally that she has time to talk to a staff member and yet uses the non-verbal gesture of checking her watch constantly, she

CULTURAL COMPETENCE IN ACTION

Preferred Forms of Address
Healthcare providers are taught to respect client wishes with respect to preferred forms of address.

Rita, a registered nurse, worked on a unit with several elderly clients and always referred to the clients by their titles and last names (e.g., Mr. X or Mrs. Y). One client, Robert Smith, indicated that he preferred to be called Bob and shared this preference with Rita directly. Rita was from a South Asian background and had grown up in a culture where elders were rarely referred to by first names, and thus had difficulty using first names for her elderly clients. However, she respected the client's preference and agreed to use his first name, only to slip back into calling him Mr. Smith.

After Bob's third request that she use his first name, Rita decided to explain her difficulty to the client and shared with him her background and the subsequent difficulty in using first names for clients who reminded her of her elders. To Rita, the formality of address was a form of respect and not meant to introduce distance into the relationship or to disregard the client's preference. Once Bob became aware of the meaning of the address for Rita, he said: "Oh, in that case, you call me Mr. Smith—I kind of like that."

This scenario illustrates the influence of the healthcare provider's personal culture, the dilemma it can create, and the importance of developing shared meanings.

is likely to indicate to the staff that she really doesn't have time, and the verbal response is interpreted to be polite but untrue. In another situation, a wave of the hand may suffice as a greeting, with no words needed. Common non-verbal methods of communication include the following:

- Facial expressions
- Touch
- Gestures

Touch

While all human beings have a need to be touched, cultural norms and contexts determine what is considered an appropriate amount of touching. The amount of personal space we need also is strongly influenced by culture. Many cultures use touch as part of a greeting (e.g., handshakes, hugs, and kisses) (Gudykunst & Young, 1992). In cultures with greater personal distance, non-touch greeting gestures are used (e.g., bowing and/or using folded hands to indicate a greeting). Many cultures frown on public displays of affection, especially across genders.

Touch also is used to convey respect and power. Examples of differentiations in power as a message in body language are the friendly shoulder pat, the stroke over the head, the arm around the shoulder, and the bowing down and touching of feet. Gender and age rules also may dictate the circumstances under which "power-related" gestures or close physical contact (such as a hug or kiss) can occur. For example, some cultures interpret the stroke over the head as a blessing given by elders to youngsters (thus it is inappropriate for youngsters to do it to elders), while younger members may convey respect by touching the elders' feet.

Physical touch is a major part of professional life for many healthcare providers and is used to provide both physical care and emotional comfort (Chang, 2001). Experiences of touch vary depending on gender, age, parts of the body that are touched, and how the message of touch is interpreted. Although most clients interpret a healthcare provider's touch as a caring gesture, physical touch also can be interpreted as control (Mulaik et al., 1991). Overall, touch has been noted to have a comforting and calming effect on clients (Routasalo, 1999). Understanding both the provider's and the client's cultural norms around touch will not only help healthcare providers to ensure respect and caring, but also can also aid in gaining insight into the client's relationships with others.

Differences in Values that Affect Communication

Power Distance

Power distance refers to the following two ways in which power is shared in a culture:
- Vertically, with power aggregated at the top and large distances between the rich and powerful and those who are poor or at the lower end of the status ladder (high power distance)
- Horizontally, where power is shared among individuals and all individuals are regarded as equals (low power distance)
  (Goleman, 2003; Gudykunst & Young, 1992)

Members of high power distance societies tend to be more formal in their forms of address, often wait for conversations to be initiated by those in authority, are hesitant to criticize authority or offer their own opinions, and often use silence as a form of respect. They may also hesitate to ask questions to get clarification because doing so could imply that the person communicating has failed to do so clearly. Individuals with high power distances also are less likely to initiate conversations regarding conflict, and when involved in such a conversation, may indicate agreement out of respect for the other versus a commitment to the resolution or course of action.

Individualism versus Collectivism

First described by Harry Triandis, individualism/collectivism is a major dimension of cultural variability that influences many aspects of behaviour, including communication (Gudykunst & Young, 1992). **Individualism** is a social pattern in which individuals are primarily motivated by their own preferences, needs, rights, and desires, and view themselves largely as being independent of the larger collective. Individualistic cultures place greater emphasis on individual goals and achievements and promote self-realization for their members (Gudykunst & Young, 1992; Xu & Davidhizar, 2004). In contrast, collectivist cultures give greater priority to the needs of the group (family, work unit, community), and the

CULTURAL COMPETENCE IN ACTION

Cross-Cultural Communication Style Inventory

Directions:

a) Consider your own style of communicating at work (school) and indicate your preferences on the items below by placing an *X* on each line. Then connect your *X*s, forming a profile.

b) Now think of an individual from a different culture with whom you have had some interaction (maybe a client or a colleague). Put a second checkmark on each line representing the other person's style. You may wish to use a different coloured ink to highlight the difference. Draw a dotted line to connect the checkmarks to form the other person's profile. Where does your profile help or hinder you as a communicator?

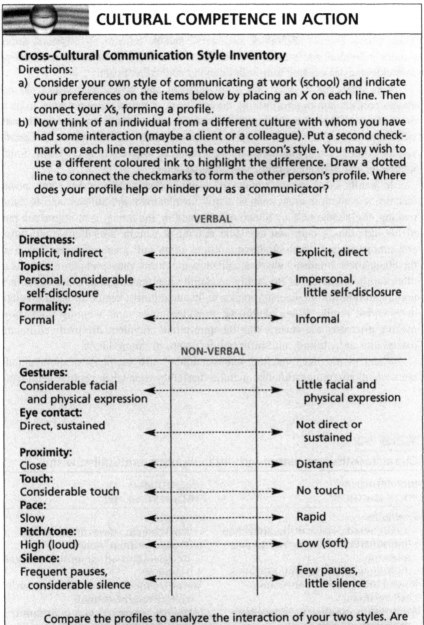

VERBAL

Directness: Implicit, indirect	Explicit, direct
Topics: Personal, considerable self-disclosure	Impersonal, little self-disclosure
Formality: Formal	Informal

NON-VERBAL

Gestures: Considerable facial and physical expression	Little facial and physical expression
Eye contact: Direct, sustained	Not direct or sustained
Proximity: Close	Distant
Touch: Considerable touch	No touch
Pace: Slow	Rapid
Pitch/tone: High (loud)	Low (soft)
Silence: Frequent pauses, considerable silence	Few pauses, little silence

Compare the profiles to analyze the interaction of your two styles. Are there areas of similarity and/or differences? Can you reflect on your past interactions and consider the impact of communication style differences on your relationship? What style shifts can you make to reconcile differences and communicate more effectively with this person?

From *The global diversity desk reference: managing an international workforce* (p. 152), by L. Gardenswartz, A. Rowe, P. Digh, and M. Bennett, 2003, San Francisco: John Wiley & Sons Inc./Pfeiffer. Reprinted with permission.

individual is expected to fit into the group. In **collectivism**, individuals see themselves as parts of one or more collectives and they are motivated primarily by group norms (versus individual pleasures) and by collectively imposed duties (versus individual preferences and desires). Table 5-2 highlights the contrasting characteristics associated with individualism and collectivism.

It is important to note that individualistic and collectivist values do not always conflict and that promoting the one form of values does not have to be at the expense of the other. Although individuals and societies can have both individualistic and collectivist tendencies, one style tends to predominate. In Canada and the United States, individualism predominates, whereas in many Asian, South American, and African cultures, collectivism does.

In health care, the influence of individualism, collectivism, and power distance is evident in areas such as family involvement in both care and decision making. For people with a collectivist orientation, the family is an important part of the individual's care, and decision making is a more consultative and time-consuming process. Individualistic cultures often will make decisions based on the client's best interests, whereas collectivist cultures may consider the needs of other family members or the family as a unit when making major decisions. It is not uncommon for the decision maker to be an authority figure in the immediate or extended family. When healthcare providers understand a family's decision-making processes and ensure that the appropriate members are involved in care discussions early, timely and informed decisions are more likely.

Members of collectivist, high-context cultures also are likely to adopt an indirect style of communication that includes hesitancy even when positive sentiments

TABLE 5-2

Characteristics Associated with Individualism and Collectivism

INDIVIDUALISM FOCUS ON THE "I"	COLLECTIVISM FOCUS ON THE "WE"
Emphasize ■ Goals, needs, views of the individual ■ Individual preferences, rights, and pleasure ■ Individual initiatives and outcomes	*Emphasize* ■ Goals, needs, views of the group ■ Shared in-group beliefs ■ Co-operation with in-group members ■ Harmony
Reward individual initiative and achievement	*Reward* support to the collective and collective achievement
Universalistic approach, where same values are applied to all	*Pluralistic approach,* where different value standards are applied to members of "in group" and "out group"
Influence of group views and values on the individual is limited in intensity and scope (group norms affect individual behaviour in very specific circumstances)	*Influence* of group views and values is greater in intensity and scope (group norms affect behaviour in many different aspects of an individual's life)

are being expressed, thus making it hard for healthcare providers to determine the degree to which something is desired or valued. When dealing with clients who use the indirect approach of communication, healthcare providers need to establish ties to the clients at the outset through community members and friends. Such clients may be reluctant to ask questions directly and are more likely to involve intermediaries in care; questions may not elicit immediate responses.

Direct talk often is associated with Western culture and its scientific and democratic attitude (Yum, 1994). Indirect talk often is associated with East Asian, Hispanic, and Aboriginal cultures (Tripp-Reimer, Choi, Kelley, & Enslein, 2001; Yum, 1994).

The direct/indirect communication style becomes particularly important in client education (Chachkes & Christ, 1996; Tripp-Reimer et al., 2001). For communities with indirect communication styles, it is important that the educator first gain credibility with the community and also frame messages in way that ensures they are offered for consideration, versus telling people what to do (Tripp-Riemer et al., 2001). Examples of the two approaches to framing messages are as follows:

- "Someone who has such a problem might do this" (consideration approach)
- "If you have this symptom, do this" (the more prescriptive approach)

Cultural values influence how conflict is both viewed and addressed. Some cultures view conflict as a positive factor, while others see it as undesirable. Canadian, American, and European cultures often prefer to deal with conflict directly, via face-to-face meetings, and with the individuals involved. In contrast, in many Eastern cultures, open conflict is perceived as embarrassing or demeaning. The preferred style of conflict management is embedded in the larger cultural values of individualism, collectivism, and power distance, and requires one to bear in mind the concept of face (see below) during negotiation.

Face

The term **face** refers to the projected image of oneself in a relational situation involving two or more parties and is associated with "honour" and related emotions such as respect, shame, pride, dignity, and guilt (Xu & Davidhizar, 2004).

In collectivist cultures, face concerns not only individuals but also the family, work unit, and community; in individualistic cultures, face tends to be limited to the individuals and/or the situation. The notion of face varies in importance across cultures, and thus preserving, maintaining, or saving face becomes a key communication principle. Using indirect speech may be a result of predominant concern for the other face, reflecting a Confucian legacy of consideration for others and human relationships (Yum, 1994). Face is a critical concept in many Asian cultures where saving, maintaining, and preserving face is of extreme importance, and may even be greater in importance than the substantive issues in the conflict situation (Xu & Davidhizar, 2004).

Understanding that conflict situations may contain both an issue of conflict and a face orientation is important for healthcare providers because there is always the potential for conflict within a team, and with students, clients, and families.

CULTURAL COMPETENCE IN ACTION

Direct Communication and Feedback
One area of practice in which the differences in direct/indirect communication and the concept of face often are evident is that of feedback. In developing clinical cultural competence, feedback is therefore an important area for healthcare providers to focus on.

The usual assumption in the West is that the best approach to providing feedback is immediate and direct. Verbal feedback is thought to be less intimidating than written feedback since the latter often is associated with progressive discipline. However, individuals—whether they are clients or part of the healthcare system—do not all perceive direct, verbal feedback in the same way.

An example of this is the experience of a Vietnamese student who reported feeling "that the teacher had shamed her by confronting her in a public place about a client's complaint. The student felt that, according to her cultural ways, the teacher should have written her a note instead. The student responded by not completing her clinical rotation and telling the teacher she was ill" (Paterson, Osborne, & Gregory, 2004).

Disclosure

Cultural variations exist with respect to disclosure of personal and intimate information. Prerequisites for disclosure include an element of trust and the establishment of both a relationship and shared values. Rogers and colleagues (2005) studied physician–client encounters involving clients with inflammatory bowel disease, and noted that although a "majority of patients had their own detailed plans for diet, eating times, and daily routines, to which they adhered to control symptoms and lead as normal a life as possible" (p. 232), these strategies were not valued by the medical staff in the same way, and thus the strategies as well as concerns often remained undisclosed by the clients (Rogers et al., 2005).

Even when there is a safe relationship, clients may be hesitant to discuss particular issues due to the provider's age, gender, and/or authority. Public healthcare nurses may be regarded as representatives of the state, for example, and thus viewed with suspicion. Clients with uncertain residency status (refugees, visitors, or those considered illegal aliens) could hesitate to disclose information for fear that doing so would affect their residency. Disclosure also may be limited in situations involving emotions, intimacy, and conflict. Providing selective information to preserve face often is a cultural expectation and is not regarded as lying by omission or being untruthful. Clients from cultures with indirect styles of communication also may feel uncomfortable during direct questioning, or consider the practice rude and not worthy of a complete response.

Within cross-cultural encounters, challenges frequently arise with respect to disclosing bad news to clients. As discussed in the context of cultural care reframing in Chapter 4, many cultures (e.g., Aboriginal peoples and Chinese and East Indian cultures) believe that speaking of future illnesses and consequences will bring them to pass; the norm in these communities is of non-disclosure (Barnes et al., 1998; Ellerby et al., 2000; Kaufert & Putsch, 1997; Kaufert et al., 1999; Tuckett, 2004; Turner, 2003). Often, family members request that the bad news not be communicated directly to the client. Following a review of the literature on truth-telling, Tuckett (2004) concluded that while most clients want truthfulness about their health, truth-telling preferences and practices are a cultural artifact and vary not only by country but also by diagnosis and age of the client. Rather than make assumptions, healthcare providers are advised to rely on therapeutic communication and ask for the client's and family's informational requirements. Alternatives such as offering truth when clients request it and maintaining hope, while respecting the choices made by the family, need to be explored (Kaufert et al., 1999).

Although the above discussion on culture and communication has focused on the client's culture, the same factors apply to healthcare providers. Research on the impact of the healthcare provider's culture is limited. Roter et al. (2002) conducted a systematic review of literature to quantify the effect of physician gender during communication visits and noted that in the studies reviewed, female physicians engaged in communication more broadly than male physicians in the following ways:

- By addressing psychosocial issues through related questioning and counselling, and through greater use of positive (agreement, encouragement, and reassurance) and emotional talk (talk reflecting inquiry about feelings and emotions)
- By seeking more client input

We have already learned in Chapter 2 (see "Myth #2") that the practice of ethnic matching—matching healthcare providers and clients with respect to background—can lead to improved communication and other benefits (Bowen, 2004; Paterson et al., 2004). However, we also discovered that ethnic matching appears to be effective for some outcomes but not for others (Bowen, 2004).

Communicating through Language

Unfamiliarity with the language is perhaps the most commonly identified communication barrier in a multicultural society. In Canada, four population groups face barriers to healthcare access due to language: Aboriginal peoples; immigrants; people who use sign language; and people who speak one of Canada's official languages but live in an area where the other language is prominent (e.g., French-speaking people in a predominantly English-speaking environment, and vice versa) (Health Canada, 2003). In the following pages, we will consider issues and strategies for working with clients who have limited proficiency in the dominant language, and in Chapter 6 we will discuss working with interpreters.

Language

Language issues are far more complex than whether or not we can speak a particular language. In every culture, many expressions and phrases that are commonly understood by members of the cultural group can be ambiguous or confusing for

CULTURAL COMPETENCE IN ACTION

Culture, Communication, and Interpretations
Below are behaviours that are frequently encountered in a variety of healthcare settings. In the middle column (A), write down what the behaviour means to you. After reflecting on your knowledge of other cultures, write down what the same behaviour might mean to someone of a different culture or background.

BEHAVIOUR	COLUMN A: WHAT IT MEANS TO ME	COLUMN B: WHAT IT MIGHT MEAN TO ANOTHER PERSON
1. Not making eye contact		
2. Saying "yes" or nodding when he or she doesn't understand		
3. Giving a soft handshake		
4. Standing very close when talking		
5. Spending time on small talk instead of getting to the reason for coming		
6. Arriving late for an appointment		
7. Bringing family members to an appointment		
8. Addressing you as Dr./Mr./Mrs./Ms./Nurse rather than by your first name		
9. Giving inaccurate or vague information		
10. Not making a decision without consulting other family members who are not present		

At the end of this exercise, discuss your answers with a colleague or in a small group. Did you have similar interpretations? Did you discover interpretations that you had not considered before? From "Diversity level II: Clinical Cultural Competence Education, Workshop I," 2005, presented by Centre for Addiction and Mental Health, March 23, 2004.

outsiders. For example, healthcare providers often use expressions such as "you are stable," "you are treading water," or "you are out of the woods," all of which may be misinterpreted by clients. For example, clients may understand "stability" as being cured, getting better, or not getting worse (Barnes et al., 1998). Familiarity with language does not ensure familiarity with associated meanings and behaviours.

Second-Language Issues

Research indicates that individuals experience first and second languages differently (Burke, 2004). First languages are seen as enabling emotional expressiveness and are associated with intimacy because speaking in the first language can be seen to signify and engender closeness. First languages often are the language for creativity (poetry, drama) and humour, and people see more of themselves in the first language. In a study of South Asian asthma clients, Hussein and Partridge (2002) noted a preference for material in the first language since this was read more quickly and likely with better comprehension. Confidence and fluency in a second language also is influenced by the social context. One may be comfortable with day-to-day needs in the second language but may not have the linguistic ability to understand medical or healthcare-related terminology. People often are reluctant to say they do not understand (they may see it as a poor reflection on themselves or may see it as being disrespectful to authority figures). Times of

CULTURAL CONSIDERATIONS IN CARE

When Providing Instructions Is Not Enough

A young Tamil couple brought their 18-month-old son to the hospital emergency room with complaints of fever and irritability. The child was also tugging on his ear. Both parents had a working knowledge of English, and interpreter services were neither requested nor offered.

Following an assessment, the parents were informed that the child had an ear infection in his right ear, and they were given a prescription for an oral antibiotic that they were instructed to give to the child every six hours. The parents were repeatedly asked if they understood the instructions, and each time they responded in the affirmative. Two days later, the parents returned to the emergency room in greater distress. They had followed the instructions carefully but the child was getting worse. The triage nurse noted a yellowish discharge from the right ear. What do you think happened?

The parents had followed the instructions, as they understood them. They had taken the prescription to a pharmacy and received a bottle of liquid medicine with a dropper to administer the medication. The instructions to give 2.5 ml every six hours were emphasized. The parents used the dropper to administer the 2.5 ml, but administered it directly into the child's right ear. This example clearly illustrates the challenges of communication. The problem did not reside in what was said but, rather, in what was assumed and not said. Healthcare providers failed to be explicit that the medication had to be taken orally, and the parents assumed that the medicine was to be applied to the affected area.

One other such example involves an insulin-dependent man who was brought to the emergency room in a diabetic coma. When asked later if he was following through with the instructions he had been given to inject insulin, the man demonstrated by injecting the insulin into an orange, as he had been taught, and then he ate it. In this instance, the teaching strategy for injections had been misunderstood as the exact way to take insulin—with potentially serious consequences (Howard, Andrade, & Byrd, 2001).

crisis or stress also can compromise fluency in a second language. In the emergency room, healthcare providers often are frustrated with clients who are unable to communicate in English even though they are able to convey and understand basic information at other times. It also is important to remember that limited fluency in a second language often means individuals need more time to respond because they first have to translate the question from English into their own language, prepare an answer in their own language, and then translate the answer back into English. Unfortunately, such individuals are at risk of being labelled slow or as simply not knowing what is going on (stupid) (Paterson et al., 2004).

Working with Clients Who Have Limited English Proficiency (LEP)

When working with clients whose first language is not the dominant language of the healthcare organization or system, healthcare providers need to carefully assess the need for interpretation services. Clients often have enough language proficiency that, when it is combined with supportive strategies on the part of the healthcare provider, allows for effective communication. At other times, interpreters are either not available or not preferred by the client. Table 5-3 presents strategies for communicating effectively with limited English proficiency (LEP) clients in the absence of language interpretation.

Effective Conversations in Healthcare Settings

Elements of effective conversations should be identifiable in all clinical encounters (Goldbloom, 2003); however, cross-cultural communication requires extra vigilance. Table 5-4 (p. 118) identifies characteristics of effective conversations.

Commitment

The first step toward effective communication is a commitment to mutual communication. When healthcare providers value communication and the expression of the client's voice, they are more likely to use additional strategies to ensure that the encoded and decoded meanings agree.

Communication barriers are often attributed to the client. It is important, however, to consider the location of the "problem." Is the problem located in the client and based on culture, or is the problem located in the discriminatory attitudes and practices of the healthcare organization (Robb & Douglas, 2004; Tripp-Reimer, Brink, & Saunders, 1984)? Commitment to effective communication requires that healthcare providers individually and collectively take responsibility for addressing the "barrier," regardless of where it may be located.

Kavanagh (1992) notes that commitment to mutual communication is based on four assumptions:

1. Recognition and value of human dignity
2. Cultural relativism (recognizing that cultures need to be understood in context) as an acceptable and preferred condition

TABLE 5-3

Cultural Competence in Action: Strategies for Improving Direct Communication with Limited English Proficiency (LEP) Clients

1. *Speak slowly, not loudly.* A loud voice implies anger; and in most cultures, the healthcare provider holds a high position of respect and authority. When clients feel that the "authority figure" is angry, they tend to become anxious or feel intimidated and begin to answer questions in the way that they think will please that person rather than give the true picture of the complaint. Speaking slowly does not mean exaggerating the enunciation of words as that is often more confusing than helpful.

2. *Face the person and use non-verbal communication* such as gestures, pictures, and facial expressions. By the same token, watch the client's face, eyes, and other non-verbal communications carefully. When these don't agree with the client's words, inquire further. Don't assume that the non-verbal communication used in your culture is the same as that in the client's culture.

3. *Avoid difficult and uncommon words* and idiomatic expressions. **Idioms** are phrases or expressions that are based on culture rather than the sum of the meanings of each individual word. North American English is full of idioms such as "right on target" or "kill two birds with one stone."

4. *Be aware of frequently misunderstood words,* such as "anxiety," "depression," "dizziness," and words that describe sensations (e.g., "pins and needles").

5. *Don't complicate communication* with unnecessary words or information. More is not better in this situation. Keep what you say simple.

6. *Organize what you say for easy access.* Use short, simple sentences, starting with the subject and following it as closely as possible with the verb and a simple object. A good rule of thumb is that people tend to remember information in an inverted bell curve—what is said at the beginning and end is remembered best, while information in the middle is missed or quickly forgotten.

7. *Repeat when you have not been understood.* If something has been said as simply as possible, try repeating the same sentence again first; changing words may confuse the client.

8. *Rephrase and summarize often.* Summarize what you understand the person is saying, and check with the client to see if your understanding is correct. When giving information, ask questions, and try to say the same thing or ask the same question in at least two or three different ways.

9. *Don't ask questions that can be answered with a "Yes" or "No."* The person's answer will only tell you whether or not the question has been heard—not whether it has been understood. If you phrase questions in a way that requires the person to respond with information (what, where, when, why, and how), they can only reply sensibly if they have understood the question. Use such phrases as "tell me about."

10. *Greet the client in the client's own language* to establish a rapport.

From Breen, 1999; Gerace & Salimbene, 2002; McPhee, 2002; Putsch, 2002.

3. Willingness to alter personal behaviour in response to the communication process
4. Willingness to decrease personal resistance

Commitment to effective conversations also means a willingness to take risks. Often healthcare providers are hesitant to bring up issues or engage in

TABLE 5-4

Characteristics of Effective Conversations

- Commitment
- Respectful engagement
- Bi-directional conversation
- Responsiveness and empathy

Adapted from *Skills for culturally sensitive pediatric care*, by R. B. Goldbloom, 2003, Philadelphia: Saunders; *Promoting cultural diversity: Strategies for health care*, by K. Kavanagh, 1992, Newbury Park, CA: Sage.

particular conversations because they fear being politically incorrect or offending the client. However, avoidance is not a useful strategy. Effective conversations require a genuine desire, risk taking, and vigilance for miscommunication. Healthcare providers need to search for ways to make communication work, rather than assigning blame for its breakdown.

Respectful Engagement

The second step toward effective communication is respectful engagement. The word "respectful" implies that all views should be treated as legitimate and that respect will be integrated into the manner of conversation. The word "engagement" implies a connection between two parties.

Healthcare providers need to establish a common ground with clients with respect to desired goals for care. In a study of what constitutes effective and ineffective communication in a variety of chronic illness contexts, Thorne et al. (2004) describe three distinct dimensions of communication, as courtesy, respect, and engagement. This breakdown works as follows:

1. *The courtesy dimension:* refers to the general tone of the interaction and includes politeness, sincerity, remembering names, and accommodating office practices.
2. *Respect:* seen in expressions that show regard for the specific individuals as being intelligent consumers of healthcare information and having lives outside the context of illness. Respect is evident through behaviours such as listening, recognition of client expertise, awareness of social context, empathy, and offering information. Discounting client opinion/expertise, withholding information, and over-reliance on scientific evidence for decisions are seen as problematic attitudes or behaviours.
3. *Engagement:* described with respect to the sense of commitment—a feeling of teamwork and shared decision making—and viewed as a valuable feature of effective health care. Conversely, maintaining professional distance, disinterest/dismissal of client opinions about disease management, and blocking access to information and resources (such as complementary and alternative therapy) are seen as problematic.

Similarly, Browne (1997) documented the following characteristics of respectful interactions:

- Treating people as inherently worthy and equal
- Conveying acceptance of others
- Conveying a willingness to listen actively to clients
- Genuinely attempting to understand clients and their unique situations
- Attempting to provide adequate explanations
- Conveying sincerity during interactions

Interactions lacking respect were characterized by the following:

- Discriminatory attitudes
- Failing to consider the client's perspective
- Failing to provide privacy
- Failing to provide adequate explanations
- Demonstrating negative non-verbal behaviours through tone of voice, body posture, position relative to the client, facial expressions, and the activities that providers engage in while clients are present

In a study of doctor–client cross-cultural communication from the perspective of clients, medical residents, and faculty, authors Shapiro, Hollingshead, and Morrison (2002) noted that clients interpreted culturally competent communication generically, without much specific cultural reference. Characteristics of good communication included behaviours such as the following:

- Taking time
- Writing things down
- Being thorough, and doing all the necessary tests
- Calling with results
- Apologizing for being busy
- Answering questions
- Providing complete explanations
- Using a collaborative model of care involving the clients appropriately in decision making

Bi-Directionality

Bi-directional conversations, in which information flows from and to both parties, are effective conversations. Healthcare providers need to give as much time to listening as to talking (Goldbloom, 2003). Listening is a powerful skill that often is underused. Clients (and people in general) listen to healthcare providers (or colleagues, teachers, parents) who listen to them. Bi-directional conversations require healthcare providers to further develop their listening skills and use their minds as well as their hearts to understand not just what is being said, but also what it means to the clients, and what it reflects about the clients' views of who or what they are. All of these views and meanings need to be heard, acknowledged, and acted upon as appropriate.

Bi-directional conversations also require healthcare providers to use more inquiring responses and open-ended questions, instead of dismissive responses and closed-ended questions. **Inquiring responses** are responses that inquire into the client's perspectives and invite further conversation. Often, what we ask and how we ask can prematurely end conversations. Clients may not continue talking if they perceive that their story is not being heard or understood, or if they are afraid that their views will be judged, trivialized, or ignored.

Bi-directional conversations also require an understanding of power differences between the client and the healthcare provider, and strategies to balance the power. With children, this is reflected through behaviours such as bending down to be at the same level as the child or using language appropriate to age; with adults it may mean using privilege and authority to raise issues that are hard for a client to broach. For example, when the client has disclosed an aspect of a cultural identity, the healthcare provider can follow up with statements along the line of, "You indicated that you are Buddhist. Can you tell me what I need to know about the religion and how it could influence your care?" or "Many of my clients use or look for complementary or alternative remedies. Is there anything you are using or want to use that might be of help?" The key is not to stereotype or impose particular characteristics to a given identity, but rather to use the knowledge of patterns to assess for individual applicability and relevance. These statements are inquiring but also reflect an indication of interest and acceptance and the use of the provider's authority to legitimize the issues.

Responsiveness and Empathy

For conversations to be effective, they need to be responsive and not reflect predetermined outcomes (Goldbloom, 2003). For example, discussions of complementary and alternative therapy are mostly initiated by clients or family members and frequently are ignored by the physician (Suraez-Almazor, 2004). Clients and family members need to be treated as partners in the healthcare planning process, and a plan of care should emerge only after a healthcare provider has listened to and understood the client's perspective. Healthcare providers also need to be aware of their own biases and attitudes, which may impede the development of effective relationships (Kavanagh, 1992; Putsch, 2002).

Hatem and Rider (2004) note that while the practice of medicine is lived in stories, the place of stories in the world of medicine is uncertain. The Western, biomedical culture values scientific evidence and hard data; stories are regarded as soft data or subjective information with less relevance to care. In a biomedical culture, details of disease become more important for a healthcare provider to pursue than the details of the client's life. However, for many cultures the details of life may have considerable significance and value for the healthcare encounter. For example, Aboriginal belief systems are based on oral traditions and include the emotional, physical, spiritual, and intellectual well-being of a person.

A non-Aboriginal doctor who wants to work with an Aboriginal client must take a holistic view of the illness, be able to truly listen, and bear witness to the violence and the struggles of the Aboriginal peoples by understanding the history and the impact of colonization (Hester & Lavallee, 2002). The advice is appropriate for all clients and consistent with client-centred approaches to care. The reflection not only allows the healthcare provider to become more aware of his or her own reaction and ability to work with the client, it also enhances the ability to gather more data and develop insights that could be important to accurate diagnosis and effective healthcare management (Hatem & Rider, 2004).

Effective conversations demonstrate empathy by ensuring that the understanding of client views is reflected back in subsequent conversations and interactions (Goldbloom, 2003). If clients feel understood, they are more likely to trust the healthcare provider and the system and also are more likely to follow through with the determined plan of care. The ability to present an issue as it is perceived from another's perspective is important for the individual relationship, as well as the broader systemic advocacy, to ensure that the client does not get lost in the system (Kavanagh, 1992).

Fields et al. (2004) define empathy in client care situations as a "*cognitive* (as opposed to affective) attribute that involves *understanding* of the inner experiences of the patient combined with a capacity to *communicate* these to the patient" (p. 84). The three key terms in this definition are:

1. Cognitive attributes
2. Understanding
3. Communication of the understanding

It is not enough for healthcare providers to feel that they understand the contexts of their clients; empathic communication requires the communication of the understanding back to the clients. Cultural competence requires that healthcare providers develop both individual and systemic knowledge in order to address the complexities and inequities associated with culture and difference.

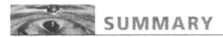 **SUMMARY**

This chapter discussed issues in communication in health care generally and more specifically with respect to cross-cultural variations. Within the healthcare environment, communication can be compromised by client physical and emotional distress as well as healthcare providers' professional jargon and time constraints. Client interviews involve three essential functions: information gathering, relationship building, as well as client education; however, in many encounters, the medical perspective dominates. Communication differences can lead to ineffective communication, which, in turn, contributes to misdiagnosis, inadequate health teaching, failure to obtain informed consent, compromised healthcare provider–client relationship, and dissatisfaction with care.

Cross-cultural communication is characterized not only by differences in communication styles (verbal and non-verbal) but also by fundamental differences in values and approach that influence how communication happens, what kind of communication happens, and with whom. The major elements of cross-cultural communication include an understanding of the role of context and power, as well as values related to individualism or collectivism and disclosure.

Barriers related to limited English proficiency can be addressed through the use of deliberate strategies on the part of healthcare providers. These include speaking slowly and directly using short simple sentences; repeating information and seeking client understanding and interpretations; and avoiding the use of jargon and idioms.

The characteristics of effective conversations remain the same across cultures and include a focus on respect, listening, empathy, inquiring responses, and, most important, recognition that effective communication is a key ingredient to all healthcare interactions. Healthcare providers must also recognize the importance of valuing their clients' perspectives.

REFERENCES

Baker, C. (2001). *Service provision by representative institutions and identity.* Halifax: Department of Canadian Heritage.

Barnes, D. A., Davis, A. J., Moran, T., Portillo, C., & Koenig, B. A. (1998). Informed consent in a multicultural cancer patient population: Implications for nursing practice. *Nursing Ethics, 5*(5), 412–423.

Bowen, S. (2004). *Assessing the responsiveness of health care organizations to culturally diverse groups.* Winnipeg: University of Manitoba: Department of Community Health Sciences.

Breen, L. (1999). What should I do if my patient does not speak English? *Journal of the American Medical Association, 282*(9), 819.

Browne, A. (1997). A concept analysis of respect applying the hybrid model in cross-cultural settings. *Western Journal of Nursing Research, 19*(6), 762–781.

Burke, C. (2004). Living in several languages: Implications for therapy. *Journal of Family Therapy, 26*, 314–339.

Centre for Addiction and Mental Health. (2005). Diversity level II: Clinical cultural competence education, Workshop I. Toronto: presented March 23, 2004.

Chachkes, E., & Christ, G. (1996). Cross cultural issues in patient education. *Patient Education and Counseling, 27*, 13–21.

Chang, S. O. (2001). The conceptual structure of physical touch in caring. *Journal of Advanced Nursing, 33*(5), 820–827.

Coffman, M. (2004). Cultural caring in nursing practice: A meta synthesis of qualitative research. *Journal of Cultural Diversity, 11*(3), 100–109.

Cruz, M., & Pincus, H. (2002). Research on the influence that communication in psychiatric encounters has on treatment. *Psychiatric Services, 53*, 1253–1265.

Degner, L. F., Kristjanson, L. J., Bowman, D., Sloan, J. A., Carriere, K. C., O'Neil, J., Bilodeau, B., Watson, P., & Mueller, B. (1997). Information needs and decisional preferences in women with breast cancer. *Journal of the American Medical Association, 277*(18), 1485–1492.

DuPraw, M., & Axner, M. (1997). *Working on common cross-cultural communication challenges.* Topsfield Foundation and Marci Reaven. Retrieved January 20, 2005, from http://www.wwcd.org/action/ampu/crosscult.html

Ellerby, J. H., McKenzie, J., McKay, S., Gariépy, G. J., & Kaufert, J. M. (2000). Bioethics for clinicians: 18. Aboriginal cultures. *Canadian Medical Association Journal, 163*(7), 845–850.

Fields, S. K., Hojat, M., Gonnella, J. S., Mangione, S., Kane, G., & Magee, M. (2004). Comparisons of nurses and physicians on an operational measure of empathy. *Evaluation & the Health Professions, 27*(1), 80–94.

Gardenswartz, L., Rowe, A., Digh, P., & Bennett, M. (2003) *The global diversity desk reference: Managing an international workforce.* San Francisco, CA: John Wiley & Sons Inc./Pfeiffer.

Gerace, L., & Salimbene, S. (2002). Cultural competence for today's nurse part four: Communicating effectively with patients who have limited English proficiency. *Nursing Spectrum.* Retrieved June 20, 2004, from http://www2.nursingspectrum. com/ce/self-study_modules/course.html?ID=305

Goldbloom, R. B. (2003). *Skills for culturally sensitive pediatric care.* Philadelphia: Saunders.

Goleman, P. (2003). Communicating in the intercultural classroom. *IEEE Transactions on Professional Communication, 46*(3), 231–235.

Gudykunst, W., & Young, Y. K. (1992). *Communicating with strangers.* New York: McGraw-Hill.

Hatem, D., & Rider, E. (2004). Sharing stories: Narrative medicine in an evidence based world. *Patient Education and Counseling, 54,* 251–253.

Health Canada. (2003). *Equity and access in health care: Section 4: Underserved populations in Canada,* Health Care Network. Retrieved May 2, 2005, from http://www. hc-sc.gc.ca/hppb/healthcare/pubs/circumstances/partI/doc1.html

Hester, J., & Lavallee, B. (2002). Dealing with cultural differences, *Urban Aboriginal Health Centres Meeting Final Report,* 19–21. National Aboriginal Health Organization. Retrieved May 15, 2004, from http://16016.vws.magma.ca/english/ pdf/UAHCM.pdf

Howard, C. A., Andrade, S. J., & Byrd, T. (2001). The ethical dimensions of cultural competence in border health care settings. *Family and Community Health, 23*(4), 36–41.

Hussein, S., & Partridge, M. (2002). Perceptions of asthma in South Asians and their views on educational materials and self management plans: A qualitative study. *Patient Education and Counseling, 48,* 189–194.

Imai, G. (1996). *Gestures: Body language and non-verbal communication.* Pomona, CA: California State Polytechnic University, Teachers' Asian Studies Summer Institute. Retrieved December 12, 2004, from http://www.csupomona.edu/~tassi/gestures.htm

Kaufert, J., & Putsch, R. W. (1997). Communication through interpreters in healthcare: Ethical dilemmas arising from differences in class, culture, language, and power. *Journal of Clinical Ethics, 8,* 71–87.

Kaufert, J., Putsch, R. W., & Lavallee, M. (1999). End of life decision making among Aboriginal Canadians: Interpretation, mediation, and discord in the communication of bad news. *Journal of Palliative Care, 15*(1), 31–38.

Kavanagh, K. (1992). *Promoting cultural diversity: Strategies for health care.* Newbury Park, CA: Sage.

King, G. I. (2000). The implications of differences in cultural attitudes and styles of communicating on peer reporting behaviour. *Cross Cultural Management, 7*(2), 11–17.

Korac-Kakabadse, N., Kouzmin, A., Korac-Kakabadse, A., & Savery, L. (2001). Low- and high-context communication patterns: Towards mapping cross cultural encounters. *Cross Cultural Management, 8*(2), 3–24.

McJannett, M., Butow, P., Tattersall, M. H. N., & Thompson, J. F. (2003). Asking questions can help: Development of a question prompt for cancer patients seeing a surgeon. *European Journal of Cancer Prevention, 12,* 397–405.

McPhee, S. (2002). Caring for a 70-year-old Vietnamese woman. *Journal of the American Medical Association, 287*(4), 495–503.

Meleis, A. (1996). AAN Expert panel report: Culturally competent health care. *Nursing Outlook, 6,* 277–283.

Mir, G., & Tovey, P. (2002). Cultural competency: Professional action and South Asian careers. *Journal of Management in Medicine, 16*(1), 7–19.

Mulaik, J. S., Megenity, J. S., Cannon, R. B., Chance, K. S., Cannella, K. S., Garland, L. M., & Gilead, M. P. (1991). Patients' perceptions of nurses' use of touch. *Western Journal of Nursing Research, 13*(3), 306–323.

Munoz, C., & Luckmann, J. (2005). *Transcultural communication in nursing.* Clifton Park, NY: Thomson.

Olson, T. (2004). *Analysis of cultural communication and proxemics.* Lincoln: University of Nebraska.

Paterson, B., Osborne, M., & Gregory, D. (2004). How different can you be and still survive? Homogeneity and difference in clinical nursing education. *International Journal of Nursing Education Scholarship, 1*(1), article 2. Retrieved on May 16, 2005 from http://www.bepress.com/ijnes/vol11/iss1/art2

Pope, C. (2004). Concept paper: Language access services in nursing, Washington: Office of Minority Health, US Department of Health and Human Services.

Putsch, R. W. (2002). *Language access in healthcare: Domains, strategies and implications for medical education.* Washington: Office of Minority Health, US Department of health and human resources. Retrieved January 2, 2006, from http://www.think-culturalhealth.org/cccm/papers/putsch.pdf

Robb, M., & Douglas, J. (2004). Managing diversity. *Nursing Management, 11*(1), 25–29.

Rogers, A., Kennedy, A., Nelson, E., & Robinson, A. (2005). Uncovering the limits of patient centeredness: Implementing a self management trial for chronic illness. *Qualitative Health Research, 15*(2), 224–239.

Roter, D., Hall, J., & Aoki, Y. (2002). Physician gender effects in medical communication. *Journal of the American Medical Association, 288,* 756–764.

Routasalo, P. (1999). Physical touch in nursing: A literature review. *Journal of Advanced Nursing, 34*(4), 843–850.

Shapiro, J., Hollingshead, J., & Morrison, E. H. (2002). Primary care resident, faculty, and patient views of barriers to cultural competence, and the skills needed to overcome them. *Medical Education, 36,* 749–759.

Sue, S (1998). In search of cultural competence in psychotherapy and counseling. *American Psychologist, 53,* 440–448.

Suraez-Almazor, M. (2004). Patient-physician communication. *Current Opinions in Rheumatology, 16,* 91–95.

Thorne, S. E., Harris, S. R., Mahoney, K., Con, A., & McGuiness, L. (2004). The context of health care communication in chronic illness. *Patient Education and Counseling, 54,* 299–306.

Tripp-Reimer, T., Brink, P. J., & Saunders, J. M. (1984). Cultural assessment: Content and process. *Nursing Outlook, 32*(2), 78–82.

Tripp-Reimer, T., Choi, E., Kelley, L. S., & Enslein, J. (2001). Cultural barriers to care: Inverting the problem. *Diabetes Spectrum, 14*(1), 13–22.

Tuckett, A. (2004). Truth telling in clinical practice and the arguments for and against: A review of the literature. *Nursing Ethics, 11*(5), 500–513.

Turner, L. (2003). Bioethics in a multicultural world: Medicine and morality in pluralistic settings. *Health Care Analysis, 11*(2), 99–117.

Xu, Y., & Davidhizar, R. (2004). Conflict management styles of Asian and Asian American Nurses: Implications for nurse managers. *The Health Care Manager, 23*(1), 46–53.

Yum, J. O. (1994). The impact of Confucianism on interpersonal relationships and communication patterns in East Asia. In L. A. Samovar & R. Porter (Eds.), *Intercultural communication* (pp. 75–86). Belmont, CA: Wadsworth.

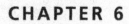

CHAPTER 6

Working with Interpreters in Healthcare Settings

RANI SRIVASTAVA

LEARNING OBJECTIVES

At the end of this chapter, the learner will be able to:

- Distinguish between translation, linguistic interpretation, and cultural interpretation
- Explain the pros and cons of using an untrained professional versus a trained interpreter, and describe situations in which each would be most appropriate
- Describe the techniques required to work effectively with professional interpreters
- Describe the techniques required to work effectively with untrained interpreters
- Differentiate between the roles of the healthcare provider and the interpreter in a healthcare interview
- Identify the multiple roles that interpreters often play
- Discuss common interpretation errors and appropriate strategies that the healthcare provider can use to overcome them

KEY TERMS

Ad hoc interpreters	Linguistic interpretation
Back translation	Pre-session
Bicultural	Remote interpreting
Bilingual	Telephonic interpreting
Consecutive interpreting	Translation
Cultural interpretation	Triadic communication
Interpretation	

Communicating successfully with clients who do not speak the same language as the healthcare provider requires serious advance planning. Language differences are the most commonly identified problem area for multicultural health care (Baker, 2001). Interpreters can greatly reduce the language gap; however, being able to find a suitable interpreter when needed and making the most effective use of **interpretation** services remains an ongoing challenge. This chapter discusses five basic steps that are critical to working effectively with interpreters (see Table 6-1).The discussion is largely framed with respect to spoken language interpretation, but many of the issues and strategies also apply to working with clients who depend on sign language. For detailed information about sign language interpretation, which is beyond the scope of this chapter, readers are referred to the Canadian Hearing Society (see "Online Learning Resources" at the end of this chapter).

Canada is rapidly transforming from a bilingual to a multilingual country, where more than 100 languages are spoken. Although the term **bilingual** generally describes a person with proficiency in two languages (National Council on Interpreting in Health Care, 2001), bilingualism in Canada refers to the ability to speak the country's two official languages, English and French. According to the 2001 census, one in six Canadians has a mother tongue other than English or French, and about 2 percent speak neither of the two official languages (Statistics Canada, 2002). Language often is considered a key aspect of culture and is thought to have a greater role than ethnicity or socio-economic status in accounting for differences in health status, use of services, and satisfaction with the healthcare system among minority populations (Bowen, 2004). Language difficulties are experienced by immigrant groups as well as many Aboriginal clients (particularly the elderly or those from isolated areas), clients who depend on sign language, and even some of the clients who speak one of Canada's official languages depending on where in Canada they seek health care (e.g., French-speaking clients in predominantly English-speaking environments) (Bowen, 2004).

A significant amount of research has documented the negative impact of language barriers on client health care (Baker, 2001; Bowen, 2004; Jacobs, 2002; Pope, 2004; Putsch, 2002; TriAd Research, Inc., 2002). In a comprehensive review of the literature related to language access, Bowen (2004) analyzed research evidence from a Canadian perspective and concluded that there was "strong evidence from Canadian programs that patients who do not speak an official language often do not receive the same standard of ethical care as other Canadians" (p. 53). Differences in care also have been noted with respect to the degree of client choice provided and the amount of healthcare teaching done with clients who do not speak English (Srivastava, 1997).

Language has an impact on the following areas of health care:
- Ability to obtain care
- Participation in preventive and screening activities
- Perceived health status
- Extent to which healthcare providers are trusted
- Satisfaction with care
- Protection of client rights
  (Baker, 2001; Bowen, 2004)

TABLE 6-1
Five Steps to Working Effectively with Interpreters

STEP 1: Recognize the need for an interpreter.
STEP 2: Seek out the appropriate type of interpreter.
STEP 3: Clarify the role of the interpreter and that of the healthcare provider.
STEP 4: Maintain control and engage in direct conversation with the client.
STEP 5: Be vigilant for errors in interpretation.

Language barriers also have been noted to lead to the following negative outcomes:
- Miscommunication
- Misdiagnosis
- Inappropriate client treatment
- Reduced comprehension and adherence to treatment
- Clinical inefficiency
- Malpractice injury
- Death
    (Bowen, 2004; Institute of Medicine, 2002; Masi, 1988; Office of
    Minority Health Resource Center, 2001)
Similarly, research from Britain has documented that healthcare providers caring for language minority populations experience difficulties in their relationships with clients and an increased focus on physical tasks. Clients report feeling lonely, isolated, and excluded (Pope, 2004).

Despite compelling evidence of the need for language support, healthcare organizations do not have a consistent way of approaching the issue. Individual healthcare organizations and coalitions have introduced programs to train and employ cultural interpreters for the healthcare context, but overall, inconsistencies exist in terms of expectations, requirements, and supports available (Baker, 2001; Bowen, 2004).

In the United States, where there are national standards to address inequities in health care, four of fourteen standards address the issue of language access (Office of Minority Health Resource Center, 2001). Canada, however (with the exception of interpretation services for deaf clients), has not categorically established the rights of clients to trained health interpretation. There is no overall legislative framework that requires the provision of language access to all language communities, and the different language constituencies (official languages, First Nations and Inuit languages, visual languages, and "immigrant" languages) often operate in isolation and competition with each other. The specific requirements are governed by different legislation and often are the responsibility of different government departments (Bowen, 2004). Consequently, considerable variation exists in the availability of services and in the development of standards and accountabilities across healthcare organizations and provincial jurisdictions.

CULTURAL CONSIDERATIONS IN CARE

Close Encounters with Disaster

Misunderstandings in a medical office or an emergency ward could have grave consequences, as the following examples show:

A pregnant Spanish-speaking client seemed to be asking about an abortion, and the obstetrician concerned decided to contact a community-based multicultural healthcare service. The doctor wanted to know about support services to which he could refer the woman. A bilingual, bicultural worker contacted the client, and the pregnant woman was horrified to learn of the doctor's concerns. She did not want to end the pregnancy; instead, she was worried about a miscarriage. In Spanish, the word for spontaneous abortion is used to describe both a spontaneous abortion or miscarriage and a planned abortion (Kelly, 2005).

In the second example, an untrained community interpreter was working with an immigrant client in a hospital emergency department but had to leave due to other commitments. A program co-ordinator from the hospital (who did not have the responsibility to provide interpretation services but was fluently bilingual) volunteered to interpret. At this time, in addition to the complaint for which the client was being treated, two issues were brought to the attention of the interpreter. First, hospital records indicated that the client had an appointment for a pregnancy termination; however, she claimed to have no knowledge of what procedure she had been scheduled for. Second, the client complained several times to the attending staff that she believed she had malaria and wanted to be tested for it. After several attempts, the attending physician finally responded that the test could not be done at the hospital. The staff member providing the interpretation contacted infectious diseases and was informed that not only could the test be done at the hospital but that it should be done there. The physician was subsequently contacted to clarify hospital policy and services (Bowen, 2004).

Both of these examples highlight major challenges that clients who require language support encounter: over-reliance on limited words or actions, and the difficulties in getting their voice heard when the role of the interpreter is not valued. In the second example, Bowen (2004) notes that if the volunteer community member had continued to interpret, it is unlikely that either the failure to communicate regarding the scheduled procedure or the hospital's role in malaria testing would have been clarified, resulting in risks to the individual client as well as to the hospital (Bowen, 2004).

Translation versus Interpretation

Language barriers can be addressed via translation as well as interpretation. **Translation** generally refers to written communication because translators deal with the written word. "Interpretation," on the other hand, involves the spoken word and refers to the process of mediating a verbal interaction between people who speak two different languages.

Generally, interpretation focuses purely on the spoken interaction, without omission, addition, editorializing, or any distortion in meaning (TriAd Research,

Inc., 2002). However, within a healthcare setting, understanding the meaning embedded in the words, tone, and gestures is just as important as understanding what is being said. Hence, a distinction needs to be made between the following:

- **Linguistic interpretation**, where only the spoken word is interpreted
- **Cultural interpretation**, where an interpreter may offer additional information about the culture

Linguistic interpreters understand the language but may not understand all the subtleties of the cultural context. Cultural interpreters not only understand the spoken language, but also understand and communicate the cultural context, including the meanings of looks and gestures. Cultural interpreters can provide valuable information about cultural traditions, acceptable and unacceptable topics, and interpretations associated with the situation as well as the language (Goldbloom, 2003; Wang, 2002). The extent to which an interpreter functions (or should function) as a linguistic or cultural interpreter depends on a variety of factors that will be discussed later in the chapter.

Healthcare providers who use translated materials need to be able to assess the adequacy of these materials. As noted by Jacobs (2002), this does not require knowledge of the other language but knowledge of the best method by which to ensure adequacy: back translation. **Back translation** requires two translators; one translates the document or information from English into the target language, and the other translates it back into English. Comparing the original and the translated versions allows the healthcare provider to determine whether the meaning and intent are the same, or if further refinement is needed (Jacobs, 2002). Adequacy of educational materials (particularly health promotion materials) also can be assessed by broad consultations, to determine possible cultural interpretations and responses.

Recognizing the Need for an Interpreter

The first step to working effectively with an interpreter is to recognize the need for one. Lack of effective interpretation remains a major access barrier to health care for many communities (Bowen, 2004; Tripp-Reimer, Choi, Kelley, & Enslein, 2001).

The evidence that language has an impact on health care is overwhelming. However, in the absence of established standards and requirements for interpretation, the decision as to whether to request an interpreter is frequently left to the individual healthcare provider (and, to a lesser extent, the client). Often, the need for an interpreter is clearly indicated, but on many occasions it is not addressed or the need is underestimated. Factors that contribute to a healthcare provider's underestimation of the need for an interpreter include the following:

- Overconfidence in interpretation of non-verbal behaviour
- False fluency (overestimation of one's abilities at understanding or speaking a second language) on the part of the client or the healthcare provider (Breen, 1999; Goldbloom, 2003; McPhee, 2002)

Clients and healthcare providers who have limited proficiency in a language may be able to communicate effectively in social situations but often have greater difficulty in the healthcare context, which is characterized by jargon, medical terminology, and stress (Tripp-Reimer et al., 2001). In such situations, clients may not recognize their own needs or may be hesitant to indicate their difficulties because of high self-expectations or fears of being judged negatively by the system. At the same time, healthcare providers may assume fluency based on a client's background and initial presentation. The mere fact that some English words are being spoken should not give the English-speaking healthcare provider a false sense of security that accurate information transfer has taken place (Howard, Andrade, & Byrd, 2001).

Even when the need for an interpreter is recognized, healthcare providers often choose to provide care without a qualified interpreter because of the perception that working with interpreters takes too long, the view that interpreters are an avoidable expense, or because interpreters are seen as potentially problematic in the areas of accuracy and confidentiality (Srivastava, 1997). Self-overestimation, combined with a lack of knowledge regarding the impact of ineffective interpretation on healthcare experiences and outcome, results in underestimating the need for, and the use of, interpreters.

Models of Interpreting

We can overcome language barriers in a variety of ways. Examples of different kinds of interpreters found in healthcare environments include trained interpreters; multilingual healthcare providers; and bilingual staff, volunteers, friends, or family members. Interpretation also can take many forms, most notably face-to-face consecutive interpreting, telephonic interpreting, and remote interpreting. It is important for healthcare providers to be aware of the strengths and limitations of the various approaches.

Modes of Interpreting

Face-to-Face Interpretation

Face-to-face, on-site interpreting is the most frequent and desired mode of interpretation in health care. Face-to-face interpreting is also known as **consecutive interpreting,** during which the interpreter is present with the healthcare provider and the client, and uses pauses between each one's speech to transform the message into a language understood by the other (Putsch, 2002). The clear advantage of this approach is that it allows for observation and interpretation of verbal as well as non-verbal responses.

Telephonic and Remote Interpretation

Even though face-to-face interpreting is the preferred mode, there are many situations where an interpreter is not available in a timely manner. Telephonic interpretation and remote interpretation in general are particularly useful in such situations.

Remote interpreting refers to situations in which the interpreter is not in the presence of the speakers (National Council on Interpreting in Health Care, 2001), and interpretation usually is done via a telephone (**telephonic interpreting**). Telephonic and other remote styles of interpretation, using telephone lines, speakerphones, and headsets, rely on technology to provide language support. The most popular service of this nature in Canada and the United States is the language line, which offer multiple languages, 24-hour access, and interpreters who are trained and certified for the healthcare context. The clear advantage of telephonic interpretation is that it can provide access to a trained interpreter within minutes, regardless of where (geographically) or when (time of day) the language support is needed. Emergency services frequently use such services. Disadvantages to telephonic interpretation include cost and the lack of ability to assess non-verbal cues and meanings. It is estimated that a large percentage of the emotional and social meaning (as high as 65 percent) in a situation is transmitted non-verbally (Pope, 2004). Use of speakerphones also can compromise confidentiality, and thus may limit a full and frank discussion of particular topics. As technology evolves, however, such services are expected to grow, with video conferencing becoming a more workable option (Pope, 2004; Putsch, 2002).

Other methods of interpretation include using a combination of the following: translated materials, picture cards or cards with key phrases that clients can point to, and key phrases that are learned by the healthcare provider. As noted earlier, caution is needed when such strategies are employed as over-reliance on limited pictures, phrases, or gestures can lead to misinterpretation and miscommunication.

Types of Interpreters

We have already touched on the reality that even though the need for competent, professional healthcare interpreters is readily recognized in health care, the availability of such resources is frequently limited. Instead, healthcare providers rely on various other types of interpreters—family, friends, volunteers, as well as professional staff. The volunteers or professional staff may be untrained or trained, and the training they have received may vary from brief workshops to formal training programs lasting several days. It is important that healthcare providers understand the challenges associated with each category of interpreter, to make the most appropriate decision under the circumstances. Understanding these challenges also allows healthcare providers to develop strategies for minimizing the disadvantages.

Bilingual, Bicultural Healthcare Providers

Being bilingual and **bicultural** is considered ideal for a healthcare provider because it means familiarity and fluency in language and culture, as well as an understanding of healthcare terminology, methods, and procedures. When the healthcare provider is fluent in the client's language, the need for three-way communication (i.e., involving an interpreter) and the associated dynamics is eliminated. However, many Canadian cities have small numbers of individuals from different linguistic and ethnic groups, and, thus, it is not feasible to offer even primary care to all communities by a healthcare provider of the same ethnic or language background (Bowen, 2004). Even when there is support from bilingual healthcare providers, many of the communication barriers discussed in the previous chapter may still exist. Linguistic similarity cannot be equated with cultural similarity, particularly when we consider the complexity of the various cultural identities and the associated issues of power and authority.

Bilingual Healthcare Staff

Many healthcare agencies have developed volunteer interpreter services that are staffed by professional and non-professional employees of the organization. Where such services exist, staff are generally provided with some training, guidelines, and support. The advantage of using employees—particularly professional staff—is that they are easier to access, may be viewed as trustworthy by the clients, and will likely have knowledge of healthcare terminology (Jacobs, 2002).

There is a downside, though. The presence of someone who speaks the same language does not ensure ethnic or cultural compatibility. Often, support staff who have no professional knowledge of health issues or the related terminology are asked to interpret. In a study examining the effectiveness of untrained physicians and nurses, miscommunication was noted in half the encounters, with the healthcare provider misunderstanding the problem, having contending agendas, slanting explanations to undermine the patient's account in favour of the institution, and missing cultural metaphors or context (Elderkin-Thompson, Silver, & Waitzkin, 2001). Another disadvantage of this approach is that, generally, bilingual employees act as interpreters in addition to their regular work. Consequently, they may be rushed during the interpretation because they need to return to their regular work responsibilities.

Ad Hoc Interpreters

Ad hoc interpreters, also known as informal interpreters, include family, friends, and community volunteers. While they may be convenient, there are many disadvantages to using them, including a greater risk for issues related to confidentiality, disclosure, and errors in interpretation. Studies have noted the error rate with ad hoc interpreters to be between 23 and 52 percent (Flores et al., 2003; Manson, 1988).

Family and friends continue to be a frequently used type of interpreter, mainly because of easy access and sometimes due to client preference. Family and friends are appropriate to use when the information involved is factual and non-sensitive, such as personal statistics (e.g., name, age, phone numbers), information about appointments or directions, or simple instructions for procedures. Healthcare providers should always be sensitive to potential interpersonal dynamics, however, and should be alert to any signs of discomfort on the part of either the client or the interpreter.

Friends and family are frequently unprepared for the complexity or intensity of the healthcare situation. Confidentiality also is threatened, and in some instances, clients may be reluctant to disclose information of a personal nature, particularly if it implies cultural transgressions. Family members may be reluctant to relay everything the client says, because of concerns of privacy, shame, or family dynamics. Family members who act as interpreters can readily, often unintentionally, become proxy decision makers, particularly if there are questions regarding the client's capacity to make his or her own decisions (Kaufert, Putsch, & Lavalle, 1999). Healthcare providers also may start to favour the family member's perspective, which means that the client's voice remains unheard.

In many immigrant families, children become the interpreters for their parents. This places the children in awkward and potentially traumatic situations, and the role reversal can adversely affect the entire family unit. Children as interpreters

CULTURAL COMPETENCE IN ACTION

Allaying Anxiety with Direct Communication

Mrs. Giovani, a 55-year-old woman of Italian origin, was hospitalized for acute renal failure and started on dialysis. Both the client and her husband had limited English proficiency, but their 27-year-old daughter was available for regular family meetings.

Over the first week, Mrs. Giovani's condition stabilized, although she continued to experience many symptoms related to the renal failure and dialysis, including fatigue, nausea, and vomiting. The couple's anxiety level continued to increase, as indicated by the husband's constant presence in the hospital room, non-verbal expressions of anxiety and confusion, and loud verbal expressions in Italian.

The clinical team felt that the communication with the client was good because of regular family meetings, and they tried to address the couple's anxiety through reassuring words in English and through non-verbal communication such as pats on the shoulder. Little attempt was made to communicate fully with the couple in a direct way until a new nurse on the clinical team began meeting the couple regularly during daily rounds. In response to the couple's obvious distress, this nurse tried to establish a direct relationship with the client and enlisted the help of an Italian-speaking staff member in the hospital.

The first such interaction resulted in a lengthy conversation during which the husband had many questions about the treatment, medications, prognosis, and progress. After the initial concerns had been addressed, the nurse asked if the information was new to the couple or if they had heard it before through their daughter. The couple looked at each other and then the husband responded, "Of course, our daughter told us all this, about the medicines and that her mother was getting better, but what else could she say? Do you think our daughter would be able to tell us that her mother was dying?"

This clearly illustrates the need for ensuring that the communication between the client and healthcare provider is as direct as possible. If family members serve as interpreters, it is important to identify and address the issues around uncomfortable topics such as death and the dynamics around disclosure. Even when direct communication is not possible on a regular basis, attempts should be made to access professional interpreters at periodic intervals to ensure that the clients and providers have the same understanding of the situation and that there are regular opportunities for assessment and clarification of issues.

usurp the parental role of guide and decision maker. This is true regardless of the age of the children, and even parents of adult children who are acting as interpreters may feel their position or status compromised. The client also may feel that the interpretation is selective, based on the family member's desire to protect the client and minimize the concerns.

Professional Interpreters

In contrast to ad hoc interpreters, professional interpreters are able to interpret with consistency and accuracy, and adhere to a code of ethics (National Council on Interpreting in Health Care, 2001).

Professional interpreters can generally be counted on to have obtained some form of certification that usually includes language assessment, as well as training related to medical terminology, ethics, and working in healthcare teams. In Canada, where there are no clear credentialing requirements for professional interpreters, it is important for organizations and professionals seeking these services to assess the qualifications, experience, and expertise of the interpreter.

In general, the use of trained professional interpreters has been associated with positive experiences and outcomes for both clients and healthcare providers (Office of Minority Health Resource Center, 2001; TriAd Research, Inc., 2002). An evaluation of a pilot project on language and cultural facilitation with Jewish seniors in Canada noted that the seniors felt comfortable with the services provided, and that they felt that the healthcare providers had an increased understanding of their health issues, medication use, and concerns. The healthcare providers also felt that the clients were more accepting of the services provided (TriAd Research, Inc., 2002). Before the pilot project, when the interpretation generally was provided by family and friends, several challenges were noted, including the following:

- Seniors were often hesitant to ask family (too busy).
- Untrained interpreters did not always interpret word for word.
- Family and friends gave unsolicited advice to healthcare professionals and to the client.
- Confidentiality issues arose.
- Understanding medical terminology was a problem.
  (TriAd Research, Inc., 2002, p. 3)

The Interpreter Role

The basic function of a healthcare interpreter is to provide a linguistic conversion from one language system to another, in such a way that the meaning is maintained. The role of the interpreter has evolved over time and ranges incrementally from message passer to advocate, with additional roles of clarifier and cultural broker in between (see Figure 6-1).

At the most basic level, the interpreter may be viewed as a neutral party whose sole purpose is to be a conduit between the healthcare provider and the client. In this light, the interpreter is simply an instrument or a "voice box," with

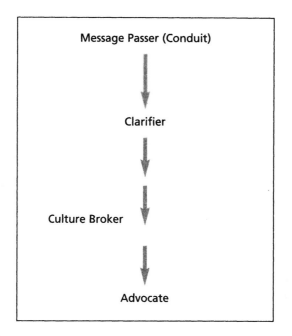

FIGURE 6-1 ■ **Increasing Complexity of Interpreter Roles**
Modified from *Language access in healthcare: Domains, strategies and implications for medical education* (p. 10), by R. W. Putsch, 2002, American Institutes for Research (AIR). Concept Paper. Retrieved May 19, 2005, from http://www.thinkculturalhealth.org/cccm/concept_papers.asp. Reprinted with permission.

messages entering in one language and coming out in another; the interpreter is expected to remain neutral and maintain a disengaged presence.

As the differences between the other two parties become more complex, the interpreter may shift to a more active role by clarifying, to see if both sides truly understand each other's meaning and intent. For example, if cultural factors or values are creating a misunderstanding about the goal of the encounter, the interpreter may intervene and alert both parties to the miscommunication while offering suggestions to promote mutual understanding (Avery, 2001). From a purist perspective, if the interpreter is viewed as a bridge, then what is brought across the bridge is up to the practitioner and not the interpreter. In reality, however, often interpreters have cultural information and insights that can greatly facilitate communication. In such circumstances, interpreters may stop or pause an interpretation session to offer their own perspective on the situation. The intent is to flag the issue for the healthcare provider, and not to usurp the position of either the healthcare provider or the client.

The role of the interpreter as an advocate occurs when an interpreter is unable to successfully fulfill his or her role as a culture broker, and sees the situation as warranting further intervention. The extent to which an interpreter will succeed in advocating further intervention (by going beyond the healthcare provider and seeking additional support, as illustrated in the in the box titled "Close Encounters with Disaster" described earlier in the chapter) depends on his or her relationship (with respect to power) to the healthcare team (Kaufert et al., 1999).

The failure of healthcare providers and administrators to recognize that interpreters can add a significant dimension to the clinical encounter has been identified as a major source of conflict during interpretation sessions involving the Canadian Aboriginal community in urban hospitals (Kaufert & Koolage, 1984; Kaufert et al., 1999).

Hatton and Webb (1993), in a qualitative study involving community healthcare nurses and interpreters, identify three styles of interactions, as follows:

1. The "voice box interpreter" is one who acts as the voice of the client and healthcare provider, without enabling or hindering the situation and the meaning of what is being said.
2. The "excluder" excludes the client and may filter information between the client and the healthcare provider.
3. The "collaborator" collaborates with both the client and the healthcare provider.

The researchers note that the collaborator is the most effective with respect to establishing rapport and subsequent assessment, planning, and delivery of services (Hatton & Webb, 1993).

Regardless of the level of intervention enacted by the interpreter, the key is to maintain transparency for all parties. This means identifying when the interpreter has to assume his or her own voice to clarify something or take on the role of the culture broker. Subsequently, if the interpreter enters into a conversation directly with either party, the interpreter must interpret this interaction as well for the benefit of all present.

Factors Affecting the Quality of Interpretation

Regardless of the type of interpreter used, many factors can affect the quality of the interpretation. Common interpreter errors include the following:

- Omission
- Substitution
- Editorialization
- Addition

Many errors—such as omitting questions regarding drug allergies or instructions on the dose, frequency, and duration of medication—could have serious clinical consequences. Lack of linguistic equivalency between the two languages is another challenge to effective interpretation (Putsch, 2002). Many commonly used medical terms (e.g., stress, allergy, mental health, and bacteria) may not have an equivalent term in other cultures; similarly, many terms and concepts from other cultures do not have parallel terms in English (Putsch, 2002). In such circumstances, clarification and verification of understanding becomes critical.

In order for an interpretation to be effective, all parties need to be knowledgeable about the issues and feel comfortable in the situation. In some instances, clients may be uncomfortable with interpreters because they do not understand the interpreter's role and also may be concerned about confidentiality. Explaining the role and the advantages of an interpreter, stressing confidentiality, and obtaining consent are effective strategies to increase client comfort with a third party in the interaction. It also is critical for healthcare providers to accurately assess their own biases and skills at working effectively with interpreters. Interpreters should be regarded as tools that provide language support to the client–provider interaction. To use the tools effectively, healthcare providers need suitable education and experience.

One uncertain experience with interpretation should not be used as the basis for making all future decisions regarding the usefulness of interpreters. It is essential that interpreters be seen as legitimate, valued members of healthcare teams, and that they be provided with some information regarding the context of the situations in which they are asked to interpret. It is equally essential that both the clients' and the interpreters' voices be heard. In health care, cross-cultural communication is frequently challenged by relationships in which the healthcare providers are dominant; this can be changed by training healthcare providers and interpreters to maintain a client-centred approach (Putsch, 2002).

The potential dynamics between the interpreter and client also need to be considered. When working with family and friends as interpreters, healthcare providers need to be aware of the potential influence of both family and interpersonal dynamics. In many cultures, role relationships between generations and genders are extremely structured and defined. There may be strong objections to even mentioning sexual organs or their functions to members of the opposite sex or members of a different generation, and clients may avoid discussing symptoms or concerns. Sometimes, interpreters may revise or omit questions thought to be inappropriate, insulting, or embarrassing. The interpreter's cultural beliefs or superstitions may influence such omissions. For example, in cultures that believe words precipitate deeds, non-professional interpreters may omit mentioning complications of surgery or other similar information. Interpreters also may offer their own advice, or may selectively interpret what the client says in order to present the culture in a positive light.

The Stress of Interpreting

When we view interpreters as neutral "language processors," their experiences tend to become invisible. The role of an interpreter is, however, extremely demanding.

Interpreters often report that their role is stressful, frustrating, and unsupported (Bowen, 2000). In addition, interpreters often deal with painful and conflictive communication, which may (particularly in the case of trauma or abuse) affect them personally. This is a very real issue for interpreters from refugee communities, many of whom have had experiences similar to those of the clients for whom they are interpreting (Bowen, 1999; Loudon, Anderson, Gill, & Greenfield, 1999; Tribe, 1999). In other cases, interpreters find themselves providing emotional support—to clients as well as providers. In some instances, interpreters may also feel personally responsible for failures in diagnosis and care (Bowen, 2004). Additionally, when staff members act as interpreters, they are expected to take time out from their regular work to provide the additional support, often in extremely intensive and emotionally draining situations. However, the emotional needs of interpreters frequently go unrecognized as they are expected to resume their regular responsibilities in a timely fashion (Srivastava, 1997).

Two important areas of support for interpreters are as follows:
1. Post-interpretation debriefing
2. Support from colleagues for time away for interpretation

Triadic Interviews

Triadic communication involves three parties. A triadic interview involves the following three individuals:
1. Healthcare provider
2. Interpreter
3. Client

In triadic communication, attention should be paid to the following (Putsch, 2002):
- Emphasis on shared meaning and understanding, including a desire to learn
- A pre-session
- Physical positioning to encourage direct interaction between the healthcare provider and client
- Unobtrusive posturing and eye contact by the interpreter
- Strategies to maximize provider–client interaction
- Use of first-person voice by the interpreter and healthcare provider
- Control by the healthcare provider

Table 6-2 provides guidelines for working with interpreters.

Emphasis on shared meanings requires an appreciation for the scope of the interpreter's role. Neutrality is traditionally emphasized in professional interpreting; in health care, differences in class, culture, expectations, trust, and power dictate that the interpreter play a more active role (Putsch, 2002). Healthcare providers need to be open to client perspectives and value the role an interpreter

TABLE 6-2

General Guidelines for Working with Cultural Interpreters

- Allow for extra time for the session.
- Use trained bilingual/bicultural interpreters.
- Never use children as interpreters.
- Consider the gender, ethnicity, language/dialect, and other characteristics, of the interpreter.
- Beware of common issues:
  - Words that can't be translated
  - Jargon or terminology
  - Being too rushed
  - Interpreter answering for the client
  - Conflict between interpreter and client (If this occurs, stop the session immediately!)
- Verify to avoid misunderstandings, mistakes, and distortions.

can play in fostering mutual understanding. A **pre-session** (a brief meeting between the healthcare provider and interpreter before the interpreted session) is a useful strategy for reinforcing the role of the interpreter on the team, as well as for clarifying the purpose of the encounter and establishing necessary ground rules and boundaries for the upcoming session (Putsch, 2002).

Throughout interpretation sessions, it is important that healthcare providers be clear on their accountability for care and that they maintain control over the session. Effective ways to accomplish this goal include the following:

- Ensuring transparency
- Ensuring proper positioning
- Using first-person speech
- Insisting that all conversations be interpreted

Direct healthcare provider–client interaction can be maximized in several ways. The health provider's use of the first-person point of view, for example, reinforces that the healthcare provider's voice should be conveyed to the client. Rather than talking to the interpreter and saying, "Please tell her that I will be asking questions about her illness," the healthcare provider needs to say, "I'd like to ask you some questions about your illness." Similarly, the interpreter's use of the first-person perspective conveys the client's voice to the healthcare provider. In some instances, interpreters may interject forms of address to communicate respect and honour. For instance, the interpreter may say, "Grandmother, the doctor says, 'I would like to . . . '" (Putsch, 2002). This is acceptable because the interaction continues to use the first person.

Positioning also can maximize healthcare provider–client interaction. Healthcare providers should face the client directly and maintain appropriate eye contact. The interpreter is encouraged to be as unobtrusive as possible, sitting beside or behind the client, to avoid having the interpreter become the focus of the exchange.

Healthcare providers frequently become concerned when interpreters give long translations to their shorter questions. It is critical that this gets addressed

CULTURAL CONSIDERATIONS IN CARE

Working with Interpreters: The Pre-Session
Whenever possible, take a few minutes to have a pre-session with the interpreter in order to:

- Introduce yourself and briefly get to know the interpreter
- Identify the objectives of the interview, topics to be covered, and time available
- Provide a brief summary of the client
- Ask the interpreter if he or she has any cautions, concerns, or issues regarding this client or the situation
- Remind the interpreter to interpret everything using the first person
- Ask the interpreter to share his or her cultural insights with you as the healthcare provider, but to differentiate these from the interpretation itself
- Reinforce confidentiality

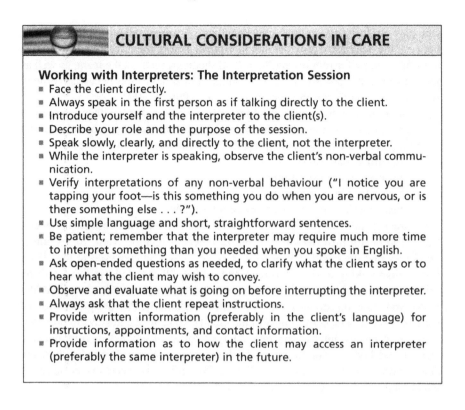

CULTURAL CONSIDERATIONS IN CARE

Working with Interpreters: The Interpretation Session
- Face the client directly.
- Always speak in the first person as if talking directly to the client.
- Introduce yourself and the interpreter to the client(s).
- Describe your role and the purpose of the session.
- Speak slowly, clearly, and directly to the client, not the interpreter.
- While the interpreter is speaking, observe the client's non-verbal communication.
- Verify interpretations of any non-verbal behaviour ("I notice you are tapping your foot—is this something you do when you are nervous, or is there something else . . . ?").
- Use simple language and short, straightforward sentences.
- Be patient; remember that the interpreter may require much more time to interpret something than you needed when you spoke in English.
- Ask open-ended questions as needed, to clarify what the client says or to hear what the client may wish to convey.
- Observe and evaluate what is going on before interrupting the interpreter.
- Always ask that the client repeat instructions.
- Provide written information (preferably in the client's language) for instructions, appointments, and contact information.
- Provide information as to how the client may access an interpreter (preferably the same interpreter) in the future.

with the interpreter immediately. Sometimes the long translation is needed to set the cultural context of the question(s), and other times the interpreter may be editorializing. It is therefore important to ask the interpreter to interpret everything as directly as possible. Healthcare providers need to know about any cultural editorializing so that they can increase their own understanding of cultural issues and also assess the quality of interpretations.

Holding a brief post-interview meeting with the interpreter could clarify information and result in discussion of relevant impressions, insights, and issues, including any difficulties that were encountered during the interpretation session. This also gives the healthcare provider another opportunity to tap into the interpreter's expertise and reinforce the valuable role interpreters can play on the healthcare team.

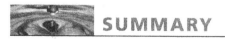

SUMMARY

The chapter began by explaining the language barriers to health care, which, if not recognized, can lead to negative health experiences and outcomes. The chapter discussed the difference between translation and interpretation, and then described five basic steps related to working effectively with interpreters (recognizing the need for interpretation; seeking out the appropriate type of interpreter;

clarifying the interpreter role; engaging in direct communication with the client by maintaining control over the interpretation; and utilizing strategies to minimize errors and miscommunication).

Different modes of interpreting were discussed, most notably face-to-face interpretation and telephonic and other remote interpretation. The types of interpreters encountered in a healthcare setting may range from untrained, ad hoc interpreters, to those who are professionally trained. The role of the interpreter also ranges, from message passer to advocate.

It is important that healthcare providers be aware of the advantages and disadvantages associated with the various types of interpreters and interpreter roles, and that they make appropriate choices based on client need. Interpreters have much to offer in a clinical encounter, and their role needs to be understood and valued for maximum effectiveness. Strategies for enhancing three-way communication between client, healthcare provider, and interpreter were explained. Regardless of the role of the interpreter, the healthcare provider must maintain control and engage in direct communication with the client. Effective interpretation is vital to effective communication in situations requiring language support.

ONLINE LEARNING RESOURCES

www.chs.ca
Developed by the Canadian Hearing Society, this Web site provides information on preventing hearing loss and enhancing the independence of deaf, deafened, and hard of hearing people. The site includes a section on frequently asked questions and provides links to related Web sites, press releases, and publications.

www.languageline.com/
This Web site provides information from a company called Language Line Services that provides language support via telephone interpretation. In addition to a description of the services available and how to access them, the site includes information on working with interpreters and offers an interpreter code of ethics.

www.ncihc.org
The National Council on Interpreting in Health Care site is a US-based organization whose mission is to promote culturally competent professional healthcare interpreting. The site features a working paper series in which a variety of issues and questions in healthcare interpreting are addressed by experts. Information about policy initiatives and healthcare interpreting associations is also available.

www.jcaho.orgs/hlc
This section of the US Joint Commission on Accreditation of Healthcare Organization's Web site provides information on a 30-month project titled "Hospitals, Language, and Culture." The project will collect information on a sample of hospitals to assess their capacity to address the issues of language and culture in order to determine realistic expectations and benchmarks. The site also provides information on standards and links to other groups addressing similar issues.

REFERENCES

Avery, M. P. B. (2001). *The role of the health care interpreter: An evolving dialogue.* Boston: National Council on Interpreting in Health Care (NCIHC).

Baker, C. (2001). *Service provision by representative institutions and identity*. Halifax: Department of Canadian Heritage.

Bowen, S. (2004). *Assessing the responsiveness of health care organizations to culturally diverse groups*. Winnipeg: University of Manitoba, Department of Community Health Sciences.

Breen, L. (1999). What should I do if my patient does not speak English? *Journal of the American Medical Association, 282*(9), 819.

Elderkin-Thompson, V., Silver, R. C., & Waitzkin, H. (2001). When nurses double as interpreters. A study of Spanish-speaking patients in a US primary care setting. *Social Science and Medicine, 52,* 1343–1358.

Flores, G., Laws, M. B., Mayo, S. J., Zuckerman, B., Abreu, M., Medina, L., & Hardt, E. J. (2003). Errors in medical interpretation and their potential clinical consequences in pediatric encounters. *Pediatrics, 111,* 6–14.

Goldbloom, R. B. (2003). *Skills for culturally sensitive pediatric care*. Philadelphia: Saunders.

Hatton, D., & Webb, T. (1993). Information transmission in bilingual, bicultural contexts: A field study of community health nurses and interpreters. *Journal of Community Health Nursing, 10* (3), 137–147.

Howard, C. A., Andrade, S. J., & Byrd, T. (2001). The ethical dimensions of cultural competence in border health care settings. *Family and Community Health, 23*(4), 36–41.

Institute of Medicine (2002). *Unequal treatment: What healthcare providers need to know about racial and ethnic disparities in health care*. The National Academies Press (Summary). 2002. Retrieved January 8, 2006, from www.iom.edu/CMS/3740/4475.aspx

Jacobs, E. (2002). *Concept paper: Language access services*. Washington, DC: American Institutes for Research (AIR). Retrieved September 19, 2004, from http://www.thinkculturalhealth.org/cccm/papers/jacobs.pdf

Kaufert, J., & Koolage, W. W. (1984). Role conflict among culture brokers. *Social Science and Medicine, 18*(3), 283–286.

Kaufert, J., Putsch, R. W., & Lavallee, M. (1999). End-of-life decision making among Aboriginal Canadians: Interpretation, mediation, and discord in the communication of "bad news." *Journal of Palliative Care, 15*(1), 31–38.

Kelly, A. (2005, April 30). Health care translates well: Interpreters bridge language gap. *The Record*, A1.

Manson, A. (1988). Language concordance as a determinant of patient compliance and emergency room use in patients with asthma. *Medical Care, 26,* 1119–1128.

Masi, R. (1988). Multiculturalism, medicine and health part I: Multicultural health care. *Canadian Family Physician, 34,* 2173–2178.

McPhee, S. (2002). Caring for a 70-year-old Vietnamese woman. *Journal of the American Medical Association, 287*(4), 495–503.

National Council on Interpreting in Health Care. (2001). *The terminology of health care interpreting: A glossary of terms*. Boston: Author.

Office of Minority Health Resource Center. (2001, March). *Assuring cultural competence in health care: Recommendations for national standards and an outcomes focused research agenda*. Retrieved September 19, 2005, from http://www.omhrc.gov/clas/index.htm

Pope, C. (2004). *Concept paper: Language Access Services in Nursing,* Office of Minority Health. US Department of Health and Human Services. Retrieved September 19, 2005, from http://www.cultureandhealth.org/rn/documents/CCNMLASConceptPaperPope_Final.pdf

Putsch, R. W. (2002). *Concept paper: Language access in healthcare: Domains, strategies and implications for medical education.* Washington, DC: US Department of Health and Human Services. Retrieved January 30, 2006, from http://www.thinkculturalhealth. org/cccm/papers/putsch.pdf

Srivastava, R. (1997). *Perceived need and utilization of interpreters in health care.* Toronto: Wellesley Central Hospital.

Statistics Canada. (2002). *Profile of languages in Canada: English, French, and many others.* (Cat. No. 96F0030XIE2001005). Retrieved June 10, 2005 from http:// www.statcan.ca/bsolc/english/bsolc?catno=96XF0030X2001005

TriAd Research, Inc. (2002). *Evaluation of the Language and Culture Facilitation Pilot Project.* Calgary: Author. Retrieved September 20, 2005, from http://www. calgaryhealthregion.ca/hecomm/diversity/EvaluationofLanguage%20andCulture FacilitationPilot.pdf

Tripp-Reimer, T., Choi, E., Kelley, L. S., & Enslein, J. (2001). Cultural barriers to care: Inverting the problem. *Diabetes Spectrum, 14*(1), 13–22.

Wang, J. (2002). Knowing the true face of a mountain: Understanding communication and cultural competence. In W. J. Lonner, D. L. Dinnel, S. A. Hays, & D. N. Sattler (Eds.), *Online Readings in Psychology and Culture,* Unit 16, Chapter 3. Bellingham: Center for Cross Cultural Research, Western Washington University. Retrieved October 15, 2004, from http://www.wwu.edu/~culture/Wang.ht

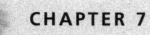

CHAPTER 7

Caring for Diverse Families

SALMA DEBS-IVALL

LEARNING OBJECTIVES

At the end of this chapter, the learner will be able to:

- Describe the family as a system
- Identify the characteristics of family diversity that influence health and illness behaviours
- Discuss individualism and collectivism in terms of the family system
- Examine his or her personal beliefs and assumptions about families
- Discuss ethical and moral dilemmas faced by healthcare providers who care for culturally diverse families
- Know how to evaluate, or assess, families when working with culturally diverse clients

KEY TERMS

Acculturation	Family system
Collectivism	Family Systems Theory
Common-law family	Generational conflict
Familism	Individualism
Family diversity	Joint family
Family roles	Nuclear family
Family structure	Skip-generation family

Cultural values, beliefs, and behaviours are learned and acquired rather than genetically inherited. We are young children when we first start to learn the behaviours that are culturally acceptable within our families and social groups (Giger & Davidhizar, 1999). Learned behaviours will likely continue throughout our lives unless we are forced to change (e.g., because we emigrate). Learned behaviours are culturally bound to our individual perception of reality and should not be isolated from the context in which they occur. Although interpretations of specific behaviour may be understandable and acceptable to those brought up within the same culture, they may never be accepted by others who exist outside that context (Giger & Davidhizar, 1999).

144

Healthcare providers bring their own cultural perspectives into the healthcare setting. In many parts of the world—including North America—healthcare providers have been socialized to attribute most illnesses to biological causes and to uphold Western medicine as the answer to all healthcare needs (Giger & Davidhizar, 1999). Generally speaking, healthcare providers believe in scientific methods and processes as the way to determine and resolve health problems. This is bound to put them in conflict with the cultural perspectives of a number of clients and their families. We have to remember constantly that everyone—clients and healthcare providers alike—looks at the world from a particular cultural viewpoint and that we each regard our views and beliefs as valid and allow them to influence our healthcare behaviour (Bernal, 1996; Giger & Davidhizar, 1999). For instance, clients from some cultures may attribute the cause of illness to evil and sin, or to the curse of a neighbour, which influences their health and illness behaviours accordingly. When caring for diverse families, it is important that healthcare providers recognize the need to adapt to the circumstances in order to be as effective as possible.

Families are an important part of the care process no matter who the client is (child, adult, or elder), no matter where care is provided (home, hospital, or community settings), and no matter what the healthcare need is. The current general philosophies associated with delivering healthcare services highlight the need for family-centred care, which requires the healthcare provider to take the "family" into account and include it in the plan of care for the client. Such an approach emphasizes the need for healthcare providers to understand and respect the family's cultural values (Hanson, 2004).

This chapter studies the concept of family, describes the composition of the family, and explains rules and roles that govern the behaviour of its members, particularly within the context of health and illness. Throughout the chapter, the need for healthcare providers to understand their own beliefs and attitudes toward families is highlighted as an important factor in the provision of family-centred care.

Family Diversity

Family diversity is defined as characteristics associated with the composition of a family that influence how members of the family respond to issues of health and illness. Friedman (1997) lists seven major areas of family diversity that require consideration:

1. Family members' race, ethnicity, and religion are of primary importance. Race relates to individual differences within the family. Ethnicity dictates the individual versus group orientation of the family members, as well as their social and cultural history. Religion can have a direct influence on the health values, beliefs, and practices.
2. Moving to a new country can be traumatic for immigrants and refugees. Often, they leave families, homes, and all that is familiar behind; then they face the pressure of adapting to the new host culture.

3. Generational difference arises due to the differences in the level of acculturation of the various members. Younger family members usually adapt relatively quickly to the host culture and adopt many of its beliefs and values.

4. The language of the host country usually is learned faster by the younger generations, sometimes at the expense of retaining the language of the original culture.

5. Socio-economic status has a great influence on family life and dynamics, producing "significant differences in a family's culture" (Friedman, 1997, p. 283). Socio-economic status also may dictate access to education, job opportunities, and appropriate housing.

6. Residential or regional differences become obvious as members of a family move between urban and rural settings, resulting in wide variations in lifestyles, values, and beliefs (Leininger, 1995).

7. The varying makeup of families is forcing a re-evaluation of the definition of the family. As the number of same-sex and common-law couples increases in Canada, family characteristics, strengths, and vulnerabilities are becoming more and more diverse.

Healthcare providers need to understand these issues and to help ensure that families participate in the process of maintaining their health and seeking healthcare services. Below, we discuss potentially challenging areas related to family diversity: family structure, roles, and rules; individualism versus collectivism; acculturation; and generational conflict.

Family Structure, Roles, and Rules

The family is considered the basic unit of society; however, the definition of family varies depending on whether we have a sociological, economic, psychological, or biological perspective. Most definitions agree on one point: that the family is a relationship community between two or more persons from similar or different kinship groups (Giger & Davidhizar, 1999). The family may also be viewed as a basic human unit that has certain generic qualities, such as the cohabitation of two or more persons involved in a continuous, permanent sharing of living quarters. The members have a perception of reciprocal obligations, a sense of commonality of values and beliefs, and a perception of certain obligations toward others in the society at large (Giger & Davidhizar, 1999).

Wright, Watson, and Bell (1996) defined the family as a group of individuals who are bound together by emotional ties and a sense of belonging, and who want to be involved in each others' lives. Perhaps the most useful definition, for the purposes of this chapter, is the one penned by Wright and Leahey (2000): "The family is who they say they are" (p. 70). This definition is based on the family's perceptions of belonging, rather than on the premise of cohabitation.

The family, as a social organization, is characterized by a steady state that has a maintained equilibrium, even as the members change (Giger & Davidhizar, 1999). The family may therefore be seen as a system or a group of interrelated parts or units that form a whole. Barry (1996) sees the **family system** as "a special type of social group that is essential to the development of all human beings" (p. 129). The family is also the primary system for the transfer of values and norms. As the family develops, a set of values, beliefs, and patterns of behaviour emerge. As the family matures, each member assumes a certain role. The members then are recognized in terms of their relationships with other family members, friends, and the society at large. Individuals within the family system are interconnected. A change affecting one member is likely to have an effect on all other members of the family. In the healthcare context, when one member of a family is affected by illness, the client's role within the family is disrupted, resulting in changes to the roles of the remaining members to compensate for the missing role responsibilities. The family members also may reach out to the extended family members, friends, or healthcare providers for support.

Wright et al. (1996) believe that, in the same way that the illness of an individual affects the whole family, the family, in turn, will affect the illness. They propose that the effect lies more in the beliefs about the illness than with the illness itself. Such beliefs might be about the diagnosis, etiology, healing and treatment, control, prognosis, and religion and spirituality, as well as the role of the illness in life. Rather than constraining family beliefs, which could cause suffering, healthcare providers are in a position to work with the family to come up with options that take their beliefs into account.

Family Structure

Family structure may be defined as an outline of the composition of the family with respect to members and their relationship to each other and the family unit. The structure of the family often shapes the rules, roles, and resources that exist within the family. It also becomes important in care processes such as consultation and consent for treatment; for example, a client may describe his same-sex common-law spouse as family, even though legislation dictates a different hierarchy for who can be a substitute decision maker for the client's care. Recognizing the potential for such conflict and developing strategies to work through it is a critical aspect of cultural competence.

Traditional Family

In twenty-first-century Canada, there is no such thing as a typical family. Still, for many people, the stereotypical view of the traditional family is that of a **nuclear family** consisting of husband, wife, and children. This family type has been on the decline in Canada, dropping from 60 percent of all couples in 1981 to only 44 percent in 2001 (Statistics Canada, 2002). Nevertheless, it remains the predominant structure in many ethnic and immigrant populations. This could be attributed in part to immigration laws that still favour family units and allow visas to certain relatives of Canadian citizens and landed immigrants. Lone-parent families are becoming more prevalent among the immigrant/refugee population as individual adults (most often women) escape the social and political turmoil of their native countries and arrive in Canada with their children. In many instances, they lack the language, financial resources, education, and training to enter the professional workforce and are forced to work in low-paying, menial jobs in order to support themselves and their children.

Common-Law Family

The **common-law family** consists of two people living together as spouses without the formality of marriage. The family also may include children. The common-law couple most frequently consists of a man and woman, but common-law spouses may be of the same sex. Census data indicates that the common-law family type is on the rise in Canada, representing 7.4 percent of all couples in 2001, compared to only 2.1 percent of all couples in 1981. Statistics on same-sex couples were captured for the first time in 2001, with 34 200 same-sex common-law couples reported, accounting for 0.5 percent of all couples. There were slightly more male same-sex couples (55 percent of all same-sex couples) than female. However, more female couples (15 percent) than male couples (3 percent) reported having children living with them (Statistics Canada, 2002). Children in gay or lesbian families could have been introduced into the household during the relationship, or could have been brought into the household initially by one or both partners from a previous relationship.

Until recently in Canada, society used to compare gay and lesbian families to the nuclear family or the stepfamily, without taking the gender composition of the couples into consideration. Even though gay and lesbian families share structural elements with heterosexual families, they share gender composition with other gay and lesbian families. This intersection of structure and gender composition makes this form of family distinct (Lynch, 2000). Gay and lesbian families have traditionally faced prejudice, discrimination, subtle forms of exclusion, and confrontations regarding their non-traditional choice of lifestyle. Despite these negative experiences and the stress they invoke on the parents, the children in such families have been found to be well-adjusted (Bos, van Balen, van den Boom, & Sandfort, 2004).

Extended and Joint Families

The extended family often is multi-generational and includes all relatives by birth or adoption. In many cultures, the extended family (also known as "kin") also includes close family friends and community members. When individuals migrate from one country to another, the loss of extended family often creates a gap in their ability to receive support, including healthcare advice and the ability to cope with the demands of an illness.

Some cultures also have the concept of a **joint family,** or a family where parents and adult children and their families live under a single roof. In a joint family, different members of the family may take on different roles. For example, some of the women may stay at home and take on the role of homemaker, including being responsible for cooking, for the entire family. The head of the household (often the oldest male member) lays down the rules and arbitrates disputes.

Other senior members of the household babysit infants and children when the mothers are working. They are also responsible for teaching the younger children their mother tongue, manners, and etiquette. In extended families, children often are raised by a number of relatives.

With the increasing numbers of lone-parent and extended families, many grandparents now find themselves taking care of grandchildren. In 2001, 6.5 percent of seniors in private households in Canada shared their household with grandchildren. Of these households, 12 percent contained only the grandparent(s) and the grandchild(ren) (Statistics Canada, 2002), indicating that the grandparent(s) had taken on the dual role of parent and grandparent. This family type is also known as the **skip-generation family.** Cultural gaps between grandparents and grandchildren are likely to exist in this family structure.

Blended or Stepfamily

Like the traditional nuclear family, the blended family is two-generational, consisting of parents and children. However, the blended family contains at least one parent who was previously married, with children from that marriage. The structure is further complicated when the new couple have children of their own. This type of family represented 12 percent of all Canadian couples with children in 2001 (Statistics Canada, 2002).

According to Lynch (2000), parents in heterosexual stepfamilies struggle to change the basic focus of the family unit from the biological parent and child to the adult couple. Interestingly, in homosexual stepfamilies, and because of the inward focus of the unit away from societal discrimination and condemnation, the focus becomes child centred.

Cultural competence in caring for diverse families means understanding and acknowledging a family's structure. It is important that healthcare providers not make assumptions about the family structure. Inclusive language is important. For example, asking about a partner or spouse instead of husband and wife will provide a more comfortable environment for a client to disclose a same-sex family structure. In some instances, visiting policies are limited to immediate family; if the healthcare provider does not allow the client to define the immediate family, the result may be exclusionary and discriminatory.

Understanding Family Rules

All families have a set of written and unwritten rules that guide their interaction within and outside the home. These rules are determined by the values and beliefs of the family members. Children learn these rules from their parents and, eventually, teach them to their own children. As the family matures and changes, family rules are modified due to life experiences, immigration, or education. However, many of the values and beliefs of the original families are retained by the new family units. These values and beliefs become a source of comfort and support for the immigrant family in the new country and a way to remain accepted within the cultural community. Immigrant families that adopt the host country's values and belief system, which could be in conflict with the "old" country's values and belief system, can be rejected and exiled from their cultural community (Giger & Davidhizar, 1999).

Table 7-1 shows contrasting beliefs, values, and practices for traditional Asian and mainstream Western families.[1]

Some of the conflict between strongly traditional and modern cultures is evident in first- and second-generation immigrant families, as children born or brought up in the host country start to break away from family rules. As children embrace Western belief systems rather than conforming to the cultural values and beliefs of their parents, generational conflict may ensue within the nuclear and extended families. This will be discussed later in this chapter under "Acculturation" and "Generational Conflict."

Interestingly, many family rules in some cultural communities are determined by religious beliefs (e.g., in the Muslim, Dutch, Mennonite, and Amish communities in Canada). These beliefs will affect decisions regarding appropriate social activities, proper attire, proximity of residence to the parents, choice of partner, and educational levels for the members of the family based on gender.

TABLE 7-1

Contrasting Family Beliefs, Values, and Practices Across Cultures

TRADITIONAL ASIAN: FAMILY-CENTRED	MAINSTREAM WESTERN: INDIVIDUAL-CENTRED
Family as primary unit	Individual as primary unit
Family solidarity, responsibility, and harmony	Individual pursuit of happiness, fulfillment, and self-expression
Continued dependence on family is fostered	Early independence is encouraged
Hierarchical family roles, ascribed status	Variable roles, achieved status
Parent–child (parental) bond is stressed	Husband–wife (marital) bond is stressed
Parent provides authority and expects unquestioning obedience, submission to structure	Parent provides guidance, support, and explanations, and encourages curiosity and critical/independent thinking
Family makes decisions for the child	Child is given many choices
Parents ask: "What can you do to help me?"	Parents ask: "What can I do to help you?"
Older children are responsible for the siblings' actions	Each child is responsible for his or her own actions

From "Families with Asian roots," by S. Chan, and E. Lee. In E. W. Lynch and M. J. Hanson (Eds.), *Developing cross cultural competence: A guide for working with children and their families* (3rd ed., p. 293), 2004, Baltimore: Paul H. Brookes Publishing Co. Reprinted with permission.

---

[1]Contemporary Asian and Western cultures can differ markedly from traditional Asian and mainstream Western cultures, and all families must be understood in their current context.

Family Function and Family Roles

Family function describes the purpose, goals, and philosophy of the family system. It is the accepted action of an individual in a given role. It depicts **family roles** and the assigned tasks for those roles. The family system serves the following five functions (Barry, 1996):

1. It generates affection in the spousal couple, between the spouses and the children, and between members of the extended family.
2. The family functions as a source of identity, security, acceptance, and support for the members.
3. The family provides a source of purpose and satisfaction for its members.
4. It provides fellowship and companionship, while guaranteeing a place in society through socialization.
5. A family provides the moral compass for right and wrong.

Illness disrupts each one of these functions. The extent of the disruption and ensuing change depends on the characteristics of the individuals and families involved (Barry, 1996).

Family roles are influenced by family structure as well as socio-cultural expectations. Roles are either assigned or acquired, and they define what each member does within the family. Family member roles will change with time, and adapt to changes within the internal and external environments. Family roles are influenced by variables such as age. Roles within the family complement one another and help preserve equilibrium within the internal environment.

Gender Roles

Certain roles are dictated by gender. For example, females can only be daughters, wives, mothers, sisters, or girlfriends; males can only be sons, husbands, fathers, brothers, and boyfriends. Other family roles (e.g., breadwinner, cook, or house cleaner) are dependent on a member's ability to perform the role. In contrast, emotional roles (e.g., nurturer, caregiver, or leader) are adopted in response to changes within the family system.

The traditional or collectivist family structure dictates gender-specific roles. These roles are regarded as complementary in their focus on maintaining the family unity (Debs-Ivall, 2002; Roberts, 2003). Women in strongly traditional societies are viewed as the nurturers and comforters. The role of mother and wife is considered the most important role for women. And even though women in these cultures are viewed as voiceless by Western or individualistic cultures, this is far from the truth. A woman in a traditionalist culture is able to advise her husband on decision making and usually is consulted in private (Roberts, 2003).

Even in Western societies, there are rules that govern how women and girls are to behave. Compared with men, women face many barriers to entering the workplace (e.g., women are viewed as having higher absenteeism rates) and to advancing in a career (Giger & Davidhizar, 1999). On the other hand, industries are making efforts to introduce policies that help prevent discrimination on the basis of gender and sexual orientation; for example, women now often have access to child-care benefits and services, and special leaves to deal with family crises (York, 1991).

The association of caregiving work with women's gender roles is widespread, regardless of whether the societal rules are those of contemporary mainstream Canada or a traditional ethnic community. As the Canadian population ages, and with the trend toward shorter hospital stays, women are increasingly finding themselves caring for family members in the home.

In traditionalist societies, men—as sons, husbands, and fathers—emerge as decision makers, protectors, and providers (Boston, 1992; Roberts, 2003). These roles may be maintained even from a hospital bed throughout the hospitalization and illness process. As fathers and husbands, men are required and expected to provide for their families, allowing the mothers to stay home and care for the children. In some cultures, it is a measure of a man's worth that he provide amply so as to allow the mother the luxury of not having to work outside the home, thus protecting the integrity of their family (Debs-Ivall, 2002).

Researchers also have explored parental roles within same-sex couple relationships. In such a study of American lesbian couples, Ciano-Boyce and Shelley-Sireci (2002) found that lesbian couples were more likely to practise equality than heterosexual couples in their division of child care, and that lesbian adoptive parents were the most egalitarian. Similar findings exist for parents in gay families, who are noted to be more open to sharing roles and responsibilities within the family unit. Being child centred in their family focus, gay fathers—whether biological or step—placed the children's needs first with respect to the family unit (Lynch, 2000).

Roles of Children

Family roles, like cultural beliefs and values, are learned and transmitted from one generation to another. Parents use example, praise, and punishment to teach children the culturally acceptable rules. These learned behaviours are generally maintained throughout life. The following excerpt illustrates just how much variation is possible in the culturally appropriate behaviours that are taught to children:

> The American child seated with his family at dinner, reaches for the salt and pepper, which is in front of his mother. The father corrects: "Does the cat have your tongue? Ask your mother for what you want, and she will pass it to you." The Afghan child seated with his family at dinner, asks his mother for the salt and pepper. The father corrects: "Don't you have hands? Don't bother your mother; reach for what you want." (Boyle and Andrews, 1989, p. 11)

In both situations, the child has learned behaviour that is culturally accepted at the dinner table. In time, such behaviour becomes ingrained and automatic. However, the two forms of behaviour above are so different that each might be considered rude or even shocking when enacted in the other person's culture.

In a traditionalist culture, young children are thought of within the context of the family rather than individually. They are kept close and their individuality is de-emphasized. Holland and Hogg (2001) cite comparative research indicating that Asian parents value conformity (including obedience and gender-specific roles) more, and self-direction less, than White British respondents. In Western cultures, where independence is valued, children are taught to think for themselves; Eastern cultures value obedience and may view the pursuit of independence as disrespectful and shocking, interpreting it as undesirable, evidence of lack of parental caring, and a threat to traditional family values and beliefs (Holland & Hogg, 2001). In Eastern cultures, independence is seen as maturing within the family rather than away from it. Children are taught respect for the authority of the parents and the elders in the family. As they mature, children in turn will take care of the parents. Traditionally, the eldest son is responsible for the financial support of the parents, while the daughters become the caregivers to their husbands' parents (Adamson & Donovan, 2004).

Valenzuela (1999) found that immigrant children, when helping their families to settle into their new countries, assume three specific roles:

1. Tutor—taking on the tasks of teaching, translating, and interpreting for their parents and younger siblings
2. Advocate—intervening or advocating on behalf of their parents and younger siblings
3. Surrogate parent—undertaking the parent-like activities of babysitting, feeding, dressing, caring, and providing for younger siblings

Healthcare providers need to be aware of the important roles that children play in the care of immigrant families.

Western cultures, on the other hand, encourage children's individual expression in the family. Parents emphasize discontinuity of relationships as a way of encouraging the children's independence and their freedom to form new families of their own (Rothbaum, Morelli, Pott, & Lui-Constant, 2000). Self-reliance is encouraged and self-esteem is valued.

Roles of Elders

In Western cultures, adult children are expected to grow away from the family and elder family members are not expected to share the same household as the adult children. This trend is changing with the increased number of young adult children living with their parents. As well, the increasing number of separations and divorces is pushing adult children—along with *their* children—to move back into the parental home (Goodman & Silverstein, 2002).

Seniors in traditionalist cultures gain generational status as they age. They are accorded respect and deference and receive physical, emotional, and financial support in their old age. Family members within these cultures expect to physically care for their elders, because multi-generational households are common (Adamson & Donovan, 2004; Debs-Ivall, 2002). Usually, the parents live with the eldest adult son, who undertakes their financial and social support. However, it is either the unmarried daughter or the daughter-in-law who assumes the informal caregiver role (Adamson & Donovan, 2004; Debs-Ivall, 2002).

Immigration to Canada may result in a disruption of the roles of the family members as they move into a more Western culture than they are used to. Older adults may have had to immigrate to a new culture so as not to be left behind when their children left the home country. Treas and Mazumdar (2002) identify several reasons why such older adults may rely more heavily than other family members on traditional role structures:

▪ They have lost a familiar background.
▪ They have heavier involvement than before in the domestic responsibilities in their children's households.
▪ They are unable to communicate in the dominant language (English or French).
▪ In many instances, they have lost financial and social status.
▪ They have less need or opportunity for acculturating experiences outside the immediate family.

This, however, could present an area of conflict with their adult children, who might see a continuation of the previous roles as difficult and inappropriate (Gelfand, 1989; Treas & Mazumdar, 2002).

Individualism versus Collectivism

Much of what we know about family members' closeness and family relatedness in cultural communities comes from research in social and cross-cultural psychology involving adults (Rothbaum et al., 2000). Much of this research, for example the work of Triandis (1995), has focused on individualistic versus collectivist outlooks (first discussed in Chapter 5) and can be applied to family systems. **Individualism** and **collectivism** within the family context should be seen only as a starting point for asking the right questions. Individualistic cultures give importance to individual rights, viewing each person as a separate entity from the group. Emphasis is placed on self-expression, personal freedom of choice, individual responsibility, and independence. Autonomy is valued, and the unit of confidentiality is the individual (Lefley, 2000; Rothbaum et al., 2000).

Family therapist Salavador Minuchin formulated the structural **Family Systems Theory,** which encourages us to consider families as interdependent subsystems, with rules and boundaries whose functions cannot be understood in isolation of one another. Interpreting the individualistic culture in view of Family Systems Theory, Rothbaum et al. (2000) labelled it romantic relatedness. They note that "in romantic relatedness, the individual subsystem and the spousal subsystem are prioritized—that is, their boundaries are relatively impermeable" (p. 345). The boundaries around the spousal pair keep the couple together and separate from the children, and thus keep the family intact. The family will also foster a "growing away" attitude toward the children (see Figure 7-1).

Collectivist cultures, on the other hand, focus on the family or group as the smallest unit in the society and give importance to social role obligations. Calling it "harmonious relatedness," Rothbaum et al. (2000, p. 345) note that in collectivist cultures the boundaries between the individual and the couple are permeable and it is the boundary around the larger family unit as a whole that is impermeable. Children are expected to "grow within" the family unit. The emphasis is placed on the group interest, propriety, social obligation, and interdependence

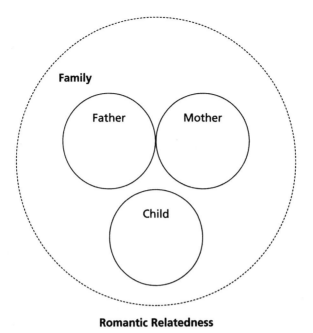

Romantic Relatedness

FIGURE 7-1 ▪ **Individualistic Culture**
Based on "Immigrant-Chinese and Euro-American parents' physical closeness with young children: Themes of family relatedness," by F. Rothbaum, G. Morelli, M. Pott, and Y. Liu-Constant, 2000, *Journal of Family Psychology, 14*(3), 334–348.

within the family. Group membership and harmony are valued, and the unit of confidentiality is the family or the group (Lefley, 2000; Rothbaum et al., 2000). Individuals may be very conscious of the obligations toward family members and the role they play in maintaining the good name and honour of the family (Holland & Hogg, 2001) (see Figure 7-2).

Researchers are becoming ever more aware that, within immigrant families, elements of individualism and collectivism—also called **familism**—could co-exist, reflecting an attempt to compromise in order to fit into the new culture. Some aspects of life in these families could resemble those of the community of choice, while others still conform to the community of origin (Rothbaum et al., 2000). Classifying cultures as either individual or group oriented would be too simplistic for the following four reasons:

1. Each category would include cultures that differ noticeably from one another in terms of what individual or group orientation means and expresses.
2. Such a broad approach is accurate only as it refers to the probability that members of one culture will act with either an individual or a group orientation in specific social situations.
3. It masks the diverse nature of social actions among members of any one culture and makes us look only at circumstances that bring about social actions that fit in with an individual or a group orientation.

4. There is a lot of similarity as well as difference between cultures. (p. 335)

Leininger (1995) found that when families move from rural into urban settings, there is a shift of family values from an emphasis on collectivism to an emphasis on individualism, materialism, and secularism. Depending on the situation, members of a family may act in ways consistent with either a group orientation or an individual orientation.

Acculturation

In the words of Miranda, Estrada, and Firpo-Jimenez (2000), **acculturation** is "a process of culture learning and behaviour adaptation that takes place as a result of exposure to a non-native culture" (p. 341). Berry (1986) described acculturation as a three-phase process:

1. Contact or an encounter with individuals from differing cultures
2. Conflict between the individual's native cultural beliefs and values and those of the new culture
3. Adaptation, which includes adopting ways to reduce conflict

In the adaptation phase, Berry (1986) describes the following types of acculturation:

▪ Assimilation into the new culture and relinquishing of the native culture

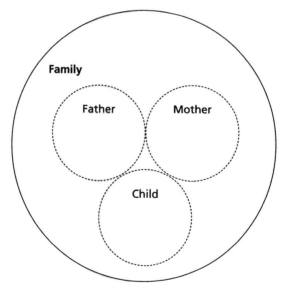

Harmonious Relatedness

FIGURE 7-2 ▪ **Collectivist Culture**
Based on "Immigrant-Chinese and Euro-American parents' physical closeness with young children: Themes of family relatedness," by F. Rothbaum, G. Morelli, M. Pott, and Y. Liu-Constant, 2000, *Journal of Family Psychology, 14*(3), 334–348.

> ## CULTURAL COMPETENCE IN ACTION
>
> **Analyze Your Own Family**
> Considering the two outlooks of individualism and collectivism discussed on these pages, examine your own family system. How many generations live in your home? Is importance placed on individual expression or family unity? Are children expected to grow away from or grow within the family? Are there solid boundaries around the spousal couple or around the whole family?

- Integration into the larger culture while maintaining the native culture's values and beliefs
- Rejection of and withdrawal from the new culture
- Deculturation, or feelings of alienation, loss of identity, and stress that lead to striking out against the new culture

Acculturation Stress

Acculturation stress refers to the difficulties, challenges, pain, and suffering involved in acculturation. Thomas (1995) identified five stressors that affect the immigrant family's acculturation process, and we discuss them briefly here:

1. *Language.* The lack of competency in the new culture's language is a major stressor for the immigrant family that may be hard to overcome, due to lack of formal education and the need to find employment quickly. Because of a higher social involvement, children and adults may attain language skills much faster than the older adults, who might not engage in social activities outside their communities.

2. *Employment and economic status.* Immigrants usually settle for menial, low-paying jobs due to lack of language skills, limited education, refugee status, or professional preparation/designation that is not accepted in the host country.

3. *Education.* Lack of education in the native culture creates a barrier to acquiring higher education in the new country, for adults and children alike.

4. *Family life.* All aspects of family life are affected when immigrants leave extended families with extensive support networks and come to a new culture where they have to function as a nuclear family. Roles change and shift as arrangements are made for babysitting, meal preparation, and new responsibilities. Both parents may have to work—sometimes at more than one job—to provide for the needs of the family, which prevents them from participating fully in their children's lives. Parents sometimes leave their children behind in the native culture, causing yet another layer of stress. Generational conflicts arise, and conflict may arise between parents as marital relationships and traditional gender roles are challenged in the new society.

5. *Socio-political and immigration status.* Political turmoil in the native culture may have been the impetus for migration, creating an additional layer of stress. Refugees may experience even more stress than immigrants do because they did not leave their native culture voluntarily. They may have also been victims of physical, emotional, or psychological oppression. As refugees, they may have to work under stressful and abusive conditions while lacking the political power to vote and affect change within their communities.

Generational Conflict

Generational conflict occurs in all cultures. As immigrant families try to adjust to the new culture and formulate a new cultural identity, they encounter generational conflicts that affect each member of the family. Conflicts arise between the children and the parents, the parents and the grandparents, and the grandchildren and the grandparents.

The parent–child relationship often is challenged by the influence on the children of the new culture's values and beliefs. In Canada, immigrant children may become more vocal and more independent as they follow the cultural norms of Canadian children. Because children acquire language skills faster than adults, English or French will become their primary language and a communication gap may develop between the children and the parents, whose mother tongue remains their primary language (Thomas, 1995). Poor communication subsequently can lead to learning and behavioural problems at school as children face conflicting messages at home and school regarding proper communication styles, helping others, and respecting authority.

Parents also may need to adjust their parenting and disciplinary skills as they learn, for example, that corporal punishment as a form of child discipline is frowned upon and/or condemned by law in the new culture (Thomas, 1995). Parents in that situation could feel that they have lost control of their children's behaviour.

In Canada, because professional bodies are reluctant to recognize international education and employers demand Canadian work experience, there is a higher concentration of immigrants in low-paying positions for which they often are over-qualified (Spitzer, Neufeld, Harrison, Hughes, & Stewart, 2003).

Women may need to enter the labour force when their husbands are unable to find adequate employment, and yet retain their gender roles of nurturer and caregiver both to the children and the grandparents. "In some societies, neglect of caregiving responsibilities—not the burden of the caregiving duties themselves—can elicit . . . negative response" (Spitzer et al., 2003, p. 269). Women are often regarded as the more appropriate caregivers and are seen as being more sensitive than men to the needs of others; men are regarded as unsuited for caregiving responsibilities. This generally prevents both genders from sharing the responsibilities equally, putting the bulk of the burden on the women and creating more conflict as women try to renegotiate their roles. As women enter the workforce, they also become aware of the economic and social opportunities available to them. They may start to challenge the traditional gender roles, creating an imbalance in the power structure of the family (Thomas, 1995).

Grandparents, on the other hand, face conflict as their status of respected wise elders and financial providers of inheritance is challenged. The knowledge that they possess may not be of use in the new country. They become dependent on their children and grandchildren, both to help them navigate through the new culture and to provide for their economic and social needs. They may perceive a loss of cultural identity as both their children's and their grandchildren's roles shift to accommodate the new culture.

How Families Affect Health Maintenance and Use of Services

Family rules and family diversity can influence the moral decisions taken by each member, as well as decisions regarding health maintenance and home treatments, illness behaviour, and the use of healthcare services (Barry, 1996).

Health Maintenance and Home Treatments

Many cultural behaviours and rituals can have a direct or indirect effect on health maintenance. Members of the Seventh-Day Adventist Church, for example, view their bodies as the temple of God and will avoid using substances that are harmful to it, such as alcohol, tobacco, caffeine, and drugs. This behaviour, even though practised for religious rather than health reasons, will still have a direct (positive) effect on health maintenance.

When clients experience symptoms, they interpret them within the context of their cultural outlook. Clients may believe that their symptoms are due to germs, a curse or magic, or a yin/yang (passive/active) imbalance. They could also view symptoms as being allowed by God as punishment for sin. The explanations that clients accept will determine the action they take to maintain health or to seek treatments.

Clients usually share their interpretation of symptoms with their families. The family, as a source of support and security, will then affect the decisions regarding health maintenance or looking for help. Some clients may be encouraged to seek home remedies, for example, while others may be steered toward healthcare providers.

Clients and their families may seek help from traditional healers or use home remedies because these therapies are viewed as more effective or more acceptable in particular circumstances. Certain categories of illness—such as psychiatric illness, human immunodeficiency virus (HIV) infections, and sexually transmitted diseases—may be stigmatized within a culture, and seeking professional help for them may not be seen as acceptable. Clients may choose alternative treatments, in the form of folk or traditional therapies, Western medical treatments, or over-the-counter preparations. When traditional remedies are used, the effectiveness of the treatment will sometimes depend on how the client "feels" rather than on the therapeutic effect. Knowing what the client is using for treatment, and why, is important for healthcare providers because although many treatments (e.g., cupping and coin rubbing) are not harmful to the client, others (e.g., some herbal remedies) may have a direct physiological effect (Bernal, 1996).

CULTURAL COMPETENCE IN ACTION

Sensitivity to Stigma Helps Reframe Problem
A 22-year-old Lebanese woman presented to the family physician with a several-week history of vise-like headaches, insomnia, weight loss, and weakness. Physical assessment and diagnostic testing revealed no physiological reason for the symptoms.

The client and her husband became visibly upset when the physician suggested a psychological cause for the symptoms. The couple, upon the recommendation of the husband's mother, sought the second opinion of a Lebanese family doctor. The Lebanese physician, being more culturally sensitive to the stigma associated with psychiatric symptoms within the Lebanese culture, was able to work with the couple to identify sources of stress upon the wife.

Apparently, the couple had been married less than a year and the wife had left her family in Lebanon and moved to Canada only recently. The husband worked all day while she stayed at home. Even though she spoke English, she had not yet made any friends within the community. The psychological label of depression was reframed as loneliness and acculturation stress. The couple agreed to continue to follow up with the physician until the symptoms were resolved.

Illness Behaviour

Family rules determine the illness behaviour of family members, such as whether clients will take an active or passive role in their illness experiences, and deciding whether they are exempt from the obligations of their roles within the family. Family rules also will determine who provides the care (a family member or a healthcare provider), how symptoms are perceived and expressed (e.g., pain), where the client will be cared for (at home, or in hospital), and how long the client should be cared for (e.g., care of the mother after childbirth) (Bernal, 1996). In many cultures, family members are expected to provide the care, while healthcare providers are expected to provide the "cure." However, healthcare providers need to be cautious in making assumptions that particular cultures "take care of their own" because this view may interfere with the exploration of other options and a specific family's need and ability to access needed services.

Use of Healthcare Services

For clients to access healthcare services, they must have symptoms that require help. Factors that determine whether the client seeks help include the type, severity, and interpretation of the symptoms, and the reaction of other family members to them (Bernal, 1996; Papadopoulos & Lees, 2004).

For members of an ethnic minority, there are further factors that influence access to health care, including the following:
- Language barriers
- Cultural barriers, including lack of culturally competent healthcare providers
- Distance to care

▪ Lack of financial resources for treatments
▪ Lack of transportation
▪ Peceptions of lack of respect, discrimination, or racism
▪ A complex healthcare system
(Bernal, 1996)

In cultures where kinship is a strong value, often family members assume the caregiver role as a way of showing gratitude to the ill relative. In a study of Thai caregivers in the United States, Limpanichkul and Magivly (2004) note that in this culture, caregiving is seen as a willingly assumed burden and an unavoidable duty reflecting the Buddhist beliefs of *karma* and fate. Further, in this study, caregiving was associated with positive outcomes such as inner growth, better understanding of life, and spirituality. While the caregivers received various types of support from family, friends, and neighbours, none of the participants reported using community services or support groups. This lack of use of community and support services may be due to such factors as the language difficulties mentioned under factors that can affect access to health care in general; or to cultural boundaries of private and public in which sharing of personal needs with strangers is not considered desirable or even acceptable. It could also be because the families lack awareness of the services or because the services are seen as culturally inappropriate (Mir & Tovey, 2002).

Implications for Healthcare Providers

Studies show that when immigrants arrive in Canada, they are generally in better health than the Canadian-born population; however, over time they become "twice as likely as Canadian born to report a deterioration in their health" (Statistics

CULTURAL CONSIDERATIONS IN CARE

A Simple Solution to Client Passivity
Client autonomy and independence are highly valued within the Western healthcare system. Often, our client education focuses on self-care practices to help clients gain back their pre-hospitalization independent status. However, in many non-Western cultures, the client is expected to assume a passive "sick role" while the family members provide the care.

An enterostomal nurse specialist felt frustrated when she encountered such passive behaviour in an elderly Italian client whom she was trying to teach how to care for his new colostomy stoma. The client kept insisting his wife needed to learn, not him.

As the healthcare provider gained some understanding of the illness behaviour of the client, she was able to negotiate an acceptable solution. When she reframed colostomy care as a normal part of everyday personal care, such as shaving and going to the washroom, the client consented to learn the skill. As long as the client viewed the colostomy care as part of his illness, he insisted that his family would take care of it. By reframing colostomy care as part of daily routines, he was able to take ownership for the colostomy routine.

Canada, 2005, p. 1). They also visit their family doctors more frequently. This could suggest that during their socialization into the Canadian culture they adopt unhealthy lifestyles and are exposed to socioeconomic factors that increase their vulnerability to poor health. Indeed, Statistics Canada indicated that immigrants were twice as likely as Canadian-born people to have an increase of 10 percent in their body mass index over an eight-year period, reflecting weight gain that could be harmful to their health (Statistics Canada, 2005). Beiser (2005) also notes that resettlement experiences can have a tremendous influence on immigrant and refugee health status over time and advocates for an integrated approach to immigrant health care that takes these factors into account.

These statistics are important for all healthcare providers who work in a diverse society. Chevannes (1997) notes: "Nurses caring for families is not new. However, effective caring for different types of families which are characterized socially, racially, and ethnically is still at a rudimentary level" (p. 163). Healthcare providers, in developing partnerships with families, must recognize that family members usually provide caring on an ongoing basis while the healthcare providers are regarded as invited, and sometimes uninvited, guests into their lives. Therefore, healthcare providers need to find ways to become part of the family system and provide care that fits with the cultural client values and beliefs of their clients (Chevannes, 1997).

Some Western-based approaches to care may produce adverse effects when used with clients from ethnic minority groups. However, approaches that incorporate family networks and use group-centred approaches are considered culturally suitable (Barrio, 2000).

Provider Attitudes toward Families

Ahmann and Lawrence (1999) challenge us to consider how we communicate not only with, but also about, families—even to other healthcare providers. Commonly used negative adjectives about families (e.g., "difficult," "demanding," "resistant," "indifferent," "non-receptive") can be detrimental to the family–healthcare provider relationship, and to the family itself. Ahmann and Lawrence (1999) advocate that the negative words, which may in turn generate negative emotions within the healthcare provider, be replaced with words and beliefs that value and respect families. It is important for healthcare providers to recognize and name the family's strengths. A policy to consider is to use the same terminology in the family's absence as one would in the family's presence. See Table 7-2 for examples of this more positive approach.

Considerations Related to Individualism versus Collectivism

Family Systems Theory suggests that all individuals in a family are interdependent and thus need to be assessed within the context of that family. Categorizing a family system as either individualistic or collectivist in outlook should be seen only as a starting point for asking the right questions.

TABLE 7-2

Better Language to Describe Families

INSTEAD OF THIS (NEGATIVE LANGUAGE)	USE THIS (POSITIVE LANGUAGE)
Demanding	Strong advocate
Controlling	Actively involved, aware of own needs
Angry	Concerned, worried
Passive, indifferent, non-participatory	May need more time
Non-compliant	Has different priorities

From "Exploring language about families," by E. Ahmann and J. Lawrence, 1999, *Pediatric Nursing, 25*(2), 221–224. Reprinted with permission.

In many collectivist cultures, decisions are made by consensus and the family may prefer to filter difficult information to the client, regardless of age (Mazanec & Tyler, 2003). Family members, in this case, could be protecting the client from the harmful effects of losing hope and also be acting within the context of social obligation and interdependence.

In individualistic cultures, autonomy is valued and the individual makes the decisions. The family in this case will act as a support system, and depending on the dynamics, may not be aware of all the specifics of the illness. Family roles also influence decision making related to care. While the mother alone may undertake the care of child in hospital, significant decisions may be taken by the father, often in consultation with extended family members such as his brother or father. The child or the mother may not be part of the decision-making process. Healthcare providers who value autonomy in decision making may find this a difficult practice to accept (Holland & Hogg, 2001). In such circumstances it is important that the family norms be respected and that the healthcare providers work with the family, sharing their experience and expertise, to allow the family to make informed choices.

Keeping in mind that family structure differs between cultures, healthcare providers need to be aware of their own views on family and determine what the client's definition of family is and how the family is to be included in any or all aspects of the care. Establishing how decisions are made and by whom is a first priority.

Family Assessment

Family assessment, or determining information about the family, should be done as part of the overall assessment of the client. A variety of cultural assessment models incorporate a section on family, and several such models are presented briefly below. Each model highlights some aspect of family diversity. In order to do a thorough family assessment appropriate to their clinical context, healthcare providers likely will use a combination of the suggested approaches, in conjunction with a holistic assessment of the client.

The Calgary Family Assessment Model

The Calgary Family Assessment Model (CFAM) has received wide recognition since it was first introduced by Lorraine Wright and Maureen Leahey in 1984. It consists of three major categories of family assessments:

1. Structural
2. Developmental
3. Functional

Healthcare providers need to establish which categories are relevant and appropriate to each family at any given time. The structural category is the most relevant to culturally diverse families and comprises five areas or classifications, which are listed along with examples of questions to ask in Table 7-3.

Even though structural context is the most relevant area of assessment for the culturally diverse family, healthcare providers also should examine the other categories in the model for areas of relevance.

Inquiry Guide

Madeleine Leininger (2002) developed a *Suggested Inquiry Guide* for use in assessing cultural care and health. Within the guide, family assessment can be explored through the area of "kinship and social factors." Leininger suggests that the healthcare provider enter the world of the client and make the inquiry natural and informal. Her suggested approach is summarized in Table 7-4.

TABLE 7-3

Structural Assessment of a Family Using the Calgary Family Assessment Model

CLASSIFICATION	SUGGESTED QUESTIONS
Ethnicity	What does health mean to you? How would you know that you are healthy? How would I know that you are healthy? Could you tell me about your cultural practices regarding illness?
Race	What differences do you notice between your relatives' child-rearing practices and your own? If you and I were the same race, how would our conversation be different? Could you help me to understand what I need to know to be most helpful to you?
Social class	How many times have you moved in the past five years? How many schools has your daughter attended? How does your money situation influence your use of healthcare resources? What impact does shift work have on your family's stress level?
Religion and spirituality	Are you involved with, a church, temple, or synagogue? Are your spiritual beliefs a source of strength for you? Have you felt that your prayer or other religious practices help you cope with your son's illness?
Environment	What community services does your family use? On a scale of 1 to 10, how comfortable are you in your neighbourhood? What would make you more comfortable so that you can continue to function independently at home?

From *Nurses and families: A guide to family assessment and intervention* (3rd ed., pp. 80–86), by L. M. Wright and M. Leahy, 2000, Philadelphia: F.A. Davis Co.

TABLE 7-4

Leininger's Inquiry Guide for Kinship and Social Factors

- I would like to hear about your family and/or close social friends and what they mean to you.
- How have your kin (relatives) or social friends influenced your life and especially your caring or healthy lifeways?
- Who are the caring or non-caring persons in your life?
- How has your family (or group) helped you stay well or become ill?
- Do you view your family as a caring family? If not, what would make them more caring?
- Are there key family responsibilities to care for you or others when ill or well? (Explain.)
- In what ways would you like your family members (or social friends) to care for you?
- How would you like nurses to care for you?

From "Culture care assessments for congruent competency practices," by M. Leininger. In M. Leininger and M. R. McFarland (Eds.), *Transcultural nursing: Concepts, theories, research and practice* (3rd ed., p. 137), 2002, New York: McGraw-Hill Companies, Inc. Reprinted with permission.

Leininger cautions that the guide lists only some of the questions that could be asked and that it is not exhaustive. The approach in the table, for example, does not determine how and by whom decisions are made within the family.

The Transcultural Assessment Model

Giger and Davidhizar (1999), in their Transcultural Assessment Model, also include a section about the social organization of the client. The items in this section are summarized in Table 7-5.

Like Leininger's (2002) inquiry guide, this model is not exhaustive and should be complemented with inquiries regarding decision making and disclosure preferences.

Cultural Assessment in Home Health Care

Taking into consideration the small amount of time a home healthcare nurse usually has to spend with a client, Narayan (1997) suggests a simple cultural assessment tool for families. It includes sections on the client's understanding of his or her illness, nutrition, pain, medication, and psychosocial assessments. She suggests four important questions pertaining to family that should be asked of all clients as part of the overall social assessment:

1. Who is the decision maker in the family?
2. What are the characteristics of the "sick role" in the client's culture?
3. Are there language barriers?
4. What are the resources available from the client's cultural community?

Even though this assessment tool includes inquiries regarding decision making, it could be strengthened to include client preferences about disclosure of diagnosis and prognosis.

TABLE 7-5

Giger and Davidhizar's Assessment of Family

Normal state of health: poor, fair, good, excellent?
Marital status?
Number of children?
Parents living or deceased?
What is your function in your family unit (what do you do)?
What is your role in your family unit (father, mother, child, advisor)?
When you were a child, what and who influenced you most?
What is your relationship with your siblings and parents?

From *Transcultural nursing: assessment and intervention* (3rd ed., pp. 10–11), by J. N. Giger and R. E. Davidhizar, 1999, St. Louis: Mosby.

Regardless of the assessment model, tool, or guide used, healthcare providers need to interactively participate in their clients' cultures in order to gain cultural knowledge about the clients and their family systems (Dunn, 2002). This knowledge must then be used to plan and implement a culturally suitable plan of care that recognizes the strengths, expertise, knowledge, and skills of the family.

Controversial Issues and Ethical Dilemmas

Conflict can arise between clients, their families, and healthcare providers on issues related to differing values and beliefs. Some of these conflicts are discussed below and, where possible, reframed within differing cultural perspectives.

Moral Issues

Differing moral values can lead to conflict. Some of these conflicts may be manifested inter-generationally within the family system. For example, parents may find themselves having to make decisions about dealing with an unwed daughter's pregnancy or dealing with the sexual orientation of an adult child. A healthcare provider who is caring for the daughter or son in one of these scenarios could be directly involved in the conflict. Recognizing that such issues could create moral dilemmas for the family will allow healthcare providers to seek support and consultation from spiritual and religious care services. Caring for the family means more than reaching decisions or helping the family support the client; it also means recognizing and supporting the needs of the family members.

Ethical Issues

Conflicts with healthcare providers may arise when there are differences in values. For example, families and clients may resist pain-control measures because they view suffering as a way to atone for past sins. This may conflict with the healthcare provider's cultural value of alleviating suffering. In such an instance, providing spiritual and emotional support rather than pain control may be the more culturally appropriate intervention.

Perhaps the most well-documented and -debated ethical dilemma facing healthcare providers when caring for clients from diverse cultural backgrounds involves full disclosure, or truth telling. The Western healthcare system advocates for full disclosure of diagnosis and prognosis to the client for the sake of truthfulness and future planning. A healthcare provider would argue that a client cannot make an informed decision in planning for the future without being provided with all the facts. This might be in direct conflict, however, with the beliefs and values of some non-Western cultures that believe that fatal diagnosis and poor prognosis should not be shared with a client but rather with the family, which then will decide how much to tell the client (Mystakidou, Parpa, Tsilika, Katsouda, & Vlahos, 2004). Within collectivist cultures, decisions are made by consensus and autonomy is not valued. Thus, decisions might not be of value unless made collectively by the family. For a client to continue to enjoy life, this cultural view dictates that he or she might need to go on as before a diagnosis was made. A client's knowledge of a poor prognosis would "condemn the person to a period of being among the dead while still alive" (Candib, Quill, & Stein, 2002, p. 213). From this cultural viewpoint, telling the client about a poor prognosis might be considered disrespectful, distressing, and unforgivable; from a Western healthcare viewpoint, not doing so is considered paternalistic and a blatant disregard of the client's personal right to know.

This conflict is further complicated with the need for end-of-life planning, such as advance directives and do-not-resuscitate (DNR) orders. Western cultures put importance on personal autonomy and the need to control the end of life, or death. It is becoming an acceptable, and even encouraged, practice to insist on decisions regarding advance directives and DNR orders with clients who face poor prognoses. Healthcare providers have seen the desperate measures taken to keep clients alive when all hope of return to a viable quality of life has been lost. They also worry about the increasing costs of such "useless" interventions.

Many non-Western traditional cultures, on the other hand, believe that talking about death with a person will hasten death upon them. Clients will lose hope and their lives will end prematurely. Some Asian cultures view discussions about advance directives as disrespectful and a portent of bad luck (Orona, Koenig, & Davis, 1994). Other cultures may mistrust any communication that would limit care and would find it threatening (Candib et al., 2002). Thus, healthcare providers caring for such clients and their families must adopt alternative, culturally suitable approaches to discussing advance directives. Presenting issues in hypothetical terms is sometimes an acceptable way of opening a dialogue and determining the family's as well as the client's comfort level regarding such discussions.

To be both client and family centred, healthcare providers need to determine how much clients want to know rather than how much they are expected to know. Once this has been determined, the clients' wishes to have decision making regarding full-disclosure and end-of-life issues should be respected, even if these wishes differ from family wishes.

Candib et al. (2002) suggest three questions that could be used to deal with end-of-life issues. The authors caution that these questions should be addressed by the family healthcare provider in advance of a diagnosis or a severe illness. The three questions are framed within a conversation that starts with a preamble

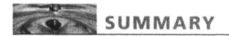

CULTURAL COMPETENCE IN ACTION

End-of-Life Issues in Your Own Environment
Try to think of a case in your practice where end-of-life issues created a conflict with a client's family. Examine how the conflict was managed. Were the client's cultural background, values, and beliefs the catalysts for the conflict? Was the client's preference regarding family involvement determined? Were decisions regarding advance directives made by the client? By the client and the family? By the family alone? Or by the healthcare team? Reflecting on the answers, how would your practice change now? What would you do differently?

addressing "future" severe illnesses and a healthcare provider's lack of knowledge about the client's specific culture and his or her need to know how to provide the best possible care. This preamble will allow the healthcare provider to determine whether family-based autonomy or personal autonomy is in effect. The three questions then tackle the following areas:

1. Determine the level of family involvement in the decision making.
2. Address the intensity of the interventions to be undertaken in case of a severe illness.
3. Address issues of disclosure.
   (Candib et al., 2002)

This culturally congruent approach will help determine a client's wishes regarding the level of involvement of the family in his or her care.

SUMMARY

Families play a pivotal role in maintaining health and seeking health care. When caring for diverse families, areas that require particular consideration include characteristics such as race, ethnicity, and religion but also migration and acculturation, generational differences, socio-economic status, and family structure. This chapter studied the family, including its composition and the rules and roles that govern the behaviour of its members, particularly within the context of health and illness.

When working with clients from culturally diverse backgrounds, healthcare providers must recognize the role families play in all aspects of the healthcare process. In the assessment phase of health care, families contribute much of the medical and social history that is analyzed for a diagnosis. In this chapter, we examined several cultural assessment models that incorporate a section on family assessment.

In the planning phase of health care, families help provide the context for the interventions. Family members should be included in all the aspects of client education and decision making. Healthcare provider attitude toward families is another area for consideration and intervention.

When implementing and evaluating the care plan, families provide the care, support, and, in many instances, the compass by which accomplishments of goals or outcomes is measured. The family's expertise and involvement must be recognized, acknowledged, and used throughout the process.

REFERENCES

Adamson, J., & Donovan, J. (2004). Normal disruption: South Asian and African/Caribbean relatives caring for an older family member in the UK. *Social Sciences and Medicine, 60*, 37–48.

Ahmann, E., & Lawrence, J. (1999). Exploring language about families. *Pediatric Nursing, 25*(2), 221–224.

Barrio, C. (2000). The cultural relevance of community support programs. *Psychiatric Services, 51*(7), 879–884.

Barry, P. (1996). *Psychosocial nursing: Care of physically ill patients and their families* (3rd ed.). Philadelphia: Lippincott-Raven.

Beiser, M. (2005). The health of immigrants and refugees in Canada. *Canadian Journal of Public Health, 96*, S30–45.

Bernal, H. (1996). Delivering culturally competent care. In P. Barry (Ed.), *Psychosocial nursing: Care of physically ill patients and their families* (3rd ed.). Philadelphia: Lippincott-Raven.

Berry, J. W. (1986). The acculturation process and refugee behavior. In C. L. Williams & J. Westermeyer (Eds.), *Refuge mental health in resettlement countries.* (pp. 25–37). Washington: Hemisphere Publishing Corporation.

Bos, H. M. W., van Balen, F., van den Boom, D.C., & Sandfort, Th. G. M. (2004). Minority stress, experience of parenthood and child adjustment in lesbian families. *Journal of Reproductive and Infant Psychology, 22*(4), 291–304.

Boston, P. (1992). Understanding cultural differences through family assessment. *Journal of Cancer Education, 7*(3), 261–266.

Boyle, J. S., & Andrews, M. M. (1989). *Transcultural concepts in nursing care.* Glenview, IL: Scott, Foresman & Company.

Candib, L. M., Quill, T. E., & Stein, H. F. (2002). Truth telling and advance planning at the end of life: Problems with autonomy in a multicultural world. *Families, Systems & Health, 20*(3), 213–228.

Chan, S., & Lee, E. (2004). Families with Asian roots. In E. W. Lynch & M. J. Hanson (Eds.), *Developing cross cultural competence: A guide for working with children and their families* (3rd ed.). Baltimore: Paul Brookes Publishing Co.

Chevannes, M. (1997). Nurses caring for families—issues in a multi-racial society. *Journal of Clinical Nursing, 6,* 161–167.

Ciano-Boyce, C., & Shelley-Sireci, L. (2002). Who is mommy tonight? Lesbian parenting issues. *Journal of Homosexuality, 43* (2), 1–13.

Debs-Ivall, S. (2002). *The meaning of social support: The perspective of Arab-Canadians with congestive heart failure.* Unpublished thesis. University of Ottawa, Ottawa, Ontario.

Dunn, A. M. (2002). Culture competence and the primary care provider. *Journal of Pediatric Health Care, 16,* 105–111.

Friedman, M. (1997). Teaching about and for family diversity in nursing. *Journal of Family Nursing, 3*(3), 280–294.

Gelfand, D. E. (1989). Immigration, aging, and intergenerational relationships. *The Gerontologist, 29*(3), 366–372.

Giger, J. N., & Davidhizar, R. E. (1999). *Transcultural nursing: Assessment and intervention* (3rd ed.). St. Louis: Mosby.

Goodman, C., & Silverstein, M. (2002). Grandmothers raising grandchildren: Family structure and well-being in culturally-diverse families. *The Gerontologist, 42* (5), 676–689.

Hanson, M. (2004). Ethnic, cultural, and language diversity in service settings. In E. Lynch & M. Hanson (Eds.). *Developing cross cultural competence: A guide for working with children and their families* (3rd ed.). Baltimore: Paul H. Brookes Publishing.

Holland, K., & Hogg, C. (2001). *Cultural awareness in nursing and health care.* London: Arnold.

Kumorek, M. (1978). *Afghanistan: A cross-cultural view.* Unpublished manuscript.

Lefley, H. P. (2000). Cultural perspectives on families, mental illness, and the law. *International Journal of Law and Psychiatry, 23*(3–4), 229–243.

Leininger, M. (1995). *Transcultural nursing: Concepts, theories, research and practice* (2nd ed.). New York: McGraw-Hill.

Leininger, M. (2002). Culture care assessments for congruent competency practices. In M. Leininger & M. R. McFarland (Eds.). *Transcultural nursing: Concepts, theories, research and practice* (3rd ed., pp. 117–143) New York: McGraw-Hill.

Limpanichkul, Y., & Magilvy, K. (2004). Managing caregiving at home: Thai caregivers living in the United States. *Journal of Cultural Diversity, 11*(1), 18–24.

Lynch, J. M. (2000). Considerations of family structure and gender composition: The lesbian and gay stepfamily. *Journal of Homosexuality, 40* (2), 81–95.

Mazanec, P., & Tyler, M. K. (2003). Cultural considerations in end-of-life care: How ethnicity, age and spirituality affect decisions when death is imminent. *American Journal of Nursing, 103*(3), 50–58.

Mir, G., & Tovey, P. (2002). Cultural competency: Professional action and South Asian carers. *Journal of Management in Medicine, 16*(1): 7–19.

Miranda, A. O., Estrada, D., & Firpo-Jimenez, M. (2000). Differences in family cohesion, adaptability, and environment among Latino families in dissimilar stages of acculturation. *The Family Journal: Counseling and Therapy for Couples and Families, 8*(4), 341–350.

Mystakidou, K., Parpa, E., Tsilika, E., Katsouda, E., & Vlahos, L. (2004). Cancer information disclosure in different cultural contexts. *Support Cancer Care, 12,* 147–154.

Narayan, M. (1997). Cultural assessment in home healthcare. *Home Healthcare Nurse, 15(10),* 663–670.

Orona, C. J., Koenig, B. A., & Davis, A. J. (1994). Cultural aspects of non-disclosure. *Cambridge Quarterly of Healthcare Ethics, 3,* 338–346.

Papadopoulos, I., & Lees, S. (2004). Cancer and communication: Similarities and differences of men with cancer from six different ethnic groups. *European Journal of Cancer Care, 13,* 154–162.

Roberts, K. S. (2003). Providing culturally sensitive care to the child-bearing Islamic family: Part II. *Advances in Neonatal Care, 3*(5), 250–255.

Rothbaum, F., Morelli, G., Pott, M., & Liu-Constant, Y. (2000). Immigrant-Chinese and Euro-American parents' physical closeness with young children: Themes of family relatedness. *Journal of Family Psychology, 14*(3) 334–348.

Spitzer, D., Neufeld, A., Harrison, M., Hughes, K., & Stewart, M. (2003). Caregiving in transnational context: "My wings have been cut; where can I fly?" *Gender & Society, 17*(2), 267–286.

Statistics Canada. (2002). Profile of Canadian families and households: Diversification continues. Retrieved February 23, 2005 from http://www12.statcan.ca/english/census01/products/analytic/companion/fam/96F0030XIE2001003

Statistics Canada (2005, February 23). Dynamics of Immigrant's Health in Canada: Evidence from the National Population Health Survey. *The Daily.* Retrieved February 23, 2005, from http://www.statcan.ca/Daily/English/050223/d050223c.htm

Thomas, T. N. (1995). Acculturative stress in the adjustment of immigrant families. *Journal of Social Distress and the Homeless, 4*(2), 131–142.

Treas, J., & Mazumdar, S. (2002). Older people in America's immigrant families: Dilemmas of dependence, integration, and isolation. *Journal of Aging Studies, 16*(2002), 243–258.

Triandis, H. (1995). *Individualism and collectivism.* Boulder, CO: Westview.

Valenzuela, A. (1999). Gender roles and settlement activities among children and their immigrant families. *American Behavioral Scientist, 41*(4) 720–742.

Wright, L. M., & Leahey, M. (2000). *Nurses and families: A guide to family assessment and intervention* (3rd ed.). Philadelphia: F. A. Davis Company.

Wright, L. M., Watson, W. L., & Bell, J. M. (1996). *Beliefs: The heart of healing in families and illness.* New York: Basic Books.

York, C. (1991). The labour movement's role in parental leave and child care. In J. Shibley-Hide & M. Essex (Eds.). *Parental leave and child care: Setting a research and policy agenda.* Philadelphia: Temple University Press.

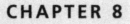

CHAPTER 8

A Working Guide to Illness Beliefs and Paths of Healing

RAJU HAJELA

LEARNING OBJECTIVES

At the end of this chapter, the learner will be able to:

- Understand the experience of health and illness in the context of culture and biophysiological, psychological, social, and spiritual dimensions
- View clients' health beliefs and practices as being moulded by, but not limited to, their cultural heritage
- Appreciate the etiological factors that the client perceives as responsible for the illness experience
- Describe a variety of approaches to treatment and healing from the world's ancient and Western cultures and traditions
- Develop a working familiarity with basic similarities and dissimilarities among the major traditions
- Understand the influence of the healthcare provider's training and cultural experiences on his or her ability to care for clients using alternative approaches to healing

KEY TERMS

Aboriginal medicine	Chiropractic
Acculturation	Curanderismo
Acupuncture	Energy medicine
Allopathic medicine or biomedicine	Epidemiology
Assimilation	Health
Ayurveda and MAV	Homeopathy
Becoming	Integrative health care
Being	Naturopathic medicine
Belonging	Osteopathy
Bio-psycho-social-spiritual framework of health	Traditional Chinese medicine (TCM)

Most people take their health for granted until a problem is perceived. Seeking care is influenced by the individual's perception of the resources that are available in the form of family, friends, and professionals. Medical healthcare resources are often biologically based, oriented toward acute care, and intent on providing a standard of care fairly equally to all. A shortfall can occur when the cultural context of client is not appreciated. This could happen because the healthcare provider fails to elicit pertinent information from the client or completely communicate appropriate treatment recommendations, or because the client misunderstands treatment directions, leading to non-adherence and a less-than-optimum health outcome.

When each client is assessed broadly on bio-psycho-social-spiritual dimensions of health, the resulting understanding of the illness experience is more complete.[1] This approach allows the health provider to take into account cultural nuances that may be critical for treatment and healing. A healthcare provider's familiarity with diverse beliefs about illness and injury is extremely useful. Nevertheless, it is still essential to assess each client as an individual rather than as a stereotypic representation of her or his racial or cultural heritage. Today's intermixing of cultures and ease of international mobility create a lot of individual variation in terms of how we view ourselves, our illness experience, and the traditions of healing.

The significance of an injury, crisis, or illness experience to a client greatly influences her or his perception of the acuteness and seriousness of the problem. Psycho-social-spiritual considerations become invaluable beyond the biophysiological examination. Clients may also turn to other approaches for treatment, such as Aboriginal medicine, traditional Chinese medicine, and Ayurveda, depending on their prior experience with these paths and/or frustration with the traditional Western approaches to care. Complementary approaches to healing that have a long history in other cultures are becoming increasingly popular in North America. A Canadian Community Health Survey indicates that by 2003, 20 percent of Canadians over age 12—or about 5.4 million people—were using alternative healthcare services (Sibbald, 2005). Healthcare providers need to have a working familiarity with possible treatment choices for clients that would be culturally meaningful.

This chapter provides an overview of the concepts and practices of major health promotion ideas, illness treatment systems, and healing traditions from around the world. The aim is to provide health professionals with a working familiarity of concepts and frameworks so that they can understand the beliefs and practices a client may have grown up with or become interested in through personal exploration and experience. Even though some healthcare providers regard the West's dominant system of biomedicine or allopathic medicine as scientific and other systems as unscientific, we should bear in mind that many

---

[1]"Bio-psycho-social-spiritual" describes a holistic perspective: "bio" refers to the biological and physiological aspects; "psycho," the thinking and feeling aspects; "social," the social network, including friends and family; and "spiritual," one's beliefs and relationship to the broader universe.

systems are based on centuries of knowledge and experience. Further, scientific investigations are establishing the benefits of complementary approaches.

As discussed in Chapter 1, cultural competence does not mean simply knowing about different cultures or having expertise in all areas of beliefs about illness and ways of healing. Every healthcare provider brings strengths and limitations to the healthcare interaction on the basis of personal heritage, life experience, and training. Healthcare providers need to develop self-awareness of their own abilities and desire to be a healing force in the lives of clients who are seeking care from them. Healthcare providers need to develop an understanding of the common illness beliefs and healing traditions. It is essential to explore a client's expectations and to offer ancillary care through a team approach whenever a client wishes to incorporate other healing traditions as part of the health care process.

Culture and Health

In the preamble to the constitution of the World Health Organization (WHO), **health** is described as a state of complete physical, mental, and social well-being, not merely the absence of disease or infirmity. While the healthcare environment often zeroes in on cause and effect, risk factors, and outcomes, there is another, more dynamic approach to health promotion that has emerged during recent decades (Pederson, O'Neill, & Rootman, 1994). This approach posits health promotion as a process in which better health is a goal, with the personal, organizational, and policy factors playing a variety of roles in initiating, managing, implementing, and monitoring change. All of this occurs in a cultural context.

The study of factors that can influence human health is broadly known as **epidemiology**. Originally, epidemiology was defined as the scientific study of epidemics (usually infectious diseases). A more current definition takes into account "the distribution and determinants of health-related states and events in defined populations, and the application of this study to the control of health problems" (Last, 1987, p. 29).

In epidemiological research, culture is often defined through categorical variables (e.g., ethnicity, place of birth, and mother tongue). Anthropology, on the other hand, considers culture more qualitatively, as an array of influences that affect the lives of individuals and groups. The common features that emerge, despite the quantitative or qualitative differences, include ideas of shared beliefs and values, social norms, shared ways of individual and collective behaviour, and a way of viewing one's relationship with self and others within the universe that has meaning and purpose (Corin, 1994).

The relationship between culture and health is often inextricable. For example, Letendre (2002) notes that "traditional medicine and practices are so entrenched within Aboriginal culture, that it is insufficient to simply define traditional medicine" (p. 79). The author goes on to identify a variety of ways through which Aboriginal medicine provides for the expression and preservation of Aboriginal culture, including Aboriginal philosophy, religion, and spirituality.

In the 1980s, Trevor Hancock and Fran Perkins developed a model called "The Mandala of Health" (see Figure 8-1), which starts from the premise that the

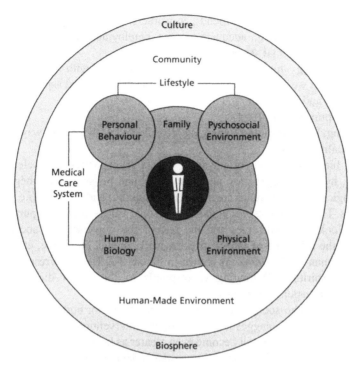

FIGURE 8-1 ▪ The Mandala of Health
From "The mandala of health: A conceptual model and teaching tool," by
T. Hancock and F. Perkins, 1985, *Health Education, 24*(1), 8–10.

client is at the centre of four key factors that influence health—human biology, personal behaviour, psychosocial environment, and physical environment. The model further incorporates the influence of family, lifestyle, medical care system, community, biosphere, and culture (Hancock & Perkins, 1985). Culture is presented as the all-encompassing sphere around the individual.

The Bio-Psycho-Social-Spiritual Model of Health and Disease

The challenge of putting the broader determinants of health into operational use and making them clinically relevant appears formidable. However, a **bio-psycho-social-spiritual framework of health** that incorporates disease, behaviour, and quality-of-life concepts offers ideas to accomplish just that (Hajela, 1994; Rootman, Brown, Raphael, & Renwick, 1994). The framework consists of three dimensions:

1. **Being**—refers to who one is as a physical, psychological, and spiritual being
2. **Belonging**—addresses how we connect with our environment and includes physical belonging (e.g., home, school, neighbourhood), social

belonging (e.g., family, friends, co-workers, intimate others), and community belonging (e.g., adequate income, employment, educational services, health and social services)

3. **Becoming**—highlights our behaviours connected with purposeful activities that we undertake to achieve our goals, hopes, and aspirations, in the short and long term

(Rootman et al., 1994)

Thus, Being, Becoming, and Belonging are reflected as the overall way we measure the quality of life.

The biophysiological, or physical, aspect incorporates such elements as nutrition, hygiene, biogenetics, and anatomical and physiological integrity. The psychological aspect includes cognitive (i.e., thinking) and affective (i.e., feeling) processes. The spiritual aspect embodies personal values, meaning, purpose, and how we look upon ourselves and the rest of the universe. The social aspect addresses the influence of family, friends, work, media, biosphere, etc. (Hajela, 1994; Rootman et al., 1994). As shown in Figure 8-2, Being corresponds to the bio-psycho-spiritual; Belonging corresponds to the social dimension; and Becoming corresponds to behaviour.

The bio-psycho-social-spiritual framework allows for both the evaluation of health status and the suggestion of treatment interventions at each level. The robustness of this model will become even clearer as health and illness are examined within this broad framework. The model is being widely applied in a variety of settings including Alcohol Risk Assessment and Intervention (ARAI) and addiction medicine (Hajela, 2000).

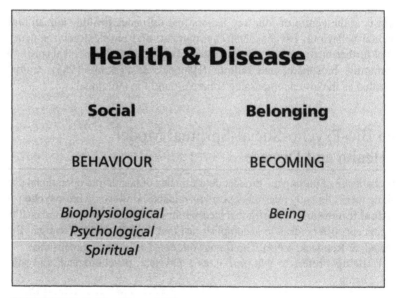

FIGURE 8-2 ■ **Health and Disease**

Faith, Spirituality, and Consciousness

That suffering is part of life is a central concept in cultures around the world. In that context, even illness can be perceived as an opportunity for change rather than simply something that has to be overcome. The commonly used metaphor of "fighting" a disease with medical weapons characterizes disease as an enemy; acceptance and "surrender to win" indicate alternative ways of framing illness that can produce more consistent, long-lasting results. This is most especially true for recovery from illnesses such as addiction. One of the most well-known stories in *Alcoholics Anonymous,* the organization's so-called big book, states:

> When I am disturbed, it is because I find some person, place or thing, or situation—some fact of my life—unacceptable to me, and I can find no serenity until I accept the person, place or thing, or situation as being exactly as it is supposed to be at this moment. Nothing, absolutely nothing happens in God's world by mistake. Until I could accept my alcoholism, I could not stay sober; unless I accept life completely on life's terms, I cannot be happy. I need to concentrate not so much on what needs to be changed in the world as on what needs to be changed in me and in my attitudes. (Anonymous, 1976, p. 449)

It has been suggested that every human comprises a unique pattern of consciousness, a manifestation of the way that person and the environment interact, within a field of absolute consciousness (Newman, 1986). Healing, in that light, can be viewed as a change in perception, with or without a measurable change in the manifest condition. Lupin (2001) describes a case in which a client was perceived by the family as ill, prior to a visit from the doctor, and better after the doctor's visit, even though the doctor could not make a definitive diagnosis. Gutowski (2001) describes an instance in which a nurse, intent on helping others, experienced a healing of her own illness—mitral regurgitation as a result of post-rheumatic heart disease—through a personal experience of spiritual power.

Cultural Heritage and Cultural Diversity

There is a tendency for healthcare providers to stereotype clients on the basis of perceived cultural heritage. While genetic factors are important to consider, health and illness behaviours are further affected by the cultural diversity clients may have been exposed to through their life experiences. **Acculturation,** we learned in Chapter 7, is the process by which people learn and adopt behaviours of a different culture as a result of close contact; it is also a dynamic phenomenon of evolution at the level of being, and it can lead to changes in vulnerabilities to specific illnesses.

Genotype (i.e., genetic predisposition) and phenotype (i.e., observable characteristics such as the expression of health or illness within given environments) are basic concepts for biological organisms. One of the classic studies in the area of coronary heart disease (CHD) examined almost 12 000 men of Japanese ancestry living in Japan, Hawaii, and California. These three settings, representing varying degrees of exposure to Western influence, were selected to examine how the occurrence of CHD was influenced in this group, given the known high rate of CHD in the United States versus a low rate in Japan (Marmot et al., 1975). The study revealed a significant gradient of increasing CHD from Japan to Hawaii to California. There were smaller differences between Japan and Hawaii than between Hawaii and California. Risk factors, such as high cholesterol, high blood pressure, and smoking, did not sufficiently explain the trend. The more likely contributors were identified as diet, occupation, and patterns of social interaction. The degree of Westernization was thus recognized as an important health determinant—which in turn highlights the role played by culture, through a proxy measure of acculturation and assimilation (Corin, 1994). **Assimilation,** or adoption of the cultural patterns of the dominant culture, is never complete, and variable degrees of integration may occur. Problems in acculturation may lead to alienation from the culture of origin and/or the dominant culture. These problems can be expected to affect social adjustment and mental health, as well as physical health. (Acculturation and acculturation stress also are discussed in Chapter 7.)

Although ethnicity can be a guide to a client's culture, a variety of factors—including potential beliefs and values, variable degrees of life experiences, acculturation, and adoption of cross-cultural behaviours—make it imperative that we not make assumptions. Rather, a more direct evaluation of clients' views of themselves and their illnesses at a very personal level is necessary. Such an evaluation takes into account not only a client's religion, but also what practices the client follows. For example, a client may identify as a Roman Catholic but not live exactly according to the Pope's pronouncements. In today's multicultural society, it is not uncommon to find children and adults who have a mixed ethnic heritage and have adopted a cultural lifestyle that differs from that of their family of origin and their ethnic background. It is essential that open-ended questions be part of a holistic assessment in which a healthcare provider can explore a client's beliefs and values, making an effort to offer care that suits the client's psycho-social-spiritual makeup in an appropriate cultural context.

Illness Beliefs and Healing Traditions

Illness in an individual or family member is often a sudden reminder of our vulnerability to factors that lie beyond our control. Reactions to illness can vary

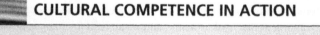

CULTURAL COMPETENCE IN ACTION

Meanings of Health and Illness
Reflect on what the meaning of health is for you. What do you do to stay healthy? Discuss your response with colleagues. Are there differences in how health, illness, and healing traditions are viewed within your group? As far as you know, is what you believe today the same as, or different from, what health means in your culture of origin? If there are differences, can you identify factors that may be influencing your current beliefs and practices?

from extremes of denial of symptoms to unrealistic expectations of how quickly the illness can be cured. The response often depends on how an individual views the particular illness, and/or the concept of illness as a whole, and what resources may be available to manage the illness experience. John Hoey (1998), editor-in-chief of the *Canadian Medical Association Journal*, has observed:

> When I practised medicine in Nigeria years ago, I often saw the botched results of the witch doctor's remedies. A common therapy for any illness in newborns was to rub cow dung on the umbilical stump, resulting in neonatal tetanus and death. On the other hand, Western-trained physicians had little to offer for most chronic conditions. Many clients came to the university centre for care, but an equal and perhaps greater number went into the bush to seek the advice of traditional healers—some of which, no doubt, was helpful. (p. 803)[1]

Medical literature has noted a significant correlation between the recovery expectations of clients and their actual health outcomes, which highlights the need to more fully explore what clients think about their illnesses and what their expectations are regarding recovery and other health outcomes (Mondloch, Cole, & Frank, 2001). Maintaining a neutral, non-judgemental stance on people's values, without necessarily rejecting them or adopting them, has been called cultural relativity (Cassidy, 1996). Remembering cultural relativity in the context of an unconditional positive regard of the client becomes essential for exploring a client's illness beliefs and expectations, which in turn may affect the assessment of illness, possible selected treatments, and health outcomes.

Indigenous systems of health care exist in countries and communities throughout the world, along with varying degrees of availability of the technologically dominated "modern" or "allopathic" medicine.[2] Healthcare providers practising in a multicultural society therefore need to be familiar with the broad, basic concepts of at least some of the world's popular healthcare systems. The rest of this chapter is therefore devoted almost exclusively to the concepts and approaches to healing in the following traditions: allopathic medicine, osteopathy, chiropractic, Aboriginal medicine, traditional Chinese medicine (TCM) and acupuncture, Ayurveda and Maharishi Ayurveda (MAV), homeopathy, naturopathic medicine, and integrative medicine. This list and discussion are not meant to be exhaustive or complete. It is simply meant to illustrate the diversity in healing traditions. Individual healthcare providers may wish to explore specific systems in greater depth, depending on their client population, level of interest, and training opportunities. Through such exploration, healthcare providers may also appreciate some similarity of ideas and unifying features across traditions, as well as dissimilar features that make integration more challenging.

---

[1]Although this excerpt offers support for the indigenous healing tradition, the phrasing "botched results of the witch doctor's remedies" may also be seen as reflective of the biases of Western-trained authoritative professionals.

[2]"Indigenous" = occurring or originating in the area where it is found.

Allopathic Medicine, or Biomedicine

Origins and Concepts

Allopathic medicine, or biomedicine, traces its roots back to the Greek physician Hippocrates (470–370 B.C.E.). Medical contributions made by him specifically, and by others from that time, were compiled in a collection called *Corpus Hippocraticum* (Lyons, 1987a). General ideas that are part of this collection include anatomy, physiology, pathology, mental illness, gynecology and obstetrics, surgery, diagnosis, prognosis, therapy, and ethics. These serve as the foundation for the Western medicine that is considered to be mainstream today.

Interestingly, the cause of illness in Hippocratic times was thought of in terms of the following:

- The four basic elements: air, fire, water, earth
- The four cardinal humors: blood, phlegm, yellow bile, black bile
- Four qualities: dry, hot, moist, cold
  (Lyons, 1987a)

When the humors were in balance within the body and environmentally, the body would be healthy, whereas an excess or deficiency would result in disease (Lyons, 1987b). The above concepts resonate with principles of Aboriginal medicine, TCM, and Ayurveda.

Allopathic medicine took on its more recognizably modern turn in the nineteenth century, when concepts related to bacterial infection as a cause of disease were promoted by the following medical pioneers:

1. Ignaz Semmelweis (1818–65) in Austria
2. Joseph Lister (1827–1912) in Scotland
3. Louis Pasteur (1822–95) in France
4. Robert Koch (1843–1910) in Germany
   (Lyons, 1987c)

The seminal work by these physicians and many others in the world has established infectious causes and their eradication as the foundation of biomedicine, such that infectious and parasitic diseases is the first category in the International Classification of Diseases system. Allopathic medicine is the dominant paradigm in the Western world; medical care is delivered through family doctors, specialist physicians, and a healthcare team that features a variety of disciplines, each of which plays a unique role in care. Thus, many healthcare providers are often needed to treat one client. Addressing the client's spiritual needs frequently does not fall within the domain of Western medical practice (Letendre, 2002).

Treatment Approaches

Western medicine's approach is analytical in nature, and the body and mind are regarded as separate entities that are treated in different areas of medicine (Letendre, 2002). Advances in knowledge related to anatomy, physiology, laboratory medicine, and diagnostic imaging have led to detailed mapping of the function of the human body and mind, together with the development of various specialties that comprise the Western medical system. The predominant emphasis on biological factors and the heavy reliance on pharmaceuticals to eradicate infection and/or restore the homeostatic balance of various body systems has often led to the neglect of psychological, behavioural, and social dimensions of illness. With the development of powerful and effective psychotropic drugs (e.g., antidepressants), even the practice of psychiatry has become more biological. This emphasis also has resulted in a system that is largely acute care oriented, and often fails miserably in the treatment of chronic conditions that are not curable within a finite length of time.

Chronic diseases generally wax and wane over a person's lifetime, due not only to biophysiological factors but also to psychological, social, and spiritual factors. Treatment of many chronic diseases (e.g., in the fields of addiction, cardiology, nephrology, and oncology) addresses the psycho-social-spiritual factors in the context of stabilizing and optimizing the quality of life of clients and their families, rather than through a single-minded focus on dealing with the anatomical lesion and/or physiological disturbance.

Osteopathy

Origins and Concepts

Osteopathy is an American system of healing that was developed by Andrew Taylor Still (1828–1917) during the nineteenth century. The founding of the American School of Osteopathic Medicine in 1892 led to the establishment of a system in which doctors of osteopathy (DOs) have come to provide healthcare to about 10 percent of the American population (Wagner, 1996). In contrast to the current American model of osteopathy, which has a strong medical component, the programs offered in Canada are focused on Traditional Osteopathy, which primarily has a manual basis. In osteopathy, the structural and mechanical integrity of the body is considered to be of prime importance in the context of proper nutrition and non-toxic environmental conditions.

The US osteopathic colleges offer four-year training programs that lead to DO degrees, much like the case for doctors of medicine (MDs). In the United States, DOs have full privileges for surgery and writing prescriptions, like MDs. In Canada, accredited training programs do not exist. However, the Canadian College of Osteopathy has been established since the 1980s and is gradually increasing the number of centres across Canada. Graduates of this five-year, part-time program are usually licensed healthcare providers who also receive a Diploma in Osteopathic Manual Practice.

Treatment Approaches

Osteopathic physicians view the client as a unit where, in addition to organ dysfunction, an osteopathic lesion is usually identified in relation to skeletal, arthrodial (refers to gliding joints), or myofascial (soft tissue) issues. Involvement of vascular, lymphatic, and neural elements is also considered. Corrective action may include:

- Skeletal manipulation
- Myofascial release
- Muscle tension/relaxation techniques
- Craniosacral manipulation
- Counterstrain
- Thrusting techniques

These are complementary to the allopathic medication, surgery, nutrition, and lifestyle issues that also may be addressed.

Chiropractic

Origins and Concepts

Like osteopathy, **chiropractic** is a healing art that originated in the United States amid controversy and reaction from the forces of allopathic medicine. Although the roots of spinal manipulation can be traced back to the Greek physician Hippocrates, the chiropractic profession was established by Daniel David Palmer in 1895. Spinal misalignment is considered to be the main problem in the chiropractic approach to healing; thus, spinal manipulation therapy (SMT) is viewed as the main treatment technique.

Canada has two chiropractic training colleges—The Canadian Memorial Chiropractic College (CMCC) in Toronto and the Université du Québec à Trois-Rivières (UQTR) in Quebec—each offering four years' training similar to that for MDs and naturopathic doctors. There are more than 6000 chiropractors in Canada, and an estimated 4.5 million Canadians seek care from them each year.

Treatment Approaches

Back pain, neck pain, and headaches are the primary neuromusculoskeletal conditions that bring clients to the chiropractor. The use of SMT for the treatment of visceral organ dysfunction (e.g., dysmenorrhea, hypertension, asthma, infantile colic, and otitis media) is being further refined (Redwood, 1996). Chiropractors are not licensed to prescribe medication, nor do they usually suggest herbal medicine.

Aboriginal Medicine

Origins and Concepts

Every culture around the world since antiquity has developed concepts related to self, health, and illness. In Aboriginal cultures, community elders and/or specifically designated healers—sometimes called shamans—minister to illness in clients and communities as a personal calling. **Aboriginal medicine** training often takes place through apprenticeship and through self-exploration in rituals that have ancient origins. Plants and minerals are often used as medicine, and healing methods include rituals that have a spiritual connection. Burning sweetgrass and tobacco, for example, are rituals for many First Nations communities in Canada; sweat lodges and spiritual imagery also figure prominently in health promotion and healing within some Aboriginal cultures.

The following two central concepts exist in most traditional Aboriginal systems of evaluating and treating illness:

1. The consideration of basic elements of nature that make up the universe of which we are a part
2. Some reference to the Circle of Life that incorporates the ideas of seasons, aging, life, and death

In Native American and Aboriginal Canadian traditions, the medicine wheel is a powerful symbol that expresses the four elements (air, fire, water, and earth), and the four directions (east, west, north, and south,). The elements and directions are considered important to human existence and to the maintenance of proper balance. Spirit is thought to be the initial impulse that brings our consciousness from the unmanifest to the manifest. Spirit permeates and weaves together the elements of air (breath of life), fire (spark and hearth of life), water (flow of life), and earth (structure of life) (McArthur, 1998). In various forms, these concepts are part of Aboriginal cultures all over the world.

The idea of maintaining "centredness" or self-awareness in the Circle of Life is also of great importance in Aboriginal cultures. It is a way of connecting with the universe. Consideration is given to all forces of nature in order to achieve balance and harmony. For example, healing-ceremony rituals involve actions aimed at both the client and a balance with Mother Earth (Morse, Young, & Swartz, 1991; Letendre, 2002).

Illness is not necessarily considered to be a bad thing; it is seen as a sign sent by the Creator to help people re-evaluate their lives. Good health is also viewed as a gift from the Creator that is to be respected and appreciated through rituals associated with Aboriginal spirituality, such as prayer and the traditional burning of sweetgrass. These religious practices also form the basis of illness treatments (Royal Commission on Aboriginal Peoples, 1996).

Treatment Approaches

As noted above, the traditional Aboriginal medicine framework supports a holistic approach to health care. Maintaining or restoring balance when it is disrupted by an illness is an essential feature of Aboriginal medicine. Various therapies, involving herbs, sound, and sacred rituals (e.g., smudging[1] and the sweat lodge[2]) attempt to restore the balance of elements and energy within the medicine wheel.

---

[1] The burning of certain herbs, such as sweetgrass, to create a cleansing smoke bath, which is used to purify people, ceremonial and ritual space, and ceremonial tools and objects. Smudging can also bring physical, spiritual, and emotional balance.

[2] A ceremonial sauna used by some Aboriginal peoples during a cleansing ceremony for the body and the spirit. The ceremony may include prayers, drumming, and offerings (e.g., tobacco) to the spirit world.

The use of herbs for medicine and health promotion is as ancient as human civilization. There is considerable variability across continents and cultures in terms of the exact practices and the specific herbs indicated for particular purposes. A herb is usually part of a shrub, tree, moss, lichen, fern, algae, seaweed, fungus, fruit, bark, seeds, roots, exudates, or flowering plant, but sometimes the entire plant is used. Many herbal traditions also use other healing agents, including animal parts, insects, secretions of organisms, worm castings, shells, rocks, metals, minerals, and gemstones (Meserole, 1996).

The Aboriginal concept of illness often considers both "natural" and "supernatural" causes, such that healing techniques use natural (i.e., herbal) and/or spiritual powers. This concept is also illustrated in **Curanderismo**, a healing tradition common in Hispanic communities. The healers, Curanderos, recognize three levels *(niveles):*

1. Material
2. Spiritual
3. Mental

(Trotter, 1996)

The material-level treatment commonly uses herbs, although objects and religious symbols with healing powers may also be used. This approach is taken for treatment of illnesses brought about by a dysfunction of the body, improper self-care by the client, and/or infection. The spiritual level rests on a belief in the existence of spirit entities that continue to exist after the death of the body, on a plane of reality separate from the physical world. The healer uses contacts with the spirits for diagnosis of "possession" and subsequent healing. The mental level uses the concept of the healer's mental energy (vibrations) to effect change.

Aboriginal medicine differs from Western medicine in its structural elements. Letendre (2002) notes that many of the traditional rituals practised by Aboriginal healers are performed outdoors and involve connecting with the spirits of nature that are thought to be responsible for whatever healing powers the healer possesses. Within traditionalist medicine, the client is the one who determines something is wrong and he or she is an active participant in healing treatment and ceremonies. In contrast, Western medicine relies on a more formal system, with services that usually limit client choices and may promote client passivity. The doctor is the healer and tends to have control over the treatment. For example, after gathering a history and compiling signs and symptoms, it is the doctor who determines if there is a problem and then prescribes the necessary treatment. There is often little encouragement for self-reliance and control on the client's part (Morse et al, 1991).

Within traditionalist medicine, health promotion is not the same as illness prevention. The Aboriginal client seeks a healer for the purposes of finding a cure for a specific ailment; going to a doctor for regular checkups to ensure normality may be viewed as unnecessary (Letendre, 2002; Morse et al., 1991).

Another difference is evident in the way treatments are administered. Traditional healers work in close contact with clients through verbal support as well as the actual administering of treatments over the course of the illness; in the biomedical model of care, the doctor spends minimal time with clients, and the duty of administering treatments is generally allocated to nurses and other healthcare providers. The discontinuity in caregiving can compromise the development of a meaningful therapeutic relationship between the healer and the client.

In Canada, the National Aboriginal Health Organization (NAHO) offers a useful Web site for advancing and sharing information related to Aboriginal medicine (see "Online Learning Resources"). Efforts of this nature are integral to personal empowerment of Aboriginal peoples in their health and well-being.

Traditional Chinese Medicine (TCM)

Origins and Concepts

Traditional Chinese medicine (TCM) views humans as part of nature, at the juncture between heaven and earth (Bienfield & Korngold, 1991). Nature is seen to be in constant motion, with cyclical patterns that are harmonic and transformative. The polar and balancing aspects of yin (passive principle) and yang (active principle) complement each other; illness is thought to arise when there is a disruption in that balance. In addition to the concept of yin and yang, the concept of energy and vitality—qi—is central to TCM.

TCM views the human body in terms of channels, called meridians, through which qi flows. Health and illness are defined in terms of a free flow or blockage in these meridians. **Acupuncture** is a technique in which special needles are manipulated to allow the free flow of qi and so improve health.

When qi flows freely through the meridians, the body is balanced and healthy, but if the energy flow is blocked, stagnated, or weakened, the result can be physical, mental, or emotional ill health. Imbalances can result from excessive emotional response (e.g., anger and grief), as well as environmental factors (e.g., cold, heat, dampness, and excessive work). Meridian channels are associated with specific organs, and meridian diagrams of the human body guide the healer in delineating where to access the blockages, depending on the particular diagnoses arrived at through a clinical assessment. Figure 8-3 illustrates the location of the meridian points in the body.

The TCM framework is built around the concept of Five Phases (*wu xing*) that are also translated as the five elements—earth, metal, water, wood, and fire. These correspond to organs and their physiological function, and to the mind, season, time of day, and direction (Ergil, 1996). The Five Phases are thought to maintain a dynamic, interactive pattern of production and restraint (see Table 8-1).

Each organ in the body is classified as yin, if it is solid, or yang, if it is hollow. The yin organs are considered more crucial in function, whereas the yang organs serve as physiological way stations for substances traversing the body (Aung, Benjamin, Berman, & Jacobs, 1997).

The liver, classified as a wood organ, is considered the authoritative yin organ that collects and directs the qi through the blood. The gallbladder assists the liver (as its yang partner) through the secretion of bile, which in turn helps turn food into proper nourishment and eliminate unnecessary substances through the intestines and colon. The heart, as a fire and yin organ, propels the blood; the

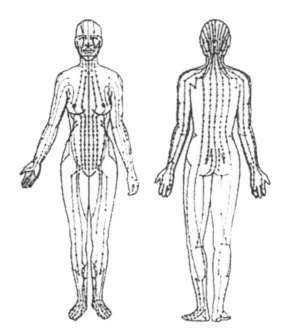

FIGURE 8-3 ▪ **Location of Meridians and Acupuncture Points in the Body**
From "Channels or meridians in acupuncture: The invisible pathways of qi," on
Holisticonline.com. Retrieved August 30, 1995, from http://www.holistic-online.
com/Acupuncture/acp_meridians.htm

small intestine, its paired yang organ, separates out the useful components of
digested food and directs the waste to the kidneys and large intestine. The heart
and small intestine support the spleen, an earth organ that regulates metabolism
and adjustment of the viscosity of blood and fluids in the vascular and lymphatic
systems. The yang pairing for the spleen is the stomach, which extracts essence
from the food that is ingested. The lungs—metal, yin organs—extract "essence"
from air and distill it into qi, combining it with nutritious substances from the
spleen and stomach. The lungs also exhale unnecessary by-products. The yang
partner of the lungs is the large intestine, which helps eliminate the waste products of digestion and metabolism. The water yin organs are the kidneys, which
accept and support the qi from the lungs. They support the reproductive organs
and the bone marrow that in turn regulates brain, spinal cord, bones, and blood.
The yang partner of the kidneys is the bladder. Together, the kidneys and bladder
regulate the retention and release of waste products—urine and stool. The cycle
then repeats, starting back at the liver as the kidneys and bladder animate the
spirit (spark for the fire) to activate the liver and spleen. The details and depths of
these interactions are thought to govern the maintenance of health or dysfunction
in various parts of the client, leading to illness (Aung et al., 1997).

Acupuncture and TCM training programs are becoming increasingly more
available in Canada. Some jurisdictions within Canada (e.g., British Columbia,

TABLE 8-1

Five Phase Correspondences

CATEGORY	WOOD	FIRE	EARTH	METAL	WATER
Viscus	Liver	Heart	Spleen	Lungs	Kidney
Bowel	Gallbladder	Small intestine	Stomach	Large intestine	Urinary bladder
Season	Spring	Summer	Late summer	Autumn	Winter
Time of day	Before sunrise	Forenoon	Afternoon	Late afternoon	Midnight
Climate	Wind	Heat	Damp	Dryness	Cold
Direction	East	South	Centre	West	North
Development	Birth	Growth	Maturity	Withdrawal	Dormancy
Colour	Cyan	Red	Yellow	White	Black
Taste	Sour	Bitter	Sweet	Pungent	Salty
Sense organ	Eyes	Tongue	Mouth	Nose	Ears
Odour	Goatish	Scorched	Fragrant	Raw fish	Putrid
Vocalization	Shouting	Laughing	Singing	Weeping	Sighing
Tissue	Sinews	Vessels	Flesh	Body hair	Bones
Mind	Anger	Joy	Thought	Sorrow	Fear

From "China's traditional medicine," by K. V. Ergil. In M. S. Micozzi (Ed.), *Fundamentals of complementary and alternative medicine* (2nd ed., p. 313), 2001, Philadelphia: Churchill Livingstone.

Alberta, and Ontario) either regulate or are considering regulation of TCM and acupuncture practitioners. More information is available through the College of Traditional Chinese Medicine Practitioners and Acupuncturists of British Columbia; the Alberta College of Acupuncture and Traditional Chinese Medicine, which offers training in collaboration with the Beijing University of Chinese Medicine; and Dr. Steven Aung (see "Online Learning Resources").

Treatment Approaches

The diagnostic methods in TCM include the following:
- Taking the client's history
- Listening
- Smelling
- Inspecting
- Palpating acupuncture points
- Feeling the pulse

The pulse diagnosis includes a three-point palpation of the radial arteries in both wrists to collect information about the organs and channels (Ergil, 1996).

Restoration of balance and health in TCM is achieved through the use of herbs, diet, and practices such as tai chi or qigong, to counteract the external disease-causing factors (wind, heat, damp, dryness, and cold) that interact with the internal emotional factors (anger, joy, pensiveness sorrow, and fear) (Leung, 2004). Cultural patterns of not expressing strong emotions in public may lead a client of Chinese heritage to somatize (express psychological distress through physical symptoms) in terms of organ pathology, and/or to deny symptoms of depression, anxiety, adjustment disorder, or even gambling addiction. The therapeutic effect of acupuncture is to regulate the flow of qi through the manipulation of fine needles at established meridian points.

TCM herbs such as ginseng, *ma huang,* and green tea are readily available in health-food stores for clients to use for their health and well-being. Internet sites such as Numark Pharmacists (see "Online Learning Resources") offer guidance for specific conditions.

Ayurveda and Maharishi Ayurveda

Origins and Concepts

Ayurveda is a Sanskrit word that can be most closely translated as the knowledge (*veda*) of life or lifespan (*ayur*). Although the literary sources known as the *Rigveda* and the *Atharvaveda* are thought to be more than 3000 years old, the consciousness-based concepts they describe imply that this knowledge has always existed and can be experienced directly from the cosmos around us. The fundamental connections between the macrocosm and microcosm are central to Vedic tradition, in which everything arises from and is composed of five basic elements:

1. Space (*akasha*)
2. Air (*vayu*)
3. Fire (*agni*)
4. Water (*jala*)
5. Earth (*prithvi*)

Even these fundamental elements are said to arise from consciousness interacting with itself, which gives rise to the concepts of an observer (*rishi*), the process of observation (*devata*), and the object of observation (*chhandas*).

Practising Ayurveda involves examining the reflection of the five elements in the human body in terms of three vital energies (*doshas*)—*vata, pitta,* and *kapha*—together with the seven tissues (*dhatus*) listed here:

1. Fluids of digestion (*rasa*)
2. Blood (*rakta*)
3. Muscle (*mamsa*)
4. Fat (*meda*)
5. Bone (*asthi*)
6. Marrow (*majja*)
7. Sexual/reproductive fluids (*shukra*)
   (Zysk, 1996)

In addition, three waste products (*malas*) exist: urine, feces, and sweat (Zysk, 1996).

A revival of Ayurveda was brought about several decades ago by Maharishi Mahesh Yogi, founder of the transcendental meditation movement, in accordance with the classical texts and in collaboration with leading Ayurvedic scholars and physicians (called *Vaidyas*). This specific reformulation considers consciousness to be of primary importance for optimal health and uses meditation techniques to develop a more integrated and coherent functioning of the nervous system and human physiology that is known as **Maharishi Ayurveda (MAV)** (Sharma, 1996).

Further elaboration concerning digestive, metabolic, and distributive processes involves consideration of the following three types of enzymatic processes:

1. *Jatharagni*—the process that breaks down food
2. *Bhutagnis*—the five liver enzymes corresponding to the assimilation of the five elements
3. *Dhatvagnis*—the seven enzymes involved in the synthesis of the seven *dhatus*
   (Zysk, 1996)

Problems in the enzymatic processes lead to the accumulation of improperly digested food that is collectively called *ama*. Internal diseases are thought to begin by accumulation of *ama* in the various channels called *srotas*, whereas external diseases are thought to increase the tendency of the body to produce *ama*. The evaluation of the physical and mental constitution is done in concert with the three *doshas* (physical energies) and the three *gunas* (psychic energies): *sattva*, *rajas*, and *tamas*. Within the MAV framework, further links of the *doshas* and *gunas* with *rishi*, *devata*, and *chhandas* are also considered. The important factor of balanced digestion and metabolism is called *ojas*, which is also produced through the mental processes of happiness and awareness of consciousness, including the connectedness with all aspects of the universe (Sharma & Clark, 1998). Methods of health promotion and treatment aim to reduce *ama* and increase *ojas*.

In the sequence of the manifestation of difficulties at the mental level, another central concept involves the evolution of the ego (*ahamkara*) from the subtle mind (*manas*) through the process of the intellect (*buddhi*). The parallels to observer (mind), observing (intellect), and observed (ego) highlight the hypothesis of *pragya-aparadh*, meaning the mistake of the intellect (i.e., dysfunction at the level of *buddhi*), which results in over-identification with the ego and sensory objects. *Pragya-aparadh* itself is considered to be a *rishi*-level problem, whereas the *devata*- and *chhandas*-level causes of disease are *asatmyaindriyartha samyoga* (untruthful interaction between senses and their objects) and *kala parinama* (the influence of time, seasons, and external factors, respectively). Table 8-2 provides a summary of the *doshas*, including their characteristics and effects of imbalance.

Treatment Approaches

A central evaluation tool in Ayurveda and MAV is pulse diagnosis—a three-point examination of the radial pulse (usually left wrist for women, right wrist for men). It considers imbalances related to the three *doshas* and the seven *dhatus* mentioned earlier. Treatment recommendations are made on the basis of imbalances detected to increase *ojas*, reduce *ama*, clear *shrotas* (microcirculatory channels), and generally create balance among *vata*, *pitta*, and *kapha*. Herbs are a common part of the treatment. Daily routine and dietary recommendations figure prominently in recommendations made by a healer or *Vaidya*. The evaluations establish the *prakriti,* or nature of the client, in terms of the *doshas* and *vikriti*,

TABLE 8-2

Summary of *Doshas*

	VATA	PITTA	KAPHA
Characteristics	Quick-moving, irregular appetite and digestion; tendency to worry, sleep lightly, be forgetful	Moderate in activity; sharp appetite (cannot skip meals); enterprising	Slow and methodical in activity; slow digestion; tranquil personality
Effect of balanced *dosha*	Clear and alert mind; healthy immunity; vitality	Lustrous complexion; contentment; balanced intellect	Strong body; affectionate and courageous
Effect of imbalances	Dry, rough skin; anxiety; arthritis; hypertension; insomnia	Excessive body heat; sweating; digestion problems; inflammation	Cold; lethargic; asthmatic; weight problems; depression
Aggravating factors	Excessive exercise, fear, grief, agitation, cold, pungent foods	Anger, hot weather, spicy foods, alcohol, sour or salty foods	Heavy food, excessive sleep, sugar, milk products
Taste and food preferences	Sweet, sour, and salty: breads, yogourt, cheese, honey	Sweet, bitter, and astringent: cold foods, dairy products, beans, vegetables	Pungent, bitter, and astringent: peppers, ginger, cumin, spinach, beans, barley, corn
Time	0200–0600 and 1400–1800	1000–1400 and 2200–0200	0600–1000 and 1800–2200
Season	Late autumn and winter	Midsummer and early autumn	Spring and early summer

known collectively as the *doshic* imbalances. The aim is to maintain and/or restore balance among the three *doshas.*

MAV specifically emphasizes transcendental meditation and the TM-Sidhi program (advanced meditation techniques). Neuromuscular integrative techniques (yoga) and neuro-respiratory techniques (*pranayama*) are part of the practice for health promotion and healing. Yoga on its own has been gaining wide popularity among Canadians (see *Ascent Magazine* under "Online Learning Resources").

Clients of East Indian origin, even those explicitly unaware of Ayurvedic medicine, may subscribe culturally to many of the above concepts related to seasonal and dietary routines. Inquiry into diet and behavioural routines is critical to understanding the clients' views on illness and healing. Further, Ayurveda and MAV have experienced a resurgence around the world in recent years, so many more people now have some familiarity with the concepts. Many clients benefit greatly when these techniques are incorporated into the overall evaluation and treatment, as a complement to Western medical treatment.

Homeopathy

Origins and Concepts

The term **homeopathy** was coined by the German physician Samuel Hahnemann (1755–1843); the central concept is the Law of Similars, which encapsulates Hahnemann's observations that remedies can resonate with the illness to stimulate the body to achieve a cure. This is in stark contrast to the allopathic system of eradicating symptoms through a superior force. Further, the remedies are thought to increase in power with additional dilutions. This idea is totally counterintuitive to the usual Western need to use more of a substance to increase its effectiveness (the dose effect). Homeopaths still consider this increase in power to be a mystery, but they rely on its effects on clients and their illness. Some people consider this practice to be a form of energy transfer, whereas homeopathy's detractors regard the remedies as placebos. Homeopathic remedies are symptom-based and individualized for each client. For this reason, they are difficult to evaluate using the traditional clinical research protocols in which treatment effectiveness is established by giving a standard dose and regimen of medications to a number of clients with the same illness.

The Canadian Academy of Homeopathy offers programs for healthcare professionals, including a 500-hour advanced home-study course.

Treatment Approaches

The homeopathic pharmacopia has been established over the years through a systematic evaluation of symptoms produced by specific substances in normal humans, and includes more than 2000 remedies. The remedies are of plant, animal, and mineral origin (Jacobs & Moskowitz, 1996).

Homeopathy has significant appeal worldwide among care providers and clients who want to make use of the body's own healing mechanisms. Chronic conditions such as high blood pressure, arthritis, and multiple sclerosis may well be amenable to homeopathic treatment. A skilled practitioner conducts a detailed assessment and tailors the remedy to the individual client's needs. Homeopathy is likely not appropriate for acute fractures, conditions requiring emergency surgical interventions, and chronic illnesses with advanced tissue damage that is unlikely to heal by way of the body's internal mechanisms alone.

Naturopathic Medicine

Origins and Concepts

Central concepts in **naturopathic medicine** establish it as a philosophy of life in which, given the proper opportunity, the body is expected to heal itself using the healing power of nature and operating within the laws of nature (*Vis Medicatrix Naturae).* Health promotion involves living in harmony with nature. Naturopathy's vitalistic approach maintains that the symptoms of diseases typically are not caused by offending agents (e.g., bacteria or viruses); rather, they represent the intrinsic reaction of the body/mind in an attempt to defend and/or heal itself (Pizzorno, 1996).

The training of naturopathic physicians is very broad and tends to include a variety of diagnostic systems, investigations, treatments, and healing systems from around the world, including conventional basic medical sciences that encompass such fields as anatomy, physiology, biochemistry, pathology, microbiology, and laboratory diagnosis. Accredited schools and licensing authorities exist in both Canada and the United States. The Canadian College of Naturopathic Medicine or CCNM (2003) identifies the key tenets of naturopathic practice as:

1. Identify and treat the causes
2. First do no harm
3. Doctor as teacher
4. Treat the whole person
5. Emphasize prevention
6. Support the healing power of the body

Treatment Approaches

Naturopathic doctors (NDs) incorporate a variety of approaches in healing, including acupuncture, homeopathy, herbal medicine, TCM, and Ayurveda, depending on their personal interests and training expertise. The demand for naturopathic services is growing rapidly in the Western world as people look toward taking charge of their health and wellness. Individuals seek care from naturopathic practitioners both as an alternative to conventional medicine and as a complement. Naturopathic medicine is sometimes called herbal medicine because herbs are often recommended instead of prescription drugs.

The emphasis in naturopathic medicine is often on lifestyle factors and personal empowerment. Generically speaking, Aboriginal medicine concepts may well be incorporated into naturopathic medicine, depending on the experience and training of the healthcare provider and/or the interest of the client. Health-food stores and even traditional pharmacies now carry herbal remedies and supplements that customers choose themselves, based on the recommendations of friends or informed store staff, or on suggestions made by healthcare providers. Headaches, cold symptoms, and menstrual disorders (including menopausal symptoms) are common conditions for which clients turn to herbal remedies. The Internet provides easy access to information for those who want to make their own choices.

Energy Medicine

Origins and Concepts

Energy medicine is a collection of techniques and systems based on the central tenet that humans are energy systems that manifest the universal life force. The concept of seven energy centres, or chakras, in the human body can be traced back to ancient Indian or Vedic roots. The seven chakras—root, sacral, solar plexus, heart, throat, third eye, and crown—also correspond to the respective colours red, orange, yellow, green, blue, indigo, and violet. The chakras are located along a central axis parallel to the spine of the physical body (Bruyere, 1994). Healers evaluate energy blockages and use their own consciousness to channel universal energy to release blockages to promote more harmonious function that translates into optimal health.

Treatment Approaches

Energy medicine treatment usually involves some form of chakra balancing, through specific hand movements or massage. In addition to faith healing, which uses touch for therapeutic, spiritual purposes, several methods are used for hand-mediated healing, such as therapeutic touch (TT), polarity therapy, reiki, jin shin jyutsu, reflexology, and shiatsu massage (acupressure) (Slater, 1996). They all involve different techniques of touching or massaging various points or parts of the body that ultimately influence the client's energy balance. The techniques are used for both health promotion the treatment of imbalances that manifest as dysfunction or disease.

TT actually does not involve touching the body; rather, it is a set of prescribed hand motions over a person's energy aura. While research evidence may be equivocal regarding the effectiveness of these techniques, the number of health providers involved and the number of satisfied recipients is increasing. In many Canadian hospitals, TT is becoming a competency for nurses to develop and use independently, with the client's consent, as a complementary therapy in the management of pain or as a health-promotion strategy. The training programs can be quite extensive, involving multiple levels of preparation.

Ways of Healing: Commonalities and Challenges

Each of the systems of health care discussed thus far incorporates methods of treatment that are consistent with the conceptualization of illness. The methods may be physical, herbal, pharmaceutical, behavioural, and/or psychotherapeutic. Because the most crucial element is the individual clients, assessments must include clients' own ideas about what may be wrong with them. This is essential, to get a sense of the framework in which they view their illness, but also to obtain a sense of their culture and past experiences with the healthcare system. Although biomedicine may dominate Western health care, clients in our society are increasingly more conversant with other healing traditions from their countries of origin, or with what they have adopted from their own investigations and experiences.

In Canada, although provincial healthcare coverage is often limited to diagnostic and treatment methods associated with biomedicine, clients frequently seek out chiropractic care. Naturopathic doctors, homeopaths, Ayurvedic *Vaidyas*, acupuncturists, and TCM practitioners are also sought out by clients who are familiar with these healers and/or want to explore beyond the limitations of allopathic medicine. By the mid-1990s, at least 15 percent of Canadians aged 15 and over were estimated to have used some form of alternative health care in the previous year (Millar, 1997). The use of alternative health care was found to be more prevalent among women, higher income earners, clients aged 45 to 64, and those with three or more chronic conditions. Although many health insurance plans now provide limited coverage for some of the alternative ways of healing, costs of treatment—including costs associated with herbal supplements—remain a major barrier to the use of these services.

We have been looking at the many differences among the various healing traditions, but there is also considerable similarity. It is interesting to note that a number of characteristics—such as the concept of balance, relationship with the elements, and a close connection between the physical and spiritual realm—are part of several healing traditions. Although many of the alternative ways of healing continue to be viewed with skepticism, in many instances physicians (MDs), nurses, and other health professionals have completed additional training to incorporate complementary methods into their practices. Ayurvedic concepts, for example, can be readily integrated into discussions about behaviour modification in individual and group psychotherapy. Depending on individual interest, clients may delve deeper into meditation or the use of dietary and/or herbal supplements. The blending of approaches by healthcare providers and clients seeking out complementary care has led to more integration of services from a variety of cultural sources and systems of health care.

Integrative Health Care

Integrative health care is based on the belief that offering the combined knowledge of old and new healing methods—which gives the client more choice from

---

CULTURAL COMPETENCE IN ACTION

Integrative Therapy Case Report
A 47-year-old married man, originally from South Africa, sought care from a psychotherapist because of marital dysfunction. Some concerns were raised regarding his alcohol use, and he expressed a wish to moderate his drinking. A referral to an addiction medicine specialist clarified the diagnosis to be alcohol dependence, such that definitive treatment required a goal of abstinence from alcohol.

The client was unable to abstain from alcohol until he started a prescription for naltrexone. This prescription drug is an opioid antagonist that decreases the craving for alcohol and diminishes the positive reward experience. The client also expressed an interest in Maharishi Ayurveda (MAV). An assessment revealed that he needed to follow a diet and routine for vata and pitta pacification. A referral was also made to a transcendental meditation (TM) teacher.

The client stopped the naltrexone after being stable in an abstinence-based recovery program for three months. He attended weekly group psychotherapy for some years and continues to remain in individual psychotherapy monthly or bi-monthly to continue to work through his feelings. More than five years later, he still practises TM twice a day and attributes a large part of his stability to this practice.

a personal perspective—is ultimately better than single-model approaches to health and wellness. **Integrative health care** refers to a blending of conventional and complementary approaches to health that address the body, mind, and spirit, as well as the relationship with the environment and others. Integrative health deals with the whole person and is considered both a client-centered and a client-empowering approach to health and healing (Boon, 2002).

There is increasing evidence that integrative approaches may offer greater benefits than single-minded approaches. For example, the Institute for Clinical Evaluative Sciences (ICES) offers an evidence-based summary of non-estrogen therapies for hot flashes that includes suggestions for herbal supplements and explores other alternatives, while single-path trials currently do not show definitive benefits (Kelsall, 2004). As the popularity of herbal remedies increases for varied illnesses such as arthritis, depression, and diabetes, healthcare providers are being urged to consider the side effects of herbs, potential drug interactions, and the lack of standardization and control that can contribute to contamination and toxicity of certain products (Borins, 1998).

Cultural Competence in Healthcare Delivery

Health disparities in access to and use of care, along with adaptation difficulties, are well known in immigrant and marginalized populations (Beiser, 2005). Lack of culturally appropriate psychosocial services is thought to be a significant factor in health disparity. For example, a low breastfeeding rate (8 percent) and prevalent iron deficiency anemia (12 percent) were identified among Chinese newborns at a pediatric practice in Montreal. Since then, the development of an interdisciplinary, culturally appropriate allied health service has resulted in a much higher breastfeeding rate (48 percent) and a decreased incidence of iron deficiency (2.8 percent) among newborns of Chinese ethnicity (Chan-Yip, 2004).

Although some ethnocultural groups already favour particular complementary healing approaches for specific health problems, the wider population of

---

CULTURAL CONSIDERATIONS IN CARE

Mix-and-Match Case Report

A 60-year-old female medical doctor, originally from England, felt that her increasing problems with arthritis and hypertension were not adequately being addressed through biomedicine. She sought help from a homeopath and an acupuncturist.

She is happy with the care she is receiving from both complementary healthcare providers. In addition to the two alternative brands of expertise that this client benefits from, she appreciates the warm, caring manner and more emotional–spiritual conversation she experiences with the complementary healthcare providers, as opposed to the matter-of-fact visits with her family doctor.

The case report that appears just before this one illustrates an active role; this one illustrates a supportive role.

countries around the world is being exposed to diverse traditions and healing approaches through migration, the mass media, Internet/rapid telecommunication, and multicultural friendships and marriages (Kirmayer, 2004). Providing health care in a global, multicultural society means recognizing the illness behaviours and ways of healing across cultures.

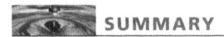 SUMMARY

It is essential that every healthcare provider approach clients as unique individuals who present with a history of prior experience of how they view themselves as individuals, members of families, and members of their community. This personal perception and experience, clients' beliefs about illness and ways of healing, and expectations of what they require to restore health and well-being are essential components of what the healthcare provider needs to know before embarking on investigations, diagnoses, and treatments.

While there is great diversity among different cultures from around the world, there are also similarities. The bio-psycho-social-spiritual model of health and illness is an integral template that can be used by all healthcare providers as part of their assessment so that they can ascertain the different dimensions of the client's health or illness experience. Healthcare providers cannot be expected to be adept at all languages, cultures, or healthcare systems of the world, but a working familiarity with the most common approaches and an attitude of unconditional positive regard for the client's belief system is the foundation for the development of cultural competence and the provision of culturally suitable care.

It is generally accepted that the most crucial ingredient in the success of any treatment is the client–provider relationship, regardless of the treatment methods used. Technical skills are of great value, but their acceptability in the particular community requires leadership that is culturally sensitive, dedicated to serving the needs of all (particularly poor and marginalized individuals), committed to working in a team, and responsive to dialogue with the people being served (Rohde, 2002).

Seeking to understand the client within her or his own perceptual framework and showing compassion for the client's suffering are essential ingredients in any client–provider interaction. The ultimate benefit of striving toward cultural competence is the enrichment of experience and skill of the healthcare provider.

ONLINE LEARNING RESOURCES

www.acatcm.com
Alberta College of Acupuncture and Traditional Chinese Medicine

www.ascentmagazine.com
Ascent Magazine

www.osteopathiecollege.com
Canadian College of Osteopathy

www.cmcc.ca
Canadian Memorial Chiropractic College (CMCC)

www.ctcma.bc.ca
College of Traditional Chinese Medicine Practitioners and Acupuncturists of British Columbia

www.homeopathy.ca
The Canadian Academy of Homeopathy

www.ccachiro.org
The Canadian Chiropractic Association

www.ccnm.edu
The Canadian College of Naturopathic Medicine (CCNM)

www.aung.com
Dr. Steven Aung

www.thehealingspectrum.com
The Healing Spectrum

www.naho.ca
National Aboriginal Health Organization

www.numarkpharmacists.com
Numark Pharmacists

www.tm.org
The Transcendental Meditation (TM) Program

www.uqtr.ca
Université du Québec à Trois-Rivières (UQTR)

REFERENCES

Anonymous. (1976). Doctor, alcoholic, addict. In AA Services (Eds.), *Alcoholics Anonymous* (3rd ed., pp. 439–452). New York: Alcoholics Anonymous World Services, Inc.

Aung, S. H., Benjamin, S., Berman B., & Jacobs, J. (1997). Alternative medicine— Exploring other healthcare systems. *Patient Care Canada, 8*(12), 36–52.

Beiser, M. (2005). Reducing health disparities: A priority for Canada. *Canadian Journal of Public Health 96*(Suppl. 2), 4–5.

Bienfield, H. & Korngold, E. (1991). *Between heaven and earth—A guide to Chinese medicine*. Toronto: Random House, Inc.

Boon, H. (2002). Integrative health care: Defining and operationalizing the fundamental elements. University of Toronto. Retrieved November 20, 2004, from http://www.hc-sc.gc.ca/sr-sr/finance/hprp-prpms/final/2002-integrative_e.html

Borins, M. (1998). The dangers of using herbs—What your patients need to know. *Postgraduate Medicine, 104*(1), 91–100.

Bruyere, R. L. (1994). *Wheels of light*. New York: Simon & Schuster, Inc.

Canadian College of Naturopathic Medicine (2003). About CCNM. Retrieved November 25, 2004, from http://www.ccnm.edu/about.html

Cassidy, C. M. (1996). Cultural context of complementary and alternative medicine systems. In M. S. Micozzi (Ed.), *Fundamentals of complementary and alternative medicine* (pp. 9–34). New York: Churchill Livingstone Inc.

Chan-Yip, A. (2004). Health promotion and research in the Chinese community in Montreal: A model of culturally appropriate health care. *Paediatric Child Health, 9*(9), 627–629.

Corin, I. (1994) The social and cultural matrix of health and disease. In R. G. Evans, M. L. Barer, & T. R. Marmor (Eds.), *Why are some people healthy and others not? The determinants of health of populations* (pp. 93–132). Hawthorne, NY: Aldine de Gruyter.

Ergil, K.V. (1996). China's traditional medicine. In M. S. Micozzi (Ed.), *Fundamentals of complementary and alternative medicine* (pp. 185–224). New York: Churchill Livingstone Inc.

Gutowski, W. D. (2001). An experience. *Canadian Medical Association Journal, 164*(3), 385–386.

Hajela, R. (1994). Health, behaviour and disease: A bio-psycho-social spiritual perspective. In M. W. Rosenberg (Ed.), *Health and Behaviour 1994* (pp. 137–145). Kingston, ON: Queen's University.

Hajela, R. (2000). *Definitions in addiction medicine.* Kingston, ON: Canadian Society of Addiction Medicine.

Hancock, T., & Perkins F. (1985). The mandala of health: A conceptual model and teaching tool. *Health Education, 24*(1), 8–10.

Hoey, J. (1998). The arrogance of science and the pitfalls of hope. *Canadian Medical Association Journal, 159*(7), 803–804.

Jacobs, J., & Moskowitz R. (1996). Homeopathy. In M. S. Micozzi (Ed.), *Fundamentals of complementary and alternative medicine* (pp. 67–78). New York: Churchill Livingstone Inc.

Kelsall, D. L. (Ed.). (2004). Hot tips—Non-estrogen management of hot flashes. *Informed, 10*(4), 6–7.

Kirmayer, L. J. (2004). The cultural diversity of healing: Meaning, metaphor and mechanism. *British Medical Bulletin, 69*, 33–48.

Last, J. M. (1987). *Public health and human ecology.* East Norwalk, CT: Appleton & Lange.

Letendre, A. (2002). Aboriginal traditional medicine: Where does it fit? *Crossing Boundaries—An Interdisciplinary Journal, 1*(2), 78–87.

Leung, L. (2004). The Sino–Canadian perspective. *Parkhurst Exchange, September,* 23.

Lupin, A. J. (2001). The miracle. *Canadian Medical Association Journal, 164*(3), 383–385.

Lyons, A. S. (1987a). Hippocrates. In A. S. Lyons, & R. J. Petrucelli (Eds.), *Medicine: An illustrated history* (pp. 207–218). New York: Harry N. Abrams, Inc.

Lyons, A. S. (1987b). Medicine in Hippocratic times. In A. S. Lyons, & R. J. Petrucelli (Eds.), *Medicine: An illustrated history* (pp. 195–206). New York: Harry N. Abrams, Inc.

Lyons, A. S. (1987c). Infection. In A. S. Lyons, and R. J. Petrucelli (Eds.), *Medicine: An illustrated history* (pp. 549–564). New York: Harry N. Abrams, Inc.

Marmot, M. G., Syme, S. L., Kagan, A., Kato, H., Cohen, J. B., & Belsky J. (1975). Epidemiological studies of coronary heart disease and stroke in Japanese men living in Japan, Hawaii and California. Prevalence of coronary and hypertensive heart disease and associated risk factors. *American Journal of Epidemiology, 102*, 514–525.

McArthur, M. (1998). *Wisdom of the elements.* Freedom, CA: The Crossing Press, Inc.

Meserole, L. (1996). Western herbalism. In M. S. Micozzi (Ed.), *Fundamentals of complementary and alternative medicine* (pp. 111–120). New York: Churchill Livingstone Inc.

Millar, W. J. (1997). Use of alternative health care practitioners by Canadians. *Canadian Journal of Public Health, 88*(3), 154–158.

Mondloch, M. V., Cole, D. C., & Frank, J. W. (2001). Does how you do depend on how you think you'll do? A systematic review of the evidence for a relation between patients' recovery expectations and health outcomes. *Canadian Medical Association Journal, 165*(2), 174–179.

Morse, J., Young, D., & Swartz, L. (1991). Cree Indian healing practices and Western health care: A comparative analysis. *Social Science Medicine, 32*(12), 1361–1366.

Newman, M. A. (1986). *Health as expanding consciousness.* St Louis: Mosby.

Pederson, A., O'Neill, M., & Rootman, I. (1994). *Health promotion in Canada.* Toronto, ON: W. B. Saunders.

Pizzorno, J. E. (1996). Naturopathic medicine. In M. S. Micozzi (Ed.), *Fundamentals of complementary and alternative medicine* (pp. 163–181). New York: Churchill Livingstone Inc.

Redwood, D. (1996). Chiropractic. In M. S. Micozzi (Ed.), *Fundamentals of complementary and alternative medicine* (pp. 91–110). New York, NY: Churchill Livingstone Inc.

Rohde, J. (2002). Conclusion: Toward the next Alma-Ata. In J. Rohde, & J. Wyon (Eds.), *Community-based health care* (pp. 309–321). Boston, MA: Management Sciences for Health, Inc. (Harvard School of Public Health).

Rootman, I., Brown, I., Raphael, D., & Renwick, R. (1994). A new approach to conceptualizing and measuring quality of life. In M. W. Rosenberg (Ed.), *Health and behaviour 1994* (pp.179–187). Kingston, ON: Queen's University.

Royal Commission on Aboriginal Peoples. (1996). *Gathering Strength,* Volume III. Ottawa, ON: Minister of Supply and Services.

Sharma, H. (1996). Maharishi Ayurveda. In M. S. Micozzi (Ed.), *Fundamentals of complementary and alternative medicine* (pp. 243–257). New York: Churchill Livingstone Inc.

Sharma, H., & Clark, C. (1998). *Contemporary Ayurveda.* New York: Churchill Livingstone.

Sibbald, B. (2005). Alternative choice. *Canadian Medical Association Journal, 172*(9), 1170.

Slater, V. E. (1996). Healing touch. In M. S. Micozzi (Ed.), *Fundamentals of complementary and alternative medicine* (pp. 121–136). New York: Churchill Livingstone Inc.

Trotter, R. T. (1996). Curanderismo. In M. S. Micozzi (Ed.), *Fundamentals of complementary and alternative medicine* (pp. 259–277). New York: Churchill Livingstone Inc.

Wagner, G. N. (1996) Osteopathy. In M. S. Micozzi (Ed.), *Fundamentals of complementary and alternative medicine* (pp. 79–89). New York: Churchill Livingstone Inc.

Zysk, K. G. (1996). Traditional Ayurveda. In M. S. Micozzi (Ed.), *Fundamentals of complementary and alternative medicine* (pp. 233–242). New York: Churchill Livingstone Inc.

Specific Cultural Considerations

In this section, which examines cultural considerations in specific populations, individual authors highlight how culture shapes the issues in the context of their practice. The discussion is not exhaustive and should be considered as a starting point toward achieving cultural competence in caring for specific populations. The chapters also show a variety of ways that populations can be grouped, which reflects the reality of our healthcare services. Sometimes healthcare services are organized by clinical specialties; at other times by clinical issues, such as pain management or developmental stage of life (e.g., prenatal, children, elderly); and on occasion by special populations, such as immigrant women.

This section shows that the specific cultural knowledge that will be most useful to healthcare providers depends on the nature of their practice and the population they serve. Key concepts such as family, communication, and decision making are raised in several chapters, illustrating once again the need to bring an understanding of generic cultural knowledge to the specific populations.

Chapters 9 and 10 present a developmental approach with respect to life stages. The authors raise issues that are critical to consider at the beginning of life (perinatal period) and end of life, but they also stress the importance of seeking out and applying cultural knowledge geared to individual clients. In Chapter 11, the authors discuss cultural considerations specific to one clinical area of practice: mental health. Some of the issues they raise are similar to those for other populations; however, they also highlight issues that are specific to mental health. Similar approaches can be taken with other clinical populations, though, such as those in cardiac care and oncology.

The population under discussion in Chapter 12 is very broad. Although there are services specific to the care of women in general and immigrant women in particular, healthcare providers encounter immigrant women across practice areas. The authors here have highlighted key issues that will need consideration. Healthcare providers working with immigrant women need to understand how the identity of individual clients intersects with ethnicity and other characteristics, along with the demands of the illness and care processes.

Chapter 13 also discusses a population that exists across practice areas, but this time the focus is on a clinical issue. As the author notes in her opening paragraph, pain is a universal human experience. The chapter goes on to examine how culture influences the meaning, expression, and response to pain.

Finally, Chapter 14 builds upon the discussion of complementary and alternative therapies contained in Chapter 8. The first half of the chapter presents an overview of complementary therapies, while the second offers a glimpse into the author's practice as a complementary therapy practitioner. Cultural competence is about exploring and examining what we see with our own eyes as well as through another's cultural lens.

CHAPTER 9

The Beginning of Life (The Perinatal Period)

NANCY WATTS AND CLAIRE McDONALD

Several contributors shared their experience and expertise in the preparation of this chapter: Lori Robson, RN, PNC(C) in Mother Baby Care at London Health Sciences Centre (LHSC); Valerie Rousom, RN, Director of NICU at St. Joseph's Health Care London; and Kathy Wodrich RN, PNC(C), Co-ordinator of the Birthing Centre at LHSC. Special thanks to Elaine Pollett, RN, MScN, Client Centred Care Consultant, LHSC, for contributing to and co-ordinating the group effort.

Gratitude is also expressed to the women whose narratives or examples appear in the chapter. The women participated in a one-day workshop titled the Integrating Cultural Diversity Conference, held in June 2004, in London, Ontario, and generously shared their experiences and ideas with perinatal and family-centred care nurses from the area. The names that appear in the chapter have been changed to protect the womens' identities, and only first names are used per the conference.

LEARNING OBJECTIVES

At the end of this chapter, the learner will be able to:

- Explore an assessment plan that addresses the role culture plays in the perinatal experience of women and their families
- Understand the importance of cultural norms, values, and preferences as the basis for providing culturally appropriate perinatal care
- Identify methods for providing culturally appropriate care during the perinatal period
- Identify the importance of culture in the grief experience of parents and families during the perinatal period

KEY TERMS

Birth plan

Birth stories

Bonding/infant attachment

Cultural reciprocity

Female circumcision

Perinatal loss

Perinatal period

Culture and care are holistic ideas that can help us get to know and understand women and their families and assist them in attaining full and meaningful lives (Leininger, 2002). Pregnancy, childbirth, and the transition to the role of parent are a time of both joy and suffering—physically as well as emotionally—for women and families. The **perinatal period** is medically defined as the time between the twenty-eighth week of gestation and the end of the first week after birth. Wallerstedt, Lilley, and Baldwin (2003) indicate that they regard the perinatal period as beginning at conception and continuing through a child's first year. For the purpose of this chapter, the perinatal period includes pregnancy through the first 28 days of a newborn's life.

Around the world, healthcare providers work with populations, families, and individual clients to promote and support people's capacity for coping with health challenges and maintaining well-being (Willis, 1999). In Canada, they work with women and families of different races, socio-economic backgrounds, and sexual orientation, as well as members of many ethnic groups. Healthcare providers are in a unique position to provide culturally integrated care to women and their families throughout the perinatal period. This chapter outlines an approach to assessing women and their families during the perinatal period, identifying their care needs, and suggesting ways of addressing those needs in a culturally appropriate way. It also presents an approach to assist parents and families who experience loss during this time.

Assessment

Family-centred care supports the family as the primary source of knowledge about what is best for them as they work in collaboration with healthcare providers to plan care (Willis, 1999). Many hospitals encourage pregnant clients to attend pre-admission programs. This early contact provides clients with the opportunity to share their expectations about their pregnancy and the birthing process with staff. At the same time, clinical staff can begin the assessment that forms the basis for providing appropriate care. Each pregnant client is assessed to determine her health status, with the focus being on her physical and psychosocial health.

As a means of providing more holistic care, this chapter provides an assessment guide for healthcare providers to use in planning and delivering culturally competent care. See Table 9-1 and the following discussion of the questions listed in the table.

How can we best communicate with you? Do you wish to have an interpreter?
Communication between a client and her healthcare provider is extremely important during pregnancy. Many women who are recent immigrants to Canada have been separated from family and friends; therefore, they are potentially separated from their sources of information and support. While some have developed new relationships and support systems, others find this difficult, particularly if they do not speak English, have limited education, or are isolated from a community of women (Lynam, Gurm, & Dhari, 2000). A client and her family may value an interpreter as someone who can help them negotiate their way through the

TABLE 9-1

Perinatal Cultural Assessment Guide*

1. How can we best communicate with you? Do you wish to have an interpreter?
2. What does being pregnant mean to you? To your family? (E.g., Is knowing the gender of your baby important to you? Do you have a birth story to share?)
3. How are you meeting your healthcare needs during your pregnancy? (E.g., Do you have a family physician, midwife, *doula*?** Do you have a preference for a female or male caregiver?)
4. What are you doing to take care of yourself during your pregnancy? Are there certain activities you prefer to do during your pregnancy? Activities you would rather avoid? Are there certain foods you prefer to eat during your pregnancy? Foods you would rather avoid? Who will most actively support you during your pregnancy? How will you make decisions? Who will attend prenatal appointments with you?)
5. Do you have a birth plan? If not, do you wish to develop one? (E.g., Who will support you during labour? How do you prefer to cope with pain? Who will be with you during your baby's birth? How do you imagine labour? What are your preferences for birth? Who will cut the cord? How do you want your baby presented to you?)
6. Have you developed a plan for after your baby's birth? (E.g., How do you plan to feed your baby? Are there foods or food temperatures you prefer after your baby's birth? Are there customs you wish us to be aware of, after your baby's birth, while you are in hospital? Have you made plans for discharge? Who will help you with the baby after you go home? How will you get rest after you go home with your baby? What information do you require about caring for your baby?)
7. Do you wish/require information about family planning/birth control?

*This is a general guide for assessment. Details about specific tools developed for clinical use appear later in Chapter 9 (see, e.g., Table 9-2, "Key Information to Include in a Birth Plan").
**A *doula* is a woman who helps, advises, and provides emotional support to another woman during and just after pregnancy.

healthcare system and also decrease their risk of being embarrassed by miscommunication. This can be critical to a client's motivation to attend prenatal visits and to her understanding of the reasons for care.

For many female clients, having a female interpreter is very important when discussing reproductive functions (Mattson, 2000). Locating resource people who speak the major languages poses a challenge to the healthcare system. There also may be a need for interpreters who can speak the various dialects within a language. Among the eleven major Aboriginal Canadian groups, there are 58 identifiable dialects (Prodan-Bhalla, 2001). It is important to involve a knowledgeable interpreter who can understand and translate the words as well as the concepts behind them, and who also understands the culture. For example, among some Aboriginal Canadians, long silences and gaps in conversation are used for reflection. It is important for healthcare providers to not interpret these silences as indifference (Prodan-Bhalla, 2001). Healthcare providers can refer clients to community resources and public health early in pregnancy, to ensure optimal health. Many public health units have successfully recruited women from different cultural groups as lay home visitors. While they are not professional healthcare workers, they are trained to provide support and encouragement to families. Pairing recent immigrants with family or lay home visitors who speak the same language can be extremely beneficial where this service is available.

With the advent of new technology such as integrative prenatal screening (IPS) tests for spina bifida and Down's syndrome, it also is important to include family members when communicating information. Written information that is available in many languages may assist a client and family to understand the testing procedures and interpretation of the results.

What does being pregnant mean to you? To your family? (E.g., Is knowing the gender of your baby important to you or to your family? Do you have a birth story to share?)

For many clients, pregnancy is a long-awaited and planned event. For others, it is unplanned, unexpected, and/or unwanted. How clients and their families view pregnancy varies among cultural groups. In some cultures, women experience special status during pregnancy; Iranian women, for example, achieve a great deal of prestige at this time, especially at the birth of their first child, and particularly if that child is male (Purnell & Paulanka, 2003). "Naiomi," who is from Sudan, told participants at a recent healthcare conference (details mentioned in chapter acknowledgement) that in her culture, women experience childbirth as an expectation.[1]

Families who immigrate to Canada bring with them their beliefs about pregnancy and childbirth. These beliefs and practices affect the way in which they experience this major life event. In addition to being immigrants, some clients and their families have arrived in Canada as refugees. Their experiences can have a major role in the way they perceive and cope with pregnancy (Battaglini et al., 2001). Women may feel themselves to be in conflict with the dominant customs and traditions they encounter within the healthcare system. Healthcare providers have an obligation to conduct assessments and work with all families so that their expectations can be addressed. It is important that expectations are documented on the health record and that ways of addressing concerns and preferences are reached through a collaborative approach.

Across cultures, women share powerful memories of their birthing experiences with others as a way of integrating the significance of birth into their lives (Callister, 2004). They will share them with healthcare providers, if invited to do so. The rich data contained in these **birth stories** can provide strong guidance to those caring for women clients during the perinatal period.

With the availability of advanced technology, some women and families ask to know the gender of the fetus through ultrasound testing. Others, including many women of Arabic origin, may be reluctant to know the sex of the baby before birth, believing that no one knows what is in a woman's womb but God (Kridli, 2002). In many cultures there are large celebrations for infants, and this

---

[1]In this chapter, first names only are used consistently to protect privacy.

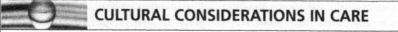

CULTURAL CONSIDERATIONS IN CARE

Birth Story: It's a Girl (Again)!
Faduma is a midwife from Saudi Arabia who faced a difficult situation while assisting a woman who desperately wanted her baby to be a boy because she already had several little girls.

When the client gave birth to yet another baby girl, Faduma says, she set the newborn aside for as long as she could and kept telling the client she had given birth to a "beautiful, healthy baby." She shared that the baby was a girl only when the client pressed her for the information. Her reasons for doing this were to give the mother time to stabilize physically before she received what she would consider disappointing news. Faduma reported that this was common practice among midwives in her country.

is particularly the case for male infants born into culture where men have higher status than women. A male infant may be given preferential standing because of his potential ability to provide physical labour, carry on the family name (as in a patriarchal society), and add to the political strength of the extended family.

The ability of a woman to provide a male heir also can increase her value and sense of worth, just as failing to meet these expectations can result in depression and affect her self-esteem. Many Arab families greet the birth of a boy with rejoicing and celebration, while the birth of a girl is received with more emotional restraint, and possibly sadness. Distributing sweets is common after birth, with more expensive candies given after the birth of a male child (Purnell & Paulanka, 2003). Some women and families perceive female infants as burdens, due to their need for protection or a future dowry. In cultures that promote arranged marriage, this may be a financial burden. However, in these cultures female infants can also be perceived more positively as the entry of a goddess into the home and family.

In other cultures, male and female infants are viewed as unique individuals who contribute equally to society. Understanding the client's and family's perception of the role of gender helps the healthcare provider prepare to provide support if needed, based on expectations at the time of birth. Healthcare providers may observe disappointment in clients or families who learn that their baby is not the gender they preferred. The caregiver may believe that the most important consideration is the birth of a healthy baby, regardless of gender. These situations demonstrate the need for caregivers to suspend their expectations and show respect for every family's preferences.

How are you meeting your healthcare needs during your pregnancy?
(E.g., Do you have a family physician, midwife, **doula***? Do you have a*
preference for a female or male caregiver?)
Many Canadian women begin their prenatal care before conception, by taking early steps to promote well-being during pregnancy. Such comprehensive care can include starting to take folic acid supplements to decrease the risk of neural

tube defects, and discussing potential family planning and/or genetic screening. Women who begin their prenatal visits later in their pregnancies do so for a number of reasons. Few Somali immigrants seek prenatal care until they begin to understand their new country and learn about the importance of health care during pregnancy (Davidhizar & Giger, 1998). The view of pregnancy as a time of wellness and health also may influence a woman's decision to delay seeking prenatal care early in her pregnancy.

Women who experience backache, fatigue, strain, worry, headache, morning sickness, and sleeping problems may perceive these as normal to pregnancy, while others see these as a reason to seek prenatal care (Bondas & Eriksson, 2001). Healthcare providers also need to ask about each client's health and/or specific concerns. Providing culturally sensitive rationales may assist clients/ families in understanding the benefits of prenatal visits.

Immigrant women may have difficulty accessing the healthcare system. Language barriers, lack of health coverage for recent immigrants, and a shortage of physicians may contribute to a delay in seeking prenatal care. After clients initiate care, there may still be barriers to their receiving the type and quality of care they require. Access to a female healthcare provider may be a preference for many women clients, especially Arab women. Attending a clinic that is staffed by both female and male physicians can thus provide constant challenges to those wishing to maintain privacy and modesty. Access to care by female midwives can help to eliminate these barriers. By mid-2006, four Canadian provinces were licensing midwives, who provide the full range of perinatal services. This enables women in these provinces to choose the caregiver they prefer.

What are you doing to take care of yourself during your pregnancy?
Are there certain activities you prefer to do during your pregnancy?
Activities you would rather avoid? Are there certain foods you prefer to eat during your pregnancy? Foods you would rather avoid? Who will actively support you during your pregnancy? How will you make decisions?
Who will attend prenatal appointments with you?
In most societies, there is an active interest in the health of a woman during pregnancy. The reason for this may be to protect the unborn child. Some cultural groups have prescriptive and restrictive beliefs for maternal behaviours during the childbearing period. Prescriptive practices identify actions a woman should take to have a health pregnancy and a healthy baby. In Canada, women are encouraged to seek prenatal health care early in pregnancy. Restrictive belief practices are behaviours that women are advised to avoid in order to ensure a healthy baby and/or childbirth experience. For example, Mexican women are discouraged from walking in the moonlight during pregnancy, due to its association with birth deformities (Purnell & Paulanka, 2003). Other practices are identified as likely to harm the baby or mother.

A woman named May Ling, who had recently immigrated to Canada from Northern China (see feature box "Birth Story: Cold Comfort"), reported at a healthcare conference (details mentioned in chapter acknowledgement) that if she had been in China during her pregnancy, she would have been encouraged to rest much of the time. In contrast, Naiomi from Sudan said that she was expected to continue working until active labour began. Healthcare providers can use open-ended questions to achieve a better understanding of health practices that are encouraged or discouraged by the client's or family's cultural group.

Sharing meals with family and friends is an important activity for women in most cultural groups. Food preparation is seen as a way of expressing love and friendship (Purnell & Paulanka, 2003). Nutrition in pregnancy is closely tied to a woman's weight gain. Guidelines for food and fluid intake during pregnancy have been developed in *Canada's Food Guide*. The focus for pregnant women includes an increased intake of the following:

- Whole grain and enriched products
- Dark green and orange vegetables and fruit
- Lower-fat milk products
- Leaner meats, poultry, and fish
- Dried peas, beans, and lentils
  (Health Canada, 1999)

Dietary practices differ among women in various cultural groups. *Canada's Food Guide* has recently undergone changes to better reflect the dietary preferences of various cultural groups.

During pregnancy, Chinese women increase their intake of meat because of a belief that their blood needs to be stronger for the fetus (Purnell & Paulanka, 2003). Korean women are expected to abstain from duck, chicken, fish with scales, and crab, as these may affect the child's appearance (Purnell & Paulanka, 2003). Exploring these beliefs with women prenatally will help the healthcare provider to understand clients' dietary intake and provide suitable instruction if health problems indicate that dietary changes are appropriate. It is important to have knowledge of the type of foods that women eat, to ensure that their nutritional needs are being met. Particular foods may also be used for managing symptoms associated with pregnancy. Where health needs dictate, clients can be referred to community or hospital-based dieticians.

Women from many cultural groups use herbal remedies and teas as therapy during pregnancy. Use of these teas depends on cultural acceptance and a woman's understanding of their purpose. Healthcare providers need information about alternative therapies to assess for potential adverse health effects for the client or baby.

Some clients prefer to be the primary decision maker regarding their care during pregnancy. Others involve family members, specifically their partners, and still others involve female members of the extended family. Social support provides a feeling of belonging and safety. A client's sense of community may determine who attends appointments with her (Health Canada, 2002). Some clients may perceive that they are better supported when their partners are actively involved throughout the care process, attending prenatal visits and testing procedures.

Do you have a birth plan? If not, do you wish to develop one? (E.g., Who will support you during labour? How do you prefer to cope with pain? Who will be with you during your baby's birth? How do you imagine labour? What are your preferences for birth? Who will cut the cord? How do you want your baby presented to you?)
This is a large issue that is addressed over several pages.

The Birth Plan

Research has been done on women's expectations, hopes and dreams for labour, birth, and postpartum months, and on their actual experiences (Health Canada, 2002). The satisfaction that women feel in respect to labour and birth is tied to the extent to which their expectations are met during the childbirth experience. As a result, the client and/or her family are encouraged to write their preferences for labour and birth in a **birth plan** so that healthcare providers can integrate the details into their care (see Table 9-2). The expectation that healthcare providers will collaborate in developing these plans emphasizes the importance and value placed on clients' and families' preferences for care.

A birth plan may cover such diverse areas as the following:
- Preference for the gender of the healthcare provider
- Pain management details
- Options for birthing positions
- The role of the support person(s) for labour or birth
- Preferences about cutting the umbilical cord at birth

Whispering a prayer into the newborn's ear may be an important welcome from a Muslim father. If healthcare providers are aware of this, it can be included in the plan of care (Roberts, 2002).

Current expectations in Western society include the pregnant client having a "support" person who comes and stays with her in a private labour room until

TABLE 9-2

Key Information to Include in a Birth Plan

1. What would you like us to know about you or your family's wishes, concerns, preferences, and fears about your labour and your baby's birth?

2. How are you going to prepare for your labour and birth? (E.g., attend classes, tour the hospital, read, view audiovisual material?)

3. The people who will be present for my labour are _____.

4. My wishes for pain management are _____.

5. The people who will be present for my baby's birth are _____.

6. The position or positions I prefer for my baby's birth are _____.

7. Immediately after my baby is born, I wish the following to be done_____.

birth is complete. In most Canadian hospitals, a nurse or midwife will stay with each client throughout her labour. In addition, family members and friends may stay, hoping to be present for the actual birth. Limiting the number of support people may be a hardship based on a client's need for "community presence" at her birth (Molina, 2001).

In China, for example, eight women may labour together in a single room with no family members for support. Liu and Moore (2000) describe the loneliness experienced among women in this situation. Orthodox Jewish women rely on female family members or close friends to provide support during labour and birth. The Orthodox Jewish husband is prohibited from touching his wife during labour or viewing the actual birth (Semenic, Callister, & Feldman, 2004). Immigrants who have personally experienced or been told stories about birthing practices in other countries may be anxious about unfamiliar practices they encounter in a Canadian hospital. The presence of a midwife can normalize the experience for many women who are familiar with female healthcare providers. Healthcare providers can assess each client's preferences for support and collaborate with her to meet these needs.

Pain Management

Childbirth has been described as a "major pain experience that accompanies the normal physiologic process of giving birth" (Callister, Khalaf, Semenic, Kartchner, & Vehvilainen-Julkunen, 2003, p. 145). Although birth is characterized by pain, it often is considered one of a woman's most positive life events. Childbirth pain also is a unique experience for each woman. Some women describe a sense of achievement and feeling of pride in their ability to cope with the pain. Finnish women often describe themselves as confident in their ability to give birth, viewing childbirth as a normal process (Callister et al., 2003).

Cultural values and beliefs shape the way clients cope with the pain and make decisions (Willis, 1999). Understanding the cultural meaning of pain is important in the care of each individual woman and family (see Chapter 13 for a closer look at this issue). A discussion with each woman regarding her perception of pain, her ability to cope, and her preferences for pain management and supportive or comfort measures is important to providing culturally appropriate care. Healthcare providers can offer comfort throughout labour in a variety of ways. Pain does not have to be eliminated for women to be comforted or to feel supported in their choices, and this decreases anxiety (Callister et al., 2003).

Another source of pain during pregnancy, labour, and birth is **female circumcision**. This practice is most common in Islamic countries but is not based on religious teachings (Davidhizar & Giger, 1998). The purpose of female circumcision is to preserve virginity, ensure marriageability, and contain sexuality. Actual procedures are completed between the ages of 9 and 12 years and range from a basic clitoridectomy (partial or complete removal of the clitoris) to complete infibulation (i.e., suturing of the labia majora, often after a clitoridectomy) (Davidhizar & Giger, 1998). Circumcision may make pelvic examinations painful, and labour and birth very difficult. Caregivers may not know in advance if a woman has been circumcised. It is important to remain non-judgemental and aware that a woman may view female circumcision as acceptable (Heatherly, 2000). The challenge also is to determine the appropriate pain management methods.

Expression of pain is another element that may be linked to cultural norms. In some cultures, verbal expression is expected and encouraged; women gain support from their faith, and may pray and cry. For other cultural groups, verbal expression may be limited so that the woman can preserve her energy for the second stage and pushing; the client would therefore be expected to remain very quiet during labour, and making loud noise could be considered shameful (Callister et al., 2003). Healthcare providers may find observation of these different expressions of pain difficult to interpret, and observation alone may not provide all the information needed to assess pain. Collaborating with each woman to determine her experience of the pain and her preferences for pain management is critical to providing good client- or family-centred care (Gerteis, Edgman-Levitan, Daley, & Delbianco, 1993).

Touch

Touch is a form of non-verbal communication that carries cultural perceptions. Some cultures are described as "high touch," while others are considered more reserved. Clarifying the meaning and desire for touch by a healthcare provider is extremely important to the relationship with the woman and family. Holding the woman's hand, patting or rubbing her back, and wiping her forehead are all possible ways to use touch and may increase the feeling or perception of support.

The touch sensation is perceived along similar nerve pathways as pain. A touch that is unexpected or unexplained can be very distressing to a woman in labour. Filipino women may increase their trust in the caregiver if a gentle touch is offered (Pasco, Morse, & Olsen, 2004). This is seen as a sign of respect. During the assessment phase, it is important to determine the type of touch seen as helpful.

The Birth

Perceptions of the birth experience also are influenced by the environment and circumstances of the pregnancy and birth. Whether this child and/or pregnancy was planned or wanted will affect the perception of the birth process for any woman. Callister et al. (2003) describe various perceptions of childbirth that include the following:

- A test of womanhood
- A test of personal competence
- A peak experience
- The first act of motherhood

Giving birth may be viewed as a time when women feel love as an empowering experience. The pain that culminates in the birth of a child may be perceived as a challenge to be overcome (Callister et al., 2003). The birth of a first child also may alter the woman's status within the family and community.

Based on cultural norms, clients may prefer positions for birth that differ from the Canadian standard. In some cultures, for example, squatting is a preferred position that has been associated with increased gravitational forces and a shorter second stage of labour. This position is infrequently used in Canadian hospitals if epidural anaesthesia is used. The more common semi-sitting position with a woman's legs in stirrups is a more open and potentially exposed position for giving birth and may be uncomfortable for those seeking modesty and privacy.

In Canada, Caesarean delivery rates increased to 21.2 percent in 2000–01, from 18.2 percent of hospital deliveries in 1991–92 (Health Canada, 2003). Statistics indicate that this increase is related to many factors:

- Convenience
- A previous Caesarean birth
- Breech position
- Medical legal considerations
- A woman's choice

Bonding, also known as **infant attachment,** is defined as the sensitive period after birth when parents have close contact with infants, to assist in the development of emotional relationships (Lowdermilk & Perry, 2003). In Canada, early mother–infant bonding is encouraged. In many families, however, the mother is expected to rest in the early days after giving birth, and the infant is cared for by the extended family. This may create conflict between staff expectations and family expectations. The boxed feature "Birth Story: The 'Slimy, Wriggling' Infant" illustrates how cultural differences can affect perceptions of the birth experience.

Healthcare providers often assess mother/parent/infant bonding by observing face-to-face contact. They may encourage this activity with families. This would be in direct opposition to the beliefs of some women and families who deliberately do not engage in face-to-face contact initially, to protect their infant from evil spirits. They also may perceive a compliment on their baby's appearance as detrimental to this infant's ability to develop humility. Determining expectations and preferences of the mother or family in advance offers the opportunity to address these issues.

 CULTURAL CONSIDERATIONS IN CARE

Birth Story: The "Slimy, Wriggling" Infant

Leona moved to Canada from El Salvador several years ago, while pregnant with her second child. She spoke little English and had no family present for her labour and birth—her husband was at home with their older child.

Leona explained that when her baby was born, the physician laid him on her abdomen. She took one look at the "slimy, wriggling" baby and promptly "passed out." She remembered waking up in her room some time later.

In El Salvador, she reported, a newborn is washed and wrapped in a blanket before being presented to the mother. She said the "Canadian" approach made the birthing experience much more traumatic than she had expected. Several years later, Leona was able to laugh at the memory, but she did not laugh at the time of her son's birth.

The umbilical cord and placenta are normally discarded by the hospital after birth; however, they are important to Aboriginal families because these products of conception reflect Earth and nature. Assisting with the transport of these items, so that the family can bury them or hang them on a tree, is extremely honouring to this cultural group (Molina, 2001).

Some families name their babies before birth, some in the first few moments of life, and others at a ceremony 30 days later. For some, it is important to not speak the baby's name until an official ceremony. The Canadian healthcare and legal systems, which focus on documentation, make the traditional custom of naming an infant challenging for these families. It is important to reinforce that this decision is the family's choice. The main problem is that without official documentation, the infant may not be able to travel outside Canada with ease.

Have you developed a plan for after your baby's birth? (E.g., How do you plan to feed your baby? Are there foods or food temperatures you would prefer after your baby's birth? Are there customs you wish us to be aware of, after your baby's birth, while you are in hospital? Have you made plans for discharge? Who will help you with the baby after you go home? How will you get rest after you go home with your baby? What information do you require about caring for your baby?)
The questions above are addressed below.

Postpartum Phase

After birth, some women feel tired and in need of rest, while others are excited and full of energy. For those clients who view labour and birth as natural processes, the recovery period will focus on physical changes leading to a restoration of health and wellness. Lynam, Gurm, and Dhari (2000) describe the first 40 days after birth as a time for new mothers to focus on their infants, recover physically from birth, and regain their strength. For mothers and babies who observe this custom, one potential benefit may be seen as a decreased exposure to airborne diseases and infections. Other women view the postpartum period as a time of illness. Korean women and families, for example, tend to see the new mother as sick, requiring care and assistance in all tasks and activities (Olds, London, & Ladewig, 2000).

In certain cultures, there is a mandatory period of rest for the mother following birth. For example, Cuban mothers are encouraged to rest for about four weeks after giving birth because of concerns that walking or moving around (ambulation), being exposed to cold, and having bare feet place the mother at risk for infection (Purnell & Paulanka, 2003). Many Chinese women are encouraged to rest for several weeks (Shah, 2004). The expectation of a postpartum rest period for mothers therefore ranges from a few days (Cuban culture) to several weeks (Chinese and South Asian women). Ideally, during this rest period female relatives provide the maternal and infant care. In the case of recent immigrants with little or no support, new fathers or partners with no experience may be required to take on this care. Including them in all postpartum educational activities is very important, to ensure their understanding of maternal and infant care. However, healthcare providers must recognize that some fathers will accept the new role with reluctance and mixed feelings, while others will embrace it with enthusiasm. Possible ways of dealing with this phase should be negotiated with family members. Healthcare providers who want to provide culturally appropriate health care could find it helpful to talk to their clients about the need for rest and the benefits of ambulation and baby care. Healthcare providers also need to be knowledgeable about resources within the community that may be available to all new families and to specific cultural groups.

Recovery after birth for the new mother includes the normal process of uterine involution. For some women, lochia is precious and seen as an important cleansing process that assists in recovery (Molina, 2001). It may be difficult for a new mother to determine if postpartum vaginal bleeding is excessive. A woman may choose a traditional method of treatment for this first and turn to a medical facility only if heavy bleeding persists (Thaddeus & Nangalia, 2004). Among the information given to new mothers, the health provider can include a time frame for postpartum follow-up as well as a list of danger signs.

The postpartum stage can be a time of worry, isolation, and depression for some women, and this can impair their ability to care for their infants. Women who are separated from their support systems or have a previous history of mental illness will benefit from a comprehensive postpartum assessment to determine their risk for postpartum depression. The intense social support that extended families and friends offer in some cultures may decrease suffering at this stage, which has been described as a time of intense misery (Bondas & Eriksson, 2001). Some researchers are exploring the possible protective effects offered by various ethnocultural childbirth rituals, in terms of preventing postpartum depression (Ross, Dennis, Robertson, Blackmore, & Stewart, 2005). Community approaches

CULTURAL CONSIDERATIONS IN CARE

Birth Story: Cold Comfort

May Ling immigrated to Canada from Northern China when she was six months pregnant. She and her husband had no family here and knew only one of her husband's colleagues. When she gave birth to her son, she reported being very concerned because she was cold.

Her concern about feeling cold was complicated by the hospital staff offering her ice water to drink. Her wish was for many blankets and only heated liquids. May Ling said the nurses and doctors did not seem to understand the importance of keeping cool air (which she saw as a source of potential illness) from blowing on her and her baby. She had acquired these preferences from listening to the birth stories of women in her home community.

May Ling faced other cultural differences in the childbearing experience. If she had been in China, for example, she would have spent about seven weeks in bed after leaving the hospital, and her son would have been cared for by other women. As her husband had to return to work immediately, this was not possible.

to promoting well-being can include home visiting, parenting groups, and prescription medication if needed.

Until relatively recently, infant care in Canada usually was delegated to the mother. The traditional role of a father or male partner has been seen as provider for the family. This role has evolved to a current expectation that fathers will be more involved with their infants (de Montigny & Lecharite, 2004). Increasingly, Canadian fathers and/or same-sex partners are more active participants in newborn care, and in many instances they share the maternity or parental leave.

Some women receive offers of support from extended family members. The new parents may see this as a mixed blessing, for at least two reasons:

1. Differing levels of acculturation between the parents and the extended family can be a source of conflict.
2. Familial role expectations may add additional demands on the new parents.

A woman named Nita told Integrating Cultural Diversity healthcare conference-goers that her parents moved in with her and her husband following the birth of their first baby. The new parents found it a challenge to balance the support offered by her parents with their need to be independent and learn about parenting on their own. Nevertheless, Nita said it was possible in the end to address everyone's needs—after considerable self-reflection and sensitivity.

Client- or family-centred care promotes the concept of choice, and healthcare providers should ensure that women can make informed choices about infant nutrition information. This is another area rich in cultural beliefs and values. Discussing the benefits of colostrum and breastfeeding may help this client or her family make informed choices. Breastfeeding is the norm among some women, while others may prefer bottle-feeding—even viewing it as a sign of affluence (Lynam, Gurm, & Dhari, 2000). Based on cultural or family information, some women expect to bottle-feed their babies for the first few days, until their milk comes in. Colostrum may be regarded as a "hot (i.e., spicy) food" which, if consumed, could disrupt the baby's equilibrium or harm the baby (Lynam, Gurm, & Dhari, 2000). Others believe that colostrum is "old milk" that is unfit for newborn infants and should be expressed and disposed of until the milk comes in on day two or three (Riordan & Gill-Hopple, 2001). The healthcare provider should not assume that a woman is uninterested in attaching to her baby if she does not breastfeed. She may be following the advice and behaviour passed to her through many generations (Mattson, 2000). Exploring her knowledge about what is right or best to do, while sharing professional knowledge, will allow for a broader range of alternatives and lead to informed choices regarding care.

Healthcare providers begin preparation for discharge during pregnancy. Table 9-3 provides an example of a mother–baby after birth care plan. These plans can be reviewed and altered, if necessary, as soon as a baby is born. During the time of recovery, there may be specific foods that new mothers prefer, while others are to be avoided. In all cultures, an emphasis on liquids during this time is extremely beneficial for breastfeeding women. Some women prefer warm broths to cold liquids. Some herbal teas used to promote milk production can cause intestinal irritation in the infant. Healthcare providers need to explore dietary practices with each woman, to determine which methods will suit both the mother and her baby.

TABLE 9-3

Mother/Baby Care Plan

1. My feeding plan for my baby is _____.

2. I prefer the following (foods or food temperatures) after my baby is born _____.

3. I prefer that you do the following while my baby is in the hospital _____.

4. _____ will help me care for my baby when I return home.

5. I will get the rest I need by _____.

6. I wish to know more about _____, so I can care for my baby at home.

7. The main concern I have about being at home with my baby is _____.

Do you wish/require information about family planning/birth control?
Cultural values and beliefs influence the choices a client makes regarding family-planning methods and returning for a postpartum visit (Jones, Bond, Gardner, & Hernandez, 2002). Describing this visit as beneficial to health and terming it a "well-woman" appointment may increase attendance (Jones et al., 2002). Linking the health of the client to her family's health, particularly to the health of her children, can result in her placing more importance on the process of seeking care.

The topic of contraception can pose a significant challenge for many clients and healthcare providers. Providing the services of a cultural interpreter and written material in a woman's language may ensure that she has adequate information regarding contraception and the various methods available to her. Building on her own knowledge and filling in the gaps is critical to a woman's decision making regarding her unique needs and preferences. Healthcare providers can discuss the benefits of a recovery time between pregnancies in terms of clients' physical well-being (Kridli, 2002). Showing understanding and respect while enabling informed choice are important aspects of client- and family-centred care for women of any culture.

Perinatal Loss

Perinatal loss is defined as an unwanted end of pregnancy during the 40 weeks of gestation (through miscarriage or stillbirth) or during the first 28 days of life (the neonatal period), and it is estimated to occur in 20 to 25 percent of all conceptions (Côté-Arsenault, 2003). In Canada in 1997, perinatal conditions were the greatest single cause of infant death, accounting for 46 percent of all such deaths. Birth defects accounted for another 27 percent (Canadian Institute of Child Health, 2000). These statistics illustrate the harsh reality that throughout pregnancy and after birth there are many times when grief and loss can occur (see Table 9-4).

Technological advances, combined with ultrasound pictures, are making earlier bonding and attachment possible by allowing increasingly earlier confirmation of

TABLE 9-4

Perinatal Situations in Which Grief Reaction Is Expected

I   Pregnancy
II Birth
   a) Normal
   b   Caesarean section
   c) Forceps
   d) Episiotomy
   e) Medicated
   f) Prolonged or short labour
   g) Place of birth
III Postpartum
   a) "Postpartum blues"
   b) Depression
   c) Psychosis
IV Abortion
   a) Spontaneous
   b) Therapeutic
   c) Elective
   d) Selective (for reasons such as genetic illness)
   e) Selective reduction (for multiple gestation)
V   Stillbirth
VI Loss of the perfect child
   a) Premature
   b) "Anomalied" (i.e., deformed) baby
   c) Sick newborn
   d) "Wrong" sex
VII Neonatal death
VIII Relinquishment (for adoption or to authorities)

From "Grief and perinatal loss," by G. B. Merenstein and S. L. Gardner. In G. B. Merenstein and S. L. Gardner (Eds.), *Handbook of neonatal intensive care* (5th ed., p. 755), 2002, St. Louis: Mosby. Reprinted with permission.

pregnancy and fetal health status. Therefore, perinatal grief can be experienced earlier as well. Perinatal death is an event for which parents are often ill prepared because it rarely is discussed in detail in education offered to women and families during pregnancy and childbirth (Malacrida, 1999).

Perinatal grief is seen as the most intense and overwhelming of all grief (Davies, 2004). It may be a response to several factors:
- The loss of a wished-for child
- The loss of innocence about pregnancy
- The damage to a woman's self-confidence about her ability to become a mother

(Côté-Arsenault & Morrison-Beedy, 2001)

A loss also may relate to the perception of the meaning of pregnancy for the woman and her family. It has been reported that 73 percent of women who experience a miscarriage or early loss believe their fetus to be a baby (Jonas-Simpson & McMahon, 2005). Some women may feel relief, while others are devastated (Swanson, 1999). Regardless of the circumstances of the loss, healthcare providers must be prepared to assist women and their families with their grieving. They need to recognize the differences in grieving patterns and provide a continuum of support and assistance that respects individuality, cultural diversity, and the reality of local social worlds (Read, Stewart, Cartwright, & Meigh, 2003).

The questions in Table 9-5 will guide healthcare providers in giving appropriate support. These questions are discussed individually in numbered form in the rest of this section of the chapter.

1. How can we best support you and your family? What information do you need?

Cultural reciprocity occurs when the client or her family feels able to share cultural needs, concerns, and feelings with healthcare providers and senses that respect and sensitivity characterize the relationship (Callister, 1995). For many, this may be their first experience with birth, death, and hospital culture.

Healthcare providers need to be aware that what differs between races and cultural groups is not so much the feelings of grief but their forms of expression (Gardner, 1999). Every family should be asked about the way they express grief. If they prefer, create an environment that allows for privacy, without isolation, and access to telephones in non-public areas for the phone calls that must be made (Thomas, 2001). Both parents should be encouraged to ask for help and support from family and friends because perceived support helps with the grieving process (Wallerstedt et al., 2003). However, if the family sees the loss as a reflection of their present or past actions, they may be reluctant to seek support. Alter visiting restrictions to allow parents to be together with their infant, family, and friends before and after death. Provide 24-hour access to spiritual care providers, social workers, and other support personnel.

TABLE 9-5

Assessment Guide to Helping Parents Facing or Experiencing Perinatal Loss*

1. How can we best support you and your family? What information do you need?
2. Do you wish to know about options for your hospital stay, or do you prefer early discharge?
3. What are your wishes regarding (palliative) care of your baby who is not expected to live?
4. Do you wish to prepare a memory box? If yes, are there particular items you wish to have included?
5. What are your wishes regarding care of your baby who has died?
6. How can we support you after you have returned to the community?

*This is a general guide for assessment. Specific tools that have been developed for clinical use (e.g., the care plan in Table 9-3) include questions that can be used for a range of language and literacy levels.

In some cultures, decision making is hierarchical. Adolescent parents may consult their own parents. The Japanese family usually looks to the eldest member for advice (Andersen, 2001). Sometimes, the father speaks for the mother, especially if the mother does not speak English. When communication barriers exist, the healthcare provider is responsible for developing a communication plan to make the client and/or family informed partner(s) in the provision of care (College of Nurses of Ontario, 1999).

Clients and/or families should be asked what they want or need. Clear, factual, and timely information must be provided, preferably to both parents at the same time. Written materials in the local community languages may be helpful for parents to refer to. The following information must be presented verbally and/or in writing as appropriate:

- Sources of community support
- Details about the process of normal grieving
- Pointers about how to recognize warning signs that indicate the need to seek medical help
- Instructions for physical care

2. Do you wish to know about options for your hospital stay, or do you prefer early discharge?

The client should be given the choice of staying in the maternal and newborn area or being transferred to another part of the hospital, with staff who are skilled in caring for families experiencing perinatal loss. She should not share a room with another mother and baby, unless she requests this (Health Canada, 2002). One strategy to help healthcare providers communicate the special needs and status of a client and family who have experienced a loss is to place a butterfly symbol(s) outside her room and on the beds of any surviving infant(s), in the case of multiple births. In North America, the butterfly is a commonly used symbol to denote perinatal loss.

Some clients may choose rapid discharge (Ellis Fletcher, 1999). To help these women maintain contact after discharge, the names and telephone numbers of key contacts (e.g., social workers, spiritual caregivers) may be provided. Follow-up care from the hospital is also helpful.

3. What are your wishes regarding (palliative) care of your baby who is not expected to live?

Parents may be culturally or personally in conflict with healthcare centres where life-extending practices are available. People of Korean background may view artificial means of sustaining life (i.e., technological advances) as reckless attempts to avoid death (Andersen, 2001). The Amish rarely consider life support to be an option (Beachy, 1997). In contrast, other families may choose every life-extending measure available. This can be a source of ethical dilemma for the healthcare team.

Conferences with the family and the extended healthcare team, including an ethicist, may be helpful to discuss medical options and related ethical issues, and to clarify the plan of care. Taking part in general decision making and the provision of care empowers families in the midst of their grieving process. What is important is honouring the meaning this baby has to the family. Christenings, blessings, saying of prayers, and preparation of the body all have a place in the grieving process. Rituals are recognized to cushion transitions in life and, therefore, often are found to be comforting. It is important to find both physical and emotional space to accommodate these practices or rituals (Irish, Lunquist, & Jenkins Nelsen, 1993).

4. Do you wish to prepare a memory box? If yes, are there particular items you wish to have included?
Creating memories of infants has been found to help with grieving and improve the long-term emotional health of grieving parents (Côté-Arsenault, 2003). Parents may be asked which mementoes, if any, would have meaning for them within their cultural context. The healthcare provider should then assist those who choose to collect mementoes and/or begin a journal (see Figure 9-1). Some families require a great deal of support and assistance with this process, due to the overwhelming grief they are experiencing, and may require more active support from staff, while others may take on a more active role themselves.

Muslim clients may not want a photographic record or to see or hold their infants because creating memories to attach significance to the loss is seen as unnecessary, and death is regarded as predestined and part of the cycle of life (Hébert, 1998). Some Latin American cultural groups believe that photographs steal the souls of the dead, which means the deceased may never rest in peace (Orb & Wynaden, 2001), and thus may refuse photographs based on these beliefs.

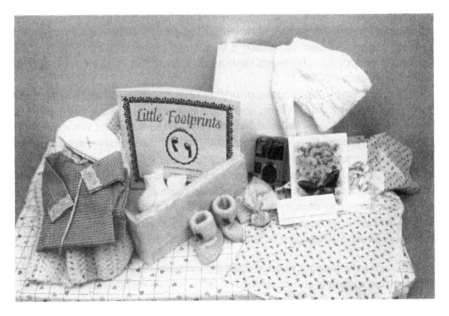

FIGURE 9-1 ■ **A Memory Box**

CULTURAL COMPETENCE IN ACTION

Birth Story: Memories of a Short Life Live On

Grace and her husband were expecting their second child. Late in her second trimester, she developed complications and was advised that her baby had mild to moderate congenital heart defects. She rested in bed at home for ten weeks. Immediately after a scheduled Caesarean section, caregivers determined that her newborn daughter had massive deformities that had not been detected through prenatal testing. She was not expected to survive.

Over the next several hours, staff provided the family with a disposable camera so they could document the infant's life with photographs. At the same time, the staff began to prepare a memory box for the family. Grace negotiated with staff to have her 4-year-old daughter visit to meet her baby sister. Many other family members visited. Photographs were taken throughout the day.

Grace's daughter died in her arms, twelve hours after birth. The following day the memory box was presented to the family. Plans also were made for Grace and her husband to have intensive follow-up with the perinatal program staff. Several days later, the family had the photo album and memory box present at the baby's memorial service. Family and friends commented on how these mementoes helped them with their grieving.

Gender and ethnicity may determine the colour preference of clothing or wraps for the infant following death. It is necessary to have clothing and wraps available in a selection of colours and ask for the family's preference.

5. What are your wishes regarding care of your baby who has died?

The role of a healthcare provider is to prepare parents for decisions they will need to make about their deceased infant. Parents may be approached to discuss the option for autopsy. Jewish parents may consult their rabbi before consenting to an autopsy (Shuzman, 2003).

The parents' feelings and comfort level regarding viewing and touching the baby must be ascertained. Time should be spent with the parents and family, to guide them in providing care for their infant. Ask who else (e.g., family, minister) they would like to help them during this period. Ensure they are not rushed through the process. They may wish to keep their infant with them for many hours after death. Allow parents to determine when they are ready for the infant's body to be transferred to the morgue. At the parents' request, allow family members or religious leaders to transport the infant's body to a funeral home or a religious establishment as per hospital policy. Some religious traditions require same-day burial following preparation of the body (Hébert, 1998).

6. How can we support you after you have returned to the community?

Supportive care needs to be offered to both parents as this affects future pregnancies and parenting. Following a loss, support may be obtained from spiritual care leaders, grief counsellors, public health units, family members, friends, and community bereavement organizations. For the computer-literate, Internet bereavement sites offer another source of information, support, and self-help. The use of support services also may be influenced by cultural beliefs. Asian cultural values emphasize that family problems or issues are private, which means participation in support or bereavement groups is not commonplace among clients with Asian backgrounds (Yick & Gupta, 2002). Muslims consider death to be the will of Allah, so it may be interpreted as disrespectful to grieve too much (Sheikh & Gatrad, 2001).

Healthcare providers also grieve the loss of the infants in their care and may require debriefing or counselling. Remember that both the personal and the professional culture of the heathcare providers will affect their grief response. It is important to involve staff in memorial events. Many organizations provide staff with educational and emotionally supportive opportunities to discuss grief, loss, ethical issues, and how to support grieving parents and families. Healthcare providers and parents can work together to identify and eliminate gaps in an organization's services and supports.

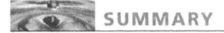 SUMMARY

Healthcare providers are required to provide culturally appropriate care to an increasingly diverse clientele during one of the most emotionally charged periods in their lives (Thomas, 2001). This chapter has outlined the role that culture plays in perinatal care, illustrating approaches healthcare providers can use in assessing and caring for clients and their families.

The phenomenon of perinatal loss was explored, in terms of determining the needs of clients and families who experience this. The chapter discussed the need to practise in a client-/family-centred way while developing skills in cultural competence. Although most healthcare providers receive little or no education about multiculturalism in educational programs, this is changing (as the study of this textbook would attest). In addition, continuing education provides the information and support that is needed to provide a high standard of care (Gonser, 2000).

We have examined some of the challenges related to the assumptions that healthcare providers make when providing care. Assumptions about clients and their families must be validated. Healthcare providers must continually challenge their own assumptions so that these do not adversely affect either the care they provide or their relationships with clients and their families.

REFERENCES

Andersen, J. (2001). Cultural competence and health care: Japanese, Korean, and Indian patients in the United States. *Journal of Cultural Diversity, 8*(4), 109–121.

Andrews, M. M., & Boyle, J. S. (1999). *Transcultural concepts in nursing care* (2nd ed.). Philadelphia: Lippincott.

Battaglini, A., Gravel, S., Poulin, C., Brodeur, J., Durand, D., & DeBlois, S. (2001). Immigration and perinatal risk. *Centres of Excellence for Women's Health Research Bulletin, 2*(2), 8–9.

Beachy, A. (1997). Cultural implications for nursing care of the Amish. *Journal of Cultural Diversity. 4*(4), 118–126.

Bondas, T., & Eriksson, K. (2001). Women's lived experiences of pregnancy: A tapestry of joy and suffering. *Qualitative Health Research, 11*(6), 824–840.

Callister, L. (1995). Cultural meanings of childbirth. *Journal of Obstetric, Gynecologic, and Neonatal Nursing, 24*(4), 327–331.

Callister, L. (2004). Making meaning: Women's birth narratives. *Journal of Obstetric, Gynecologic, and Neonatal Nursing, 33*(4), 508–515.

Callister, L., Khalaf, I., Semenic, S., Kartchner, R., & Vehvilainen-Julkunen, K. (2003). The pain of childbirth: Perceptions of culturally diverse women. *Pain Management Nursing, 4*(4), 145–154.

Canadian Institute of Child Health. (2000). *The health of Canada's children: A CICH profile* (3rd ed.). Ottawa: The Canadian Institute of Child Health.

College of Nurses of Ontario. (1999). *Practice guidelines: Culturally sensitive care.* Toronto, ON: Author.

Côté-Arsenault, D. (2003). Weaving babies lost in pregnancy into the fabric of the family. *Journal of Family Nursing, 9*(1), 23–37.

Côté-Arsenault, D., & Morrison-Beedy, D. (2001). Women's voices reflecting changed expectations for pregnancy after perinatal loss. *Journal of Nursing Scholarship, 33*(3), 239–244.

Davidhizar, R., & Giger, J. (1998). *Canadian transcultural nursing: Assessment & intervention.* Mosby: St. Louis.

Davies, R. (2004). New understandings of parental grief: Literature review. *Journal of Advanced Nursing, 46*(5), 506–513.

de Montigny, F., & Lacharite, C. (2004). Fathers' perceptions of the immediate postpartum period. *Journal of Obstetric, Gynecologic, and Neonatal Nursing, 33*(3), 328–338.

Ellis Fletcher, S. N. (1999) Cultural implications in the management of grief and loss. *Journal of Cultural Diversity, 9*(3), 86–90.

Gardner, J. (1999). Perinatal death: Uncovering the needs of midwives and nurses and exploring helpful interventions in the United States, England, and Japan. *Journal of Transcultural Nursing, 10*(2), 120–130.

Gerteis, M., Edgman-Levitan, S., Daley, J., & Delbianco, T. L. (Eds.) (1993). *Through the patient's eyes: Understanding and promoting patient-centered care.* San Francisco, CA: Jossey-Bass.

Gonser, P. A. (2000). Culturally competent care for members of sexual minorities. *Journal of Cultural Diversity, 7*(3), 72–75.

Health Canada. (1999). *Nutrition for a healthy pregnancy: National guidelines for the childbearing years.* Ottawa: Minister of Public Works and Government Services.

Health Canada. (2002). *Family-centred maternity and newborn care: National guidelines.* Ottawa: Minister of Public Works and Government Services.

Health Canada. (2003). *Canadian perinatal report.* Ottawa: Minister of Public Works and Government Services.

Heatherly, J. (2000, March). Transcultural nursing and female circumcision. *Canadian Operating Room Nursing Journal, 18*(1), 7–12.

Hébert, M. P. (1998). Perinatal bereavement in its cultural context. *Death Studies, 22*(1), 61–78.

Irish, D. P., Lundquist, K. F., & Jenkins Nelsen, V. (1993). Conclusions. In D. P. Irish, K. F. Lundquist, & V. Jenkins Nelsen (Eds.). *Ethnic variations in dying, death and grief: diversity in universality* (181–190). Washington, DC: Taylor & Francis.

Jonas-Simpson, C., & McMahon, E. (2005). The language of loss when a baby dies prior to birth: Co-creating human experience. *Nursing Science Quarterly, 18*(2), 124–130.

Jones, M., Bond, M., Gardner, S., & Hernandez, M. (2002). A call to action: Acculturation level and family-planning patterns of Hispanic immigrant women. *Journal of Maternal-Child Nursing, 27*(1), 26–32.

Kridli, S. A. (2002). Health beliefs and practices among Arab women. *Journal of Maternal Child Nursing, 27*(3), 178–182.

Leininger, M. (2002). Transcultural nursing and globalization of health care: Importance, focus and historical aspects. In M. Leininger & M. McFarland (Eds.). *Transcultural nursing: Concepts, theories, research & practice* (3rd ed. pp. 3–43). New York: McGraw-Hill.

Liu, H., & Moore, J. (2000). Perinatal care: Cultural and technical differences between China and the United States. *Journal of Transcultural Nursing, 11*(1), 47–54.

Lowdermilk, D., & Perry, S. (2003). *Maternal Nursing* (6th ed.). St. Louis: Mosby.

Lynam, M., Gurm, B., & Dhari, R. (2000). Exploring perinatal health in Indo-Canadian women. *The Canadian Nurse, 96*(4), 18–24.

Malacrida, C. (1999). Complicating mourning: The social economy of perinatal death. *Qualitative Health Research, 9*(4), 504–519.

Mattson, S. (2000). Providing culturally competent care: Strategies and approaches for perinatal clients. *AWHONN Lifelines, 4*(5), 37–39.

Merenstein, G. B., & Gardner, S. L. (2002). Grief and perinatal loss. In G. B. Merenstein, & S. L. Gardner (Eds.). *Handbook of neonatal intensive care* (5th ed., p. 755). St. Louis, Missouri: Mosby.

Molina, J. (2001). Traditional Native American practices in obstetrics. *Clinical Obstetrics and Gynecology, 44*(4), 661–670.

Olds, S., London, M., & Ladewig, P. (2000). *Maternal-newborn nursing: A family and community-based approach,* (6th ed.). Upper Saddle River, NJ: Prentice-Hall.

Orb, A., & Wynaden, D. (2001). Cross-cultural communication and health care practice. *The Australian Journal of Holistic Nursing, 8*(2), 36.

Pasco, C., Morse, J., & Olsen, J. (2004). Filipino Canadian patients. *Journal of Nursing Scholarship, 36*(3), 239–246.

Prodan-Bhalla, N. (2001). Understanding the broader context: The health of the urban Native Canadian. *Canadian Journal of Nursing Leadership, 14*(4), 20.

Purnell L., & Paulanka, B. (2003). *Transcultural health care* (2nd ed.). Philadelphia: F.A. Davis.

Read, S., Stewart, C., Cartwright, P., & Meigh, S. (2003). Psychological support for perinatal trauma and loss. *British Journal of Midwifery, 11*(8), 484–488.

Riordan, J., & Gill-Hopple, K. (2001). Breastfeeding care in multicultural populations. *Journal of Obstetrical, Gynecological and Neonatal Nursing, 30*(2), 216–223.

Roberts, K. (2002). Providing culturally sensitive care to the childbearing Islamic family. *Advances in Neonatal Care, 2*(4), 222–228.

Ross, L., Dennis, C., Robertson-Blackmore, E., & Stewart, D. (2005). *Postpartum depression: A guide for front-line health and social service providers.* Toronto: Centre for Addiction and Mental Health.

Semenic, S., Callister, L., & Feldman, P. (2004). Giving birth: The voices of Orthodox Jewish women living in Canada. *Journal of Obstetrical, Gynecological and Neonatal Nurses, 33*(1), 80–87.

Shah, M. A. (2004). *Transcultural aspects of perinatal care: A resource guide.* Tampa, FL: National Perinatal Association.

Sheikh, A., & Gatrad, A. R. (2001). Muslim birth practices. *Practising Midwife, 4*(4) 10–13.

Shuzman, E. (2003). Facing stillbirth or neonatal death. *AWHONN Lifelines, 7*(6), 537–543.

Swanson, K. (1999). Research-based practice with women who have had miscarriages. *Journal of Nursing Scholarship, 31*(4), 339–345.

Thaddeus, S., & Nangalia, R. (2004). Perceptions matter: Barriers to treatment of postpartum hemorrhage. *Journal of Midwifery and Women's Health, 49*(4), 293–297.

Thomas, J. (2001). The death of a baby: Guidance for providers in hospital and the community. *Journal of Neonatal Nursing, 7*(5), 167–170.

Wallerstedt, C., Lilley, M., & Baldwin, K. (2003). Interconceptional counselling after perinatal and infant loss. *Journal of Obstetric, Gynecologic, and Neonatal Nursing, 32,* 533–542.

Willis, W. (1999). Culturally competent nursing care during the perinatal period. *Journal of Perinatal and Neonatal Nursing, 13*(3), 45–59.

Yick, A. G., & Gupta, R. (2002). Chinese cultural dimensions of death, dying, and bereavement focus group findings. *Journal of Cultural Diversity, 9*(2), 32–42.

CHAPTER 10

The End of Life

ANN POTTINGER, ATHINA PERIVOLARIS,
AND REV. DAVID HOWES

LEARNING OBJECTIVES

At the end of this chapter, the learner will be able to:

- Describe how culture influences views on death and dying
- Identify key areas that culturally competent end-of-life care requires us to consider
- Discuss the importance of self-reflection in the provision of care
- Explore how the Western values built into the current healthcare system affect end-of-life care
- Describe how to incorporate awareness of cultural issues into end-of-life clinical care

KEY TERMS

Advance directive	Finality
Awareness	Generic cultural competencies
Bearing witness	Specific cultural competencies
Comfort	Spirituality
Faith	Suffering
Feelings	Truth telling

As is true for all aspects of life, the challenges and emotions at life's end are influenced by life experience and culture. Culture shapes values, beliefs, and practices, and its impact on these areas is intensified during death and dying.

Attitudes about end-of-life care come more from parents and grandparents than from education or socio-economic status (Back & Petracca, 2003). Attitudes and rituals around death and bereavement are shaped by family as well as by religious practices, the broader community, and cultural heritage. Within the Canadian multicultural environment, healthcare providers must have specific awareness, knowledge, and skills in order to provide culturally competent end-of-life and palliative care. This chapter presents a guiding approach that addresses cultural competence in relation to issues encountered during end-of-life care.

Cultural Competencies

We have already encountered the concept of generic and specific cultural knowledge (see Chapter 4). It follows that, for cultural competence, it is important that healthcare providers possess both specific and generic competencies (Lo & Fung, 2003). These are defined as follows:

- **Generic cultural competencies** refer to a broad set of knowledge, skills, and attitudes that enable healthcare providers to provide care to people from diverse cultural backgrounds. Such knowledge and awareness, combined with therapeutic engagement with clients, underpin clinical cultural competence.
- **Specific cultural competencies** refer to the knowledge and skills that enable healthcare providers to effectively care for clients from particular cultural groups during the end-of-life process.

(Lo & Fung, 2003).

An example of specific cultural knowledge would be the recognition that an Iranian Muslim client would likely not have been told by a physician of his impending death if he were being cared for in Iran. As well, family and friends would possibly use any means possible to conceal this information from the client (Geissler, 1998).

The danger in using culturally specific knowledge is the tendency to apply such knowledge to all clients from a particular culture. Yet such knowledge, or aspects of it, often does apply to clients and individuals who identify with the specific culture being considered. Specific knowledge applies not only to specific cultural groups but also to specific clinical populations because each population presents with some general but also some specific issues. The following are three examples of specific issues encountered during end-of-life care:

1. Advance directives
2. Organ donation
3. Rituals surrounding funerals and mourning

This chapter presents an ABC approach (*A*wareness, *B*earing witness, *C*omfort) for fostering the skills that healthcare providers need for culturally competent end-of-life care. The ABC system includes techniques for exploring key areas that need to be considered, which conveniently can be characterized as "The 4-*F*s": *f*eelings, *f*amily, *f*aith, and *f*inality. The 4-*F*s are discussed in detail later in the chapter and are intended to serve as triggers that help healthcare providers identify issues they need to explore with the client and family.

ABC: Awareness, Bearing Witness, Comfort

The three elements of the ABC approach work in synergy to promote the knowledge and skills that health providers need to provide culturally competent end-of-life care. The ABC approach provides an overview of the therapeutic relating skills required. Communication is central. In order for effective communication to occur, healthcare providers must attend to non-verbal behaviours as well as any language barriers, and may need to work with cultural interpreters (see Chapters 5 and 6) in order to accomplish this.

A = Awareness

The **awareness** aspect of competency refers to an understanding of how culture shapes the issues that are of concern to particular populations. An individual healthcare provider is unlikely to be aware of the specific cultural practices of all cultural groups. However, it is vital that healthcare providers have awareness of how culture shapes the distinct issues of concern to the population or populations that make up their clientele. Such issues include the following:

- Varying views of death and dying (including advance directives and organ donation)
- Diverse expressions of loss and grief
- Varying views on acceptable options for pain and symptom management

In addition, healthcare providers must have self-awareness of their own beliefs regarding these and other related issues and practices. An awareness of the overall healthcare system and the values inherent within it is essential, particularly as these values relate to death and dying.

B = Bearing Witness

The **bearing witness** aspect of cultural competency represents a way of "being with" clients and families to share and understand the cultural as well as health- and illness-related issues being experienced in the situation. It is indeed a skill. Bearing witness moves beyond observation. It is often not valued in practice. It is important to bear witness to how clients and families live out their values and priorities in the moment, and how they cope and manage during death and dying. Bearing witness is about being present with clients and families and listening as they share their cultural identity and what is important to them.

In order to bear witness, the healthcare provider must create opportunities in which he or she can practise authentic therapeutic relating with those involved. Clients and families need a non-judgemental therapeutic space in which to share their beliefs, customs, views on death, and struggles. It is in this kind of space that people can share specific needs around cultural practices that may be very different from those that exist in the Western, primarily Eurocentric-based, healthcare system that predominates in Canada. It is in such a space, for example, that an Aboriginal client, following a terminal diagnosis, may feel comfortable sharing his or her desire to have a traditional healer present to help restore the mind/body/spirit balance (Finkel, Leishman, Lundy, Ray, & Tonack, 2002).

Interestingly, the act and process of bearing witness to the experiences of clients from diverse cultural backgrounds increases the healthcare provider's awareness of culturally based, end-of-life care issues, which enhances competency.

C = Comfort

Comfort is both a process and an outcome. It involves promoting well-being within the physical, interpersonal, social, and spiritual domains. Healthcare providers need to establish the comfort needs of clients and to treat their pain and symptoms to an extent that is acceptable to the client and family. In some cultures, no physical pain is tolerated; in others, some pain is acceptable.

Healthcare providers need to increase their knowledge and understanding of complementary therapies such as massage, herbal remedies, topical treatments, and guided imagery. They need to understand, too, that not all clients experience talking as emotional support, and that, in some cultures, emotional support can take a more tangible form (Finkel et al., 2002). During one end-of-life encounter, for example, when a healthcare provider was working with an Asian family, the wife indicated that she needed, appreciated, and would accept support in the form of a cup of coffee or a meal, and help with the children, as well as being asked how she was doing. However, she said that it is not appropriate within her cultural background to request such support, even though she might need it. For such reasons, it is important to discuss the hospital experience, dying at home, death, and bereavement, but it is equally important to seek out what actions or resources will be of support and comfort to clients and families.

Cultural awareness and being with clients and families enable healthcare providers to establish their comfort needs. That is how the ABCs come together in synergy.

The 4-*F*s: Feelings, Family, Faith, Finality

The 4-*F*s are used to broadly impart to healthcare providers key areas for cultural exploration in the provision of end-of-life care. These are significant areas and are linked to values and decision making across cultures. Within these areas, specific cultures have specific views, but individual practices vary (Finkel et al., 2002). The provision of culturally competent end-of-life care is, therefore, complex and occurs at an intensified emotional and life-changing time for clients and families. The healthcare provider, as a cultural being, also often experiences challenges related to death and the provision of care. The areas represented by the 4-*F*s are not separate, but intertwined. Additionally, there are subcategories of focus within these areas, for example, how perspectives regarding decision making influence feelings.

F #1: Feelings

The death and dying experience represents an intense emotional time, and everyone involved experiences a variety of **feelings** (i.e., emotions that are evoked). Healthcare providers are no exception.

Strong feelings exist across cultures on issues such as the following:
- General decision making
- Disclosure of diagnosis
- Perceptions regarding the role of suffering
- End-of-life decisions
- Organ donation

The feeling of fear is universal, given the uncertainty that usually exists. However, it would be inaccurate to assume that fear is specifically related to impending death, as the nature of the fear is highly individualized. Our clinical experience and the literature (Blackhall, Frank, Murphy, & Michel, 2001; Hallenbeck & Goldstein, 1999; Kagawa-Singer & Blackhall, 2001; Lapine et al., 2001) highlight some areas that evoke strong feelings in relation to cultural values, and when there is a conflict in these values with the predominant values implicit in the Canadian healthcare system, the culture gap becomes particularly challenging. These conflicts have a negative impact on the end-of-life experience, particularly when they are unrecognized or ignored by healthcare providers. Self-awareness is critical for healthcare providers so that they can recognize their own feelings and ensure that these are not imposed on the client or on the processes of care.

Suffering

Even though the experience of **suffering** is embedded within human existence—particularly during the end-of-life period—its meaning and role varies across cultures.

Western cultures tend to resist suffering with the goal of eliminating it; the focus of end-of-life and hospice care within this paradigm tends to be on reducing suffering (Kemp, 2005). However, around the world many reasons have been given for the acceptance of suffering, such as seeing it in the following light:

- An inevitable aspect of life
- An opportunity to show strength
- A deserved punishment for sin
- A means of purification
- A redemptive experience

(Kemp, 2005; Kagawa-Singer & Blackhall, 2001)

Again, healthcare providers need to reflect on and be aware of the values within the healthcare system itself. Awareness of the potential conflict between the inevitability of suffering and the focus on reducing it is important when exploring the meaning of suffering for the client and family. Therefore, culturally competent care in relation to suffering may include the following:

- Actions or therapies to reduce suffering
- Spiritual care focused on forgiveness and acceptance
- Healthcare providers bearing witness and "remaining graceful in the presence of unrelieved suffering"

(Kemp, 2005, p. 49)

Bearing witness to suffering, without opportunity or strategies to reduce it, often is challenging for healthcare providers and can evoke strong feelings or reactions, especially if the healthcare provider lacks awareness that the notion of reducing suffering is a value embedded within the healthcare system.

Cultural beliefs, including perspectives on the role of suffering, influence several aspects of dealing with pain: the manner in which it is managed, the extent to which it is managed, or whether it is managed. Additionally, culture influences the expression of pain, with some cultures tending not to complain despite having severe pain.

Healthcare providers should be mindful of the need to pay close attention to detail when they assess pain, including a client's communication style and beliefs regarding pain. In the Latino culture, for example, pain is something you live with; clients from this background may therefore be willing to tolerate a high level of pain (University of Washington Medical Center, 2004). Pain management is discussed in greater depth in Chapter 13.

Some people hold the view that treating the suffering or pain is worse than the actual suffering, and their choices regarding pain and its management reflect this view. For instance, it is fairly common among Southeast Asian Buddhists to choose to be alert instead of having any alteration in senses that may accompany the use of pain medications. As well, the notion of suffering is a central aspect of Buddhism (Kemp, 2005; Finkel et al., 2002); the First Noble Truth is that all sentient beings suffer and all other teachings flow from this truth (Kemp, 2005).

Healthcare providers may view suffering as unnecessary or a failure of care, and thus have difficulty accepting clients' or families' views. It should also be noted that understanding the role of suffering in different populations does not negate the need for caution to ensure that individual assessments are carried out, and that care is not based on assumptions and stereotypes.

Decision Making

Making decisions is a significant aspect of the dying experience and can evoke fear and anxiety. Fear may exist on various fronts (e.g., fear of making the wrong decision, or fear of being judged) because the decisions often are difficult and made in the context of uncertainty and competing values. Decisions made regarding life support, tube feeding, organ donation, and cardiopulmonary resuscitation have significant implications for the client and family, as well as for the health care provided.

The values that guide decision making are influenced by culture. In order to begin to understand some of the feelings evoked that relate to decision making and culture, we need to take note of some of the assumptions and values within the existing healthcare culture.

It is important for healthcare providers to recognize that the North American model of individual decision making with respect to medical care may not be appropriate for ethnically diverse clients. Alternative approaches include the following:

- Family-based decision making
- Physician-based decision making
- Shared physician–family decision making
    (Searight & Gafford, 2005)

Whenever the values that influence decision making are in conflict with those reflected in our healthcare system, strong feelings are evoked. However, these conflicts are frequently not recognized as having a cultural basis and can be inappropriately labelled. For example, a family may be said to have "unrealistic expectations."

The reach of the Western values that are embedded within the Canadian healthcare system extends to healthcare providers' codes of ethics. The value of autonomy within the system arises from the value of the individual and his or her right to self-determination. This value of autonomy dictates that the individual is fully responsible for making all decisions pertaining to his or her health. However, in our multicultural society, many clients from non-Western cultures have different values pertaining to the role of the individual, the family, and society. In some Asian cultures, for example, the family is the smallest unit of identity and value is placed on interdependence as opposed to individualism (Ersek, Kagawa-Singer, Barnes, Blackhall, & Koening, 1998, p. 1683). Therefore, it would be the family that makes end-of-life healthcare decisions, and their strong desire to carry out this responsibility can evoke equally strong feelings in healthcare providers who are working within the autonomy paradigm.

In some cultures, a certain family member (e.g., the eldest son, the husband, or the oldest member) is the primary decision maker, even though the client has the capacity to make his or her own healthcare decisions. Some elderly clients may hold the view that they have earned the privilege to pass decision making on to their children and have confidence that their best interests will be protected. Another cultural perspective is the view that passing decision-making responsibility to the family is a way of acknowledging the impact of the disease on the family (Ersek et al., 1998).

The clinical implication of these values is that it is important to establish who the primary decision maker is and the role of others in decision making. Although healthcare providers should honour the existence of legal substitute decision makers and other legal requirements, having this information serves as a guide in working with clients and families in a culturally meaningful way. It is, therefore, essential for healthcare providers to ask clients questions such as, "Who or what do you need in order to help you make this decision?"

Organ Donation

Organ donation is a sensitive topic for clients and families regardless of culture because it touches upon values that are strongly influenced by culture. Since organs must be transplanted within hours after death, timely decision making, during what is often a period of intense emotional stress, is essential to ensure the success of the procedure. Cultural competence on the part of the healthcare provider can significantly influence the outcome. The aspects of culture that influence end-of-life decisions, and in turn affect organ donation, are set out below:

■ *Preference for life-sustaining treatment varies across cultural groups.* The differences are linked not to socio-economic status or access to health care, but rather to culture, religion, and perhaps a lack of trust in the medical establishment.

US literature, for example, indicates that, as a group, African Americans prefer more aggressive care at the end of life than do White Americans (Back & Petracca, 2003; Searight & Gafford, 2005). This may stem from a belief that it is God who determines when life ends and/or a fear that lack of aggressive care may actually mean a lack of care, or neglect. Searight and Gafford (2005) indicate that Black clients overall are about half as likely to accept DNR (do not resuscitate) status than Whites, and also are more likely to change DNR status to more aggressive levels of care.

Further, the literature suggests that these attitudes carry over to Black physicians, who are significantly more likely to recommend aggressive treatment to clients with brain damage and known terminal illness than are their White colleagues (Searight & Gafford, 2005).

▪ *Differences in perspective exist with respect to when life actually ends.* Although brain death is widely accepted by healthcare providers as a legitimate definition of death, from a non-medical perspective, the moment of death is not always clearly evident. The space between life and death is socially, culturally, and politically constructed and is fluid and open to dispute (Bowman & Richard, 2004). Views about when life ends can subsequently influence decisions regarding organ donation.

In Western society, which has a tendency to plan for and control major life events, there is an expectation of medical solutions to illness, and organ donation often is seen as a way of improving health as well as life, and evading death. In fact, organ donation frequently is framed as "the gift of life." In Christianity, the dominant religion in the Western world, the body is to be respected after death; however, a body without a soul is no longer considered a person. Organ donation is, therefore, viewed as an act of love and generosity. As well, communion—the symbolic giving of "the blood and body of Christ"—may have contributed to the Western acceptance of organ donation (Bowman & Richard, 2004).

▪ *There are differences in what constitutes the essence of the "person."* Again, in Western society, the locus of control is in the mind; the brain, as the home of the rational and autonomous mind, becomes synonymous with the mind. At death, the brain/mind is no longer functional in the body, and once the brain dies, the synthesis of body and mind ends. Organ procurement is, therefore, seen as an ethical practice and is reflected in the "presumed consent" stance of some European countries (Bowman & Richard, 2004; McCunn et al., 2003).

In Japanese society, Shintoism and Buddhism view death as a "natural" process which marks the end of the body we inhabit in this life, not the end of life itself. From a traditional Japanese perspective, a human is an integration of body, mind, and spirit, and the metaphoric centre of the body (kokoro) has been traditionally located in the chest. After death, the body–mind–spirit remain an integrated whole; therefore, removal of an organ from the body, especially from the chest, may be perceived as a disturbance of this integrated unit (Bowman & Richard, 2004). The notion of the dead body remaining a whole, and a subsequent discomfort with organ donation, is evident in several cultures, including among Canadian Aboriginal peoples. Gatrad and Sheikh (2002) note that persons from countries influenced by Islam have traditionally resisted organ donation and autopsy because of the importance of going to the grave with an intact body. Research indicates that in comparison to European Americans, Asian Americans hold more negative attitudes toward, and participate less frequently in, large, urban, organ-donor programs (Alden & Cheung, 2000).

An exploratory study with South Asian families in the United Kingdom, by Randhawa (1998), found that culture and religion played a much less prohibitive role in determining the level of organ donation than was previously thought. The sample included men and women from the following groups: Indian Hindu Gujrati, Indian Sikh Punjabi, Pakistani Punjabi Muslim, and Bangladeshi Sylheti Muslim. The majority of those sampled stated that they did not know what their religion prescribed in terms of organ donation. Sikhs felt confident that their religion viewed it positively, based on its humanitarian principles. Individuals of other faiths also offered similar interpretations. For example, a Hindu male noted that his religion says not to waste anything if it can be used for the good of other people. However, in general, the non-Sikh groups expressed more indecision and a desire for more discussion and clarification from religious leaders. The latter was true for Muslims, in particular.

Randhawa (1998) concludes that the main reason the South Asian population was hesitant and indecisive when it came to organ donation was that people had not given the issue much serious thought, and for Muslims particularly, because they were unsure of what their religion's stance was. The author further notes that none of the religions explicitly object to organ donation and, in fact, a recent edict, a *fatwa* issued from the Muslim Law Council, clarified that it is permissible to donate organs and accept brain-stem death as an acceptable diagnosis of death (Randhawa, 1998).

Because views about organ donation are obviously influenced by views about when death occurs and whether or not the organs are "needed" by the deceased, it is critical that discussions about organ donation begin at the community level so that there is broad and depersonalized consideration of such issues. It also is important to discuss policies and practices around organ donation with clients and families as early in the healthcare process as possible. Healthcare providers wishing to engage in such discussion, but feeling unsure of how to do this, will benefit from cultural consultations with community members and spiritual leaders.

In recent years, however, many religious scholars have re-interpreted the religious laws, and there is growing acceptance of organ donation in most communities (Kemp, 2005). These changing views point to the dynamic nature of culture.

Advance Directives

The use of advance directives is another aspect of decision making with a cultural component. An **advance directive** is a document that expresses a person's wishes about critical care or life-sustaining medical treatments in the event of incapacitation. These directives, whether formal legal documents or not, are based on the Western value of autonomy and represent a way of ensuring that the wishes and values of individual adult clients guide decision making during end-of-life discussions. However, values of individual choice and control may not be applicable to all families and/or to all cultures.

Many cultures believe that talking about death may actually hasten or bring it closer. For clients from these cultural groups, the use of advance directives may seem perplexing or even offensive, and generate strong feelings when healthcare providers directly approach them about advance directives. Some clients, such as those within the US Hispanic community, may be reluctant to appoint a specific family member to be in charge because of concerns about isolating this person or offending other relatives, opting instead for a consensually oriented approach. Furthermore, formalization through advance directives may be seen as unnecessary and potentially harmful as it may lead to increased family conflict or may hasten or "awaken" one's own death (Phipps, True, & Murray, 2003; Searight & Gafford, 2005).

Although advance directives are advocated within the Canadian healthcare system, literature indicates that only a small percentage of people of Western background have completed these directives, and the rates for minority populations are even lower (Searight & Gafford, 2005). This may be associated with a fear of premature cessation of care (including mistrust based on historical experiences), as well as a view of collective family versus individual responsibility. For all clients, many factors could potentially contribute to difficulties with advance directives. Completing and following through with advance directives brings numerous challenges. With the increasing reliance on technology, the lines between so-called ordinary care and extraordinary care are becoming more and more blurred. As well, it is difficult to clearly distinguish between the client's wishes and needs and those of the client's family.

Methods of promoting discussion and use of advance directives require careful consideration for all families. In specific cultural groups, collaboration with community members, leaders, and respected elders also may be warranted. Individuals and groups need both permission and space to explore these issues in a culturally safe manner.

Disclosure of Diagnosis and Prognosis

Truth telling including the disclosure of diagnosis and related prognosis is a significant area in which culture-related conflict often arises, and when it does, strong feelings are generated for all involved. We have already discussed that within the Canadian healthcare system, the value of individualism dictates the value for autonomy; if autonomy is to be respected, a client needs to make informed decisions. In order to make informed decisions, the client must be given information, which means that healthcare providers must engage in full disclosure and truth telling. The values and related actions are aimed at giving clients control over their health and the dying process.

Many people from non-Western cultures, however, do not place the same value on full disclosure and truth telling to the individual client, and instead value the withholding of truth, particularly when the diagnosis is terminal. The feeling may be, for instance, that the truth should be withheld in the client's best interests, in order not to be burdensome and to enable this person to maintain feelings of hope. In practice, and as is documented in the literature (Lapine et al., 2001), some family members from non-Western cultures have pleaded with healthcare providers not to disclose a diagnosis, for fear of bringing harm to the client.

In the Western value system, truth telling tends to be viewed as empowering, in that the client has the appropriate information to engage in decision making and

---

CULTURAL COMPETENCE IN ACTION

A Family Wants the Truth Withheld

Leela is a 66-year-old woman from Sri Lanka who was recently diagnosed with end-stage terminal cancer and is being cared for on a medical unit. She speaks little English. The family is present all the time and indicates that they do not want her to be told the diagnosis or prognosis.

The family has been told that Leela has less than nine months to live. Leela has been asking the nurses why she is still in hospital. The nurses do not feel comfortable with this situation; some want to be very direct, some refer to the family as being "unreasonable" and not having the right to request complicity of the team, and others want to avoid caring for this client and family.

Initial Healthcare Provider Actions

- *Awareness:* Recognize a potential conflict in values shaped by culture. Reflect upon your own values and views on death and how they influence your feelings and reactions.
- *Bearing witness:* Seek to understand the family's values and underlying feelings, instead of labelling them as unreasonable. Bear witness to their experience, needs, and struggles, and seek to understand their views on health, death, dying, and disclosure of impending death. Therefore, spend time with them and do not act upon any impulse to avoid them and the situation.
- *Comfort:* Promote comfort by carefully and non-judgementally listening to their views, wishes, and concerns, without interrupting them. Immediately disclosing the diagnosis without engaging in this process with the family will not demonstrate respect or promote comfort.
- Determine if working with a cultural interpreter would assist the healthcare provider and family in the ABC style of therapeutic engagement.

---

can develop plans. In non-Western cultures, this type of full disclosure may be seen as disempowering and burdensome to the client. The value of non-disclosure is common, not only in Aboriginal, Asian, Japanese, and African cultures, but also among people from European backgrounds, such as Bosnian Americans and Italian Americans who "perceive direct disclosure of illness as at a minimum, disrespectful, and more significantly, inhumane" (Searight & Gafford, 2005, p. 517). Doctors with Bosnian backgrounds also have been noted to "go around" the diagnosis and be indirect about serious illness, in contrast to their American colleagues, whose directness can be perceived as hurtful by both clients and colleagues (Searight & Gafford, 2005).

See the "Cultural Competence in Action" feature box on the family that wanted the truth withheld for an illustration of how the ABC approach can be used to explore feelings regarding truth telling.

In this particular situation, culturally competent care means that, following the initial actions suggested in the feature box, the healthcare provider(s) will hold a discussion with the family about the professional truth-telling obligation of healthcare providers and the values behind it. This difference in views needs to be acknowledged as a difference, not a right or wrong, and negotiation will be needed to arrive at a strategy that is acceptable to the family. The family needs to be told about plans, such as the intentions of the doctor and other healthcare team members to speak to the client through a cultural interpreter. It will be of utmost importance to ask the family who and what would be most supportive to them. Discuss with the family that the purpose of the meeting with the client is to find out her or his views and wishes, which may include disclosure of prognosis, and to determine who is to be involved in decision making, and how.

When interacting with any client, keep in mind the ABC approach. Clients should be asked about any concerns they may have, and time should be spent getting to know them. Clients should be given the opportunity to speak about their concerns and themselves without interruptions. When the time is appropriate, questions such as the following could be asked:

> Your condition requires several decisions to be made about your treatment [and care]. Is there someone, perhaps a family member, who you would like to be with you when we discuss these matters? How much of the information that needs to be discussed do you want to know? Would you feel more comfortable if I spoke primarily with _____? (Ersek et al., 1998, p. 1688)

Ersek et al. (1998) suggest we recognize that when clients freely and knowingly relinquish their responsibilities to family members, the professional obligations regarding decision making have been met. Nevertheless, it is wise to check back with clients about this—on a regular basis. This can be accomplished by asking, "Would you like me to continue speaking with your son about . . . ?"

F #2: Family

Families usually require various forms of support and are frequently important sources of information regarding cultural views and practices in relation to death and dying.

Healthcare providers have a key role in supporting families during the mourning, grieving, and planning processes. The healthcare provider should be mindful, though, that "errors in acknowledging the family are more likely to occur if the family does not fit a 'conventional' definition of family" (Kristjanson, Hudson, & Oldham, 2003, p. 271). In our healthcare culture, we have the tendency to focus on the "conventional" or nuclear family structure, as well as focus on those family members who are legally authorized to make decisions in the event that the client is not able to do so. Families, however, are diverse, and it is important to know exactly who the family members are. Some families identify friends as being part of the family.

In addition to families taking many forms, there are a variety of needs to be met within families. Healthcare providers may find it challenging to meet the needs of various family members. One dying client, for example, had been living with his same-sex partner for more than four years, but his mother, who was his next of kin and legal decision maker, had no knowledge of his sexual orientation or his living situation. For this man, it was important that the healthcare providers acknowledge his partner, and their relationship, and also acknowledge and support his mother. The healthcare providers were not to disclose to the mother the client's relationship with his partner, whom the mother viewed as a very good friend of her son's. The healthcare providers' support of these relationships was an essential component to the client's quality of dying and comfort.

Families play an important role in support and caregiving. Within the Latino culture, for example, this may mean participating in the spiritual as well as physical care of a loved one. In other cultures, families may maintain a constant presence, often in large numbers. Continuous death watching is common within the Russian community, for instance. Relatives and friends are expected to be cheerful and often bring food for the client. They also may bring gifts for the healthcare providers (University of Washington Medical Center, 2004). Although giving to healthcare providers is a common practice in many cultures, often it creates discomfort and a dilemma for healthcare providers, who may have clear policies and standards around maintaining professional boundaries and not accepting gifts from clients and families (University of Washington Medical Center, 2004). It is important for healthcare providers to explore how such gifts can be accepted without compromising their relationship with the client or family or violating organizational and professional protocols.

Clients and families also have varying preferences with respect to how, and by whom, a medical diagnosis and prognosis is disclosed. Some families prefer to hear the medical diagnosis and prognosis before the client hears it, so that they can shield the client completely or deliver the news gradually (University of Washington Medical Center, 2004).

Additional areas to explore with both client and family include their expectations around the following issues:

▪ Pain management
▪ Expectations of healthcare providers
▪ The meaning of suffering
▪ Preferred location for end-of-life care
▪ Visitors
▪ The meaning of hospice and palliative care
▪ Any potential barriers in any of the above areas

In families where there are strong expectations around family support and caregiving, options such as hospice care can be misunderstood and interpreted as the family being unable to care for the client. It is important to reframe hospice care as something that is adjunct to family members and meant to help them provide better care for their loved one, rather than being a replacement for that care (Back & Petracca, 2003). Similarly, palliative care may be seen by the family as withholding care. Again, trust and communication are critical for addressing these concerns.

Healthcare providers also need to understand what the specific cultural details are regarding the following:

▪ Death
▪ Preparation of the body
▪ Funeral arrangements

▪ Religious or spiritual practices
▪ Prolonging life
▪ Acceptable methods of providing treatment and comfort

In addition to knowing who needs to be present at the time of death, health-care providers must obtain an understanding of the role of family at that time. Procedures and practices at the time of, and following, death are strongly influenced by culture. For example, a Buddhist client from South Korea likely will need to have family members summoned to observe his or her last breath, and the family may engage in loud wailing and display intense emotion (Geissler, 1998). Making the appropriate arrangements in a timely manner to accommodate this practice is therefore a necessary component of planning care. Death rites vary across cultures, and it is important to remain aware that families usually need to preserve practices and traditions, which often are related to their faith and spiritual traditions.

F #3: Faith

Faith is an agreed-upon set of beliefs, and many people seek out comfort and direction in the dying process by drawing upon it. For many clients, faith and religion are essential components of end-of-life care (Kemp, 2005). Even if clients and families decline religious care, they rarely decline spiritual care. **Spirituality**, which may or may not encompass faith and religion, is "at the very heart of who we are" (Finkel et al., 2002, p. 12), and is manifested by our desires and what provides meaning in our lives. Therefore, clients' and families' spirituality may be reflected in their faith and religion or in their love for nature, art, or music (Finkel et al., 2002).

Issues that dying clients explore include seeking answers to the following two questions:

1. What was the meaning of my life?
2. How does dying affect the people I love and my relationships and identity with them?

Culture, faith, and spirituality influence and often shape how clients explore these areas and the meaning they derive from their exploration. Spiritual care explores issues regarding the following:

▪ Belief
▪ Identity
▪ Hope
▪ Peace
▪ Legacy
▪ Reconciliation

These are issues that affect all aspects of care, including decision making and the quality of care. Therefore, the provision of spiritual care—regardless of the healthcare provider's faith or lack of one—is part of the role of all healthcare providers who provide end-of-life care. The involvement of a multi-faith chaplain will assist members of the healthcare team in providing care that meets the specific cultural, religious, and faith needs of clients and families.

Healthcare providers must understand and acknowledge the role of faith and religion and their influence on the death and dying process. Religious teachings, and the degree to which people embrace these, will influence clients and families in several ways:

- How they cope
- What they find helpful
- Their perceptions regarding issues that arise in the end-of-life experience, such as organ donation
- If and how life should or should not be sustained by technological and other means

Major religions usually provide in-depth explanations regarding death, and dictate certain death rites and practices for followers. For instance, the Quran, the holy book of Islam, teaches that death is an inevitable part of life—a transformation of the soul from this world to another. The Muslim client often is "encouraged to repeat the 'Shahadah', a testimony of faith that affirms there is no God but Allah and Muhammad is His messenger" (Finkel et al., 2002, p. 49). Similarly, the Hindu client, at the time of death, may want to repeat verses from the Bhagavad-Gita. It is therefore important in end-of-life care to have knowledge of various practices and to be able to provide access to prayer books, prayer beads, and other religious items. As well, having timely access to various religious persons (e.g., a priest, pastor, imam, rabbi, or shaman) also is important; a multifaith chaplain can help in this regard.

Religion also influences world views with respect to living and dying. In the Greek culture, which is influenced by the Eastern Orthodox Church, death usually is viewed as a great tragedy, and many Greeks feel that every effort should be made to preserve life until God terminates it. This belief also is embraced by other cultures. In the Canadian healthcare system, end-of-life care decisions and requests guided by this belief system are often challenging for healthcare providers. This is particularly the case if healthcare providers are unaware of the belief system and lack understanding about why the client and family request "aggressive treatment," some of which may be accompanied by pain and discomfort with little or no clinical evidence that it is effective.

Again, healthcare providers need to examine implicit values within the healthcare system. In other words, in end-of-life care, the system focuses on physical comfort, quality of dying, and scientific evidence regarding treatment outcomes. For some cultures, the sanctity of life is a greater priority than quality of life, and some cultures look to God rather than science as having authority over life and death, although science may be seen as facilitating God's will. The family of a Greek man dying from terminal cancer explained:

> They say they can't do anything else for him and he is going to die . . . they don't want to do surgery because the doctors don't think it will work and he will probably die during the surgery . . . they keep asking us about the decision to resuscitate . . . but they don't understand . . . God decides when a person dies and he [the client] has to do everything to live and use all the things like surgery that God makes available . . . even if his condition is really bad we know that a miracle can happen as long as he stays alive. (Personal communication from clinical practice)

F #4: Finality

Finality—the closure of life as known and lived by a client—and its impact on families is a key area to consider in the provision of culturally competent end-of-life care. Regardless of the cultural and religious views on death and dying, finality is an aspect of the experience that is universal.

Although death may be perceived as a part of life and there may be a belief in an afterlife, life and living as known to the individual and family will change. Healthcare providers need to explore with clients and families the meaning of this experience for them and their views and beliefs regarding death. Given that dying well and dying with dignity are important worldwide, healthcare providers need to understand the hopes and desires of clients and families. The notion of dignity is highly individualized and often based on culture, spirituality, religion, and faith. What is considered a "good death" varies across cultures. For some cultures, a good death is characterized by where the death occurs (e.g., at home), the direction of the head and feet, and the nature of familial and spiritual support for the dying person. The finality component of the experience will shape care, in particular the emotional, spiritual, and physical aspects of care.

For individual clients, the emotional and spiritual care issues associated with finality frequently surface during contemplation of the following questions:

- Is there more to the experience than what I have known thus far?
- What will I leave behind?
- Do I have a legacy of some kind to leave behind?
- Will my family be all right—who will look after them?

Clients may have varying degrees of peace, hope, and emotional distress, and the experience will be influenced by individual factors as well as world views and belief systems. It is not the role of the healthcare provider to find answers to these questions and provide reassurance based on the healthcare provider's own value system. Instead, the healthcare provider encourages the client to explore his or her life experience and belief system in seeking answers to questions and in promoting reconciliation and closure based on that belief system. Although family members and friends often provide clients with support and encouragement, they themselves require care and support, specifically with regard to the finality aspect of the experience. This notion of finality, or impending finality, contributes to grief among family members.

Grieving also varies across cultures. For some, grieving is considered natural; members of a family who feel this way may not feel comfortable with the idea of receiving supportive counselling from a psychologist or psychiatrist, whom they may associate with mental illness. In other families, wailing and the demonstration of strong emotion is a sign of respect during the illness, and while the client/family may both exhibit stoicism during the time leading up to the death, this may not be maintained after death (University of Washington Medical Center, 2004).

Rituals After the Death

Rituals are an important part of the process that leads to the final rest or peace for the body and soul of the deceased. In terms of the physical aspects of finality, healthcare providers must be aware of the procedures for caring for the body at the time of, and following, death. Many such procedures and practices are related to religious beliefs, although not necessarily so.

Communicating with the client and family is essential, in addition to being aware that different cultural practices exist regarding post-death procedures. For example, the healthcare provider who knows that a client and family are of Muslim background should specifically explore with them any death rites related to Islam and how these influence the care that is expected following death. When death is near, many Muslims want clients to be directed so that their feet are facing Mecca (Finkel et al. 2002; Gatrad & Sheikh, 2002). A Hindu client may wish to be placed on the floor to be closer to Mother Earth, and the Russian client may want all the mirrors covered (University of Michigan Program for Multicultural Health, 2005).

Healthcare providers must also possess the generic knowledge that there are various culturally determined practices regarding the following:

- Who cares for the body immediately following death (the healthcare provider or certain family members)
- The gender of the person who cares for the body
- What items are to be removed, or not removed, from the body

As one example, if a Hindu client is wearing a nuptial thread around her neck or a *Bindi* (a dot on her forehead), it should not be removed (Finkel et al., 2002). Russian family members may wish to close the eyes and mouth of the deceased because to not do so is considered a bad omen. They may also want to place coins on the eyelids and a roll of cloth under the chin of the deceased (University of Washington Medical Center, 2004). In the Muslim culture, the family may wash the body and wrap it in unsewn white cloth. In Judaism, the son or nearest relative may desire to close the eyes and mouth while extending the arms and hands at the sides of the body and draping the body in a sheet (University of Michigan Program for Multicultural Health, 2005).

Traditional Buddhist beliefs view consciousness and warmth as inseparable. Dying is seen as a gradual process whereby consciousness gradually separates from the body; it is not defined by the moment when the pulse and brainwaves cease. In such a culture, death occurs when the body has completely lost its consciousness and warmth. During this process, it is important to avoid abrupt environmental changes. Thus, it is preferred that the body remain undisturbed for eight hours after death, preferably until the body has completely cooled. During this time, the body may also be accompanied by chanting, with singers present or on audiotapes (University of Michigan Program for Multicultural Health, 2005).

Clearly, many different rituals could be important during and following the period of death. No healthcare provider is expected to know, or to make assumptions about, these kinds of rituals without a discussion with the client and/or family. The discussion about the procedures that may occur at the time of death and just afterward is a difficult one to initiate, particularly in cultures where death is not openly discussed, and where speaking of impending death is in opposition to maintaining hope. Yet, in other cultures, people may want to share their practices related to death very early in the process. Hence, timing based on the existing context and use of the ABC approach of awareness, bearing witness, and comfort are of vital importance. We suggest that healthcare providers take a generic approach in initiating this discussion, and then become more specific, based on what is shared by the client and family. For example, a healthcare provider may ask the following questions, starting with generic ones and becoming more specific:

1. Please tell me about some of the practices that are important to you and others in your family, and what and who will help.
2. Many people have some specific practices that need to take place at the time of death. Please tell me about any needs you may have in this area.
3. What practices related to your _____ faith should we include in your plan of care?

Healthcare providers also can show their openness and willingness to learn from the family by making a statement such as the following:

▪ I am aware that some people of your faith (or some people of different faiths) really value _____; is that something that is important to you?

The key to the above discussion is not in the phrasing of the question but, rather, in the context and manner in which the issues are raised. A trusting, respectful relationship and an open, non-judgemental manner are necessary ingredients for an effective dialogue.

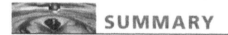 ## SUMMARY

Culture, as well as life experience, influences views on death and dying and related practices. Since "everyone has a culture" and "culture is dynamic" (College of Nurses of Ontario, 1999, p. 3), cultural sensitivity is a necessary aspect of the care provided to all clients and their families.

The ABC approach—*A*wareness, *B*earing witness, and *C*omfort—describes the interrelating processes, knowledge, and skills needed to provide culturally competent end-of-life care. Cultural knowledge, which is required to provide effective end-of-life care, means being well versed in, or sensitive to, the cultural nuances of the challenging issues that surface during this time—from the meaning of pain and suffering to the concrete preferences for rituals and spiritual acts and symbols before and after death.

The 4-*F*s—*f*eelings, *f*amily, *f*aith, and *f*inality—are key areas for consideration. Each involves specific issues that are strongly influenced by culture. The culturally competent healthcare provider who is providing end-of-life care will reflect on personal values, as well as values within the current healthcare context, that relate to life, death, and dying. Healthcare providers are encouraged to consider those clinical situations in which conflicts arose as opportunities to explore values and culture. Conflicts regarding decision making and disclosure of diagnosis and prognosis in which strong feelings are evoked often are based on values that differ from those inherent in the Western healthcare system.

It is important that healthcare providers build on culture-specific knowledge, while being ever aware of the potential danger in using such knowledge in a stereotypical manner.

REFERENCES

Alden, D., & Cheung, A. (2000). Organ donation and culture: A comparison of Asian American and European American beliefs, attitudes, and behaviours. *Journal of Applied Social Psychology, 30*(2), 293–314.

Back, A., & Petracca, F. (2003). *Cross-cultural issues in HIV/AIDS: Palliative care module contents.* University of Washington, Centre for Palliative Care Education. Retrieved August 29, 2005, from http://depts.washington.edu/pallcare/training/curriculum_pdfs/CultureModule.pdf

Blackhall, L., Frank, G., Murphy, S., & Michel, V. (2001). Bioethics in a different tongue: The case of truth-telling. *Journal of Urban Health, 78*(1), 59–71.

Bowman, K., & Richard, S. (2004). Cultural considerations for Canadians in the diagnosis of brain death. *Canadian Journal of Anesthesia, 51*, 273–275.

College of Nurses of Ontario. (1999). *Practice guideline: Culturally sensitive care.* Toronto, ON: Author.

Ersek, M., Kagawa-Singer, M., Barnes, D., Blackhall, L., & Koeing, B. (1998). Multicultural considerations in the use of advance directives. *Oncology Nursing Forum, 25*(10), 1683–1690.

Finkel, A., Leishman, M., Lundy, M., Ray, K., & Tonack, M. (2002). *Caring across cultures: Multicultural considerations in palliative care.* Toronto: St. Elizabeth Health Care.

Gatrad, R., & Sheikh, A. (2002). Palliative care for Muslims and issues after death. *International Journal of Palliative Nursing, 8*, 594–597.

Geissler, E. (1998). *Pocket guide to cultural assessment.* St. Louis: Mosby.

Hallenbeck, J., & Goldstein, M. K. (1999). Decisions at the end of life: Cultural considerations beyond medical ethics. *Generations, Spring*, 24–29.

Kagawa-Singer, M., & Blackhall, L. (2001). Negotiating cross-cultural issues at the end of life. *Journal of the American Medical Association, 286*, 2993–3002.

Kemp, C. (2005). Cultural issues in palliative care. *Seminars in Oncology Nursing, 21*(1), 44–52.

Kristjanson, L., Hudson, P., & Oldham, L. (2003). Working with families. In M. O'Connor & S. Aranda (Eds.), *Palliative nursing: A guide to practice* (2nd ed., pp. 271–283) Melbourne, Australia: Ausmed Publications.

Lapine, A., Wang-Cheng, R., Goldstein, M., Nooney, A., Lamb, G., & Derse, A. (2001). When cultures clash: Physician, patient, and family wishes in truth disclosure for dying patients. *Journal of Palliative Medicine, 4*(4), 475–480.

Lo, H. T., & Fung, K. (2003). Culturally competent psychotherapy. *Canadian Journal of Psychiatry, 48*, 161–170.

McCunn, M., Mauritz, W., Dutton, R.P., Alexander, C., Handley, C., & Scalea, T. (2003). Impact of culture and policy on organ donation: A comparison between two urban trauma centers in developed nations. *Journal of Trauma, Injury, Infection and Critical Care, 54*(5), 995–999.

Phipps, E. J., True, G., & Murray, G. F. (2003). Community perspectives on advance care planning: Report from the community ethics program. *Journal of Cultural Diversity, 10*(4), 118–123.

Randhawa, G. (1998). An exploratory study examining the influence of religion on attitudes towards organ donation among the Asian population in Luton, UK. *Nephrology Dialysis and Transplantation, 13*, 1949–1951.

Searight, H., & Gafford, J. (2005). Cultural diversity at the end of life: Issues and guidelines for family physicians. *American Family Physician, 71*(3), 515–522.

University of Michigan Program for Multicultural Health. (2005). Death and dying customs. Retrieved April 2, 2005, from http://www.med.umich.edu/multicultural/ccp/death.htm
University of Washington Medical Center. (2004). Culture clues: End-of-life care, patient and family education services. Retrieved April 2, 2005, from http://depts.washington.edu/pfes/cultureclues.html

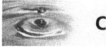

CHAPTER 11

Mental Health Practice

HUNG-TAT (TED) LO AND ANN POTTINGER

LEARNING OBJECTIVES

At the end of this chapter, the learner will be able to:

- Describe some specific and generic competencies related to the provision of mental health care
- Explain the influence of culture on the psychiatric assessment
- Explain how culture influences views on mental health and mental health care
- Describe some clinical tools, including cultural formulation, for culturally competent mental health practice

KEY TERMS

Cultural explanations	Immigrant and refugee experience
Cultural formulation	Social stressors
Cultural identity	Somatization
Cultural mindedness	

More than any other aspect of health, mental health is shaped by the pervasive influence of culture. The day-to-day experiences of interacting with the world are all subject to being filtered and interpreted through culture. Mental health assessment depends on observation and assessment techniques, which are products of the subjective experience of the assessor, with few objective tools such as radiographs or blood work.

Mental health treatment, and the setting in which it takes place, again varies from culture to culture. Its effectiveness will depend on the impact it has on the client—through complex cultural nuances—throughout care processes and at every stage of the intervention. The development of clinical competency to work effectively with clients from other cultures is an essential part of professional development for any mental healthcare provider in the increasingly diverse environments in which we work (Warren, 2000).

Cultural Competencies and Mental Health

As in other areas of practice, cultural competency in mental health requires both *generic* and *specific* competencies at various stages of the therapeutic encounter. Generic cultural competence is the knowledge and skill set required in any cross-cultural therapeutic encounter, and specific cultural competence enables clinicians to work effectively with a specific ethnocultural community (Lo & Fung, 2003, p. 161) (See Chapter 10 for detailed definitions of the two competencies, which were introduced for discussion there but in relation to end-of-life cultural care.)

Specific Competencies

Specific cultural knowledge is important to understanding the following in mental health care:
- Unique cultural symptoms and interventions
- The client's usual rules of interaction
- The client's world view or general outlook
- The client's view of mental illness

Specific cultural knowledge also includes awareness of culture-bound syndromes, such as the evil eye or *mal de ojo* in the Latino culture (American Psychiatric Association [APA], 1994; Levine & Gaw, 1995). Such syndromes are supposed to be common in various cultures, but personal clinical experience suggests that a health provider seldom encounters them unless he or she works in the country of origin. In Canada, an example of specific cultural knowledge includes being aware that the suicide rates for young people in several Aboriginal communities are higher than those for their non-Aboriginal counterparts (Kirmayer, Brass, & Tait, 2000).

The need for specific cultural competencies raises the issue of ethnic matching (discussed in Chapter 2) of healthcare provider and client, and how such matches could enhance client outcomes. However, the authors of this chapter find that in clinical reality, particularly in the diverse environment that Canada offers, it is impossible to provide ethnic matching for all clients. Furthermore, an ethnic match does not guarantee a cultural match (Sue, 1998) for reasons such as variation in ethnocultural identification and degree of acculturation (Tsang, Bogo, & George, 2003). Possessing a good knowledge of all the cultures one would encounter in one's practice also is a formidable task. It is thus imperative that all healthcare providers acquire some degree of generic cultural competence so that they can potentially provide quality and effective clinical care for any client in this multicultural country.

Generic Competencies

What follows are important points about some of the key competencies required in mental health practice. Readers are encouraged to consult additional sources on an ongoing basis for a more complete picture of each area.

Generic Knowledge of Cultures

Several classifications of generic cultural knowledge may be of note in mental health. These include:

- High- and low-context cultural features (described below)
- Cultural value orientations (i.e., how the relationship between humanity and the environment is perceived: harmony, mastery, or submission)
- Locus of control (i.e., may be external or internal depending on the degree to which individuals believe they can determine fate through their own actions)
- Emotional expression (i.e., the degree to which emotions, particularly emotional distress, are experienced and expressed openly)
- Time perspectives (discussed below)
  (Chiu, 1988; Eid & Diener, 2001; Hall & Whyte, 1960; Hsieh, Shybut, & Lotsof, 1969; Kluckhohn, 1951)

High- and Low-Context Features

As we learn about the many cultures around the world, it is increasingly evident that certain aspects of a culture often are shared by a number of other ethnocultural groups yet remain distinct from certain other groups. These are sometimes classified as high-context and low-context features (Hall & Whyte, 1960). Japanese people, as an example of a high-context culture, generally use words with meanings specific to the social situation, whereas in general North Americans, as an example of low-context culture, will use words with the same meaning regardless of the social situation. For example, in a high-context culture, depending on the situation, an individual may say "yes" or express agreement out of politeness or a desire not to openly disagree; thus, yes may mean, "Yes, I hear you," rather than, "Yes, I agree," whereas in a low-context culture, yes is more likely to mean agreement under all situations. (See Chapter 5 for further discussion of high- and low-context communication.)

Time Perspectives

Time perspectives also have been found to vary among cultures; some groups give more emphasis to the past, while others value the future, and yet others are primarily focused on the present. The predominance of the "present-oriented" focus also is a phenomenon found among refugees (Beiser & Hyman, 1997). This needs to be taken into account in planning treatment.

Shared Views of Mental Health

Some groups of cultures share similar views of both mental health and its expression. The prevalence of somatization (Kirmayer, Dao, & Smith, 1998) among many cultures is one such example. **Somatization** refers to the phenomenon where emotional or mental distress is expressed as a physical complaint. For example, in keeping with cultural norms of emotional expression, a Chinese woman suffering from depression may present with complaints of pressure on the chest, or chest compression.

Cultural views of mental health influence both the paths of help that are sought and the types of treatment that would be considered acceptable (Cheung, 1987; Herrick & Brown, 1998; Kirmayer, Galbaud du Fort, Young, Weinfeld, & Lasry, 1996).

Immigrants and Refugees

Many people in Canada are immigrants and/or refugees. The following related stressors have mental health implications:

- Adjustment
- Discrimination
- War
- Trauma
- Loss

  (Canadian Task Force on Mental Health Issues Affecting Immigrants and Refugees, 1988)

The **immigrant and refugee experience**—including events leading up to, involved in, and following the actual physical move—shapes peoples' world views. For example, a refugee client may harbour distrust toward government institutions, which should not be misinterpreted as paranoia. Even the client's time perspectives could be affected (Beiser & Hyman, 1997). Some historical and socio-political knowledge of specific immigrant communities will help in the assessment, and some knowledge of local community resources will go a long way toward formulating a plan of care. Specific cultural knowledge, like that of the refugee hearing process, also is important in working with this population (Kirmayer, 1997).

Assessments

Many aspects of the psychiatric assessment are influenced by culture (Lu, Lim, & Mezzich, 1995).

Effective communication is vital to an accurate psychiatric assessment. Styles and rules of interaction vary among cultures (Gao, Ting-Toomey, & Gudykunst, 1996). For example, the avoidance of eye contact could be one of the following:

- A show of respect
- A demonstration of shame
- A manifestation of shyness and withdrawal
- Disinterest in one's surroundings

The assessment of mood (affective) and thought disorders is particularly challenging in a cultural context. Healthcare providers are encouraged to conduct all interactions from a position of curiosity, with a willingness to ask questions about the client's background and beliefs (Andermann & Lo, 2006), and to carefully listen to the responses to these questions.

An integral part of the assessment should be an evaluation of the many aspects of culture (D'Avanzo & Geissler, 2002). This is useful even with clients who are not apparently "cultural" (Quastel & Lo, in press) since everyone has a culture. The *Diagnostic and Statistical Manual of Mental Disorders (DSM IV)* includes age, gender, and cultural considerations in many diagnostic categories, and lists religious or spiritual problems as one focus of clinical attention (APA, 1994). More important, it includes an outline for **cultural formulation**, which will be elaborated in the next section of this chapter (Mezzich, 1995).

Healthcare providers also need to understand the influence of social processes on clients. Racism has been identified as a factor contributing to misdiagnosis and inferior treatment of members of Black communities in many countries (Fernando, 1991). Similarly, to be ignorant of, disregard, or minimize the impact of colonialism on the mental and physical health of Aboriginal people will lead to inadequate care and further marginalization. Aboriginal populations have a high prevalence of mental health concerns that are linked to cultural oppression and marginalization (Kirmayer et al., 2000).

According to a 2005 national survey, approximately one in six surveyed Canadian adults indicated that they have been the victim of racism (Ipsos Reid Survey, 2005). Perceived racial discrimination has been linked to depression among Korean immigrants residing in Toronto (Noh & Kasper, 2003) and Southeast Asian refugees in Canada (Noh, Beiser, Kaspar, Hou, & Rummens, 1999). Awareness of such issues and experiences is important if a health provider is to provide competent care.

The concept of diversity goes beyond ethnocultural groups. Gay, lesbian, and transgendered individuals, for example, also can be considered a cultural group with shared values and concerns, including stress related to issues such as identity, the coming out process, and substance use (Sue & Sue, 2003). These may lead to depression and low-self esteem in response to stigma and internalization of society's view of their sexual identities.

Language support is another important aspect of care. Even when the client speaks some English, often it is desirable to work with a cultural interpreter to promote full expression (Andermann & Lo, 2006). It is important for interpreters to have training in mental health and for healthcare providers to have training in working with interpreters (Marcos, 1979). It also needs to be recognized that interpreters are cultural beings with their own feelings about the client and/or the healthcare provider, as well as their own views of mental illness. Healthcare providers should consider using interpreters for the purpose of deciphering behaviours outside of formal assessments. For example, if a hospitalized client is talking aloud to himself or herself in another language, the healthcare provider might call on an interpreter, rather than automatically labelling the behaviour as psychotic or mere "babbling."

In addition to an interpreter, often it is helpful to have the assistance of cultural consultants. They are professionals who are familiar with the client's cultural background and are able to help the healthcare provider contextualize behaviours and ideas within the client's ethnocultural background. They may be involved in the assessment or provide consultation to the healthcare provider afterward. Without this understanding, it may be impossible to conduct accurate mental health assessments. Working with cultural consultants has helped in many complex situations to address cultural and systemic factors in a manner that honoured the client's strengths and values, leading to the negotiation of treatment and care plans (Kirmayer et al, 2003).

Psychiatric Treatment and Care

Cultural competence is an essential aspect of providing effective mental health care (Campinha-Bacote, 1994). Cultural considerations may require modification in treatment methods such as psychopharmacology and psychotherapy. Treatment plans may need to be devised specifically with the help of cultural resources—for instance, by working with healers and traditional medicines.

It is important to appreciate that the area of psychopharmacology has developed with little recognition of cultural variances. Drug trials only now are beginning to include considerations of cultural groupings in sampling. However, there is an increasing body of knowledge of ethno-psychopharmacology and a recognition that drug metabolism may be influenced by genetic and racial characteristics (Ruiz, 2000). This may manifest as unexpected side effects for a low dose of antipsychotic medication in a young Asian man, or inversely as a lack of progress despite a high dose in a slim Mexican woman. As well, the way in which medication is viewed varies among cultures and needs to be taken into account.

Psychotherapy is a cultural product of nineteenth-century Europe and still may be looked upon with suspicion by many cultures. On the other hand, many spiritual practices that have fallen by the wayside in developed countries still may hold sway in other cultures. To practise psychotherapy competently, the healthcare provider is well advised to consider the complex cultural issues involved (Lo & Fung, 2003; Tseng & Streltzer, 2001). Family therapy (Ho, 1987) and group therapy (Tsui & Schultz, 1988) also needs to be practised with such cultural considerations.

Sometimes, it may be necessary to make use of cultural resources in order to customize the treatment; this may include the use of herbal remedies or the involvement of shamans and healers. The healthcare provider needs to become knowledgeable and comfortable with such practices and able to negotiate in a respectful and thoughtful manner (Jilek, 1993). In addition to having knowledge of cultural resources and complementary therapies, the healthcare provider needs to consider related factors such as professional standards, competence, organizational policies, and scope of practice in determining the extent to which he or she will be involved in such therapies or practices.

Working with Families and Communities

The meaning of family and the role of individuals within families vary among cultures. Culture shapes all aspects of family life, including communication and decision-making processes. In many cultures, it is the norm for an individual to sacrifice autonomy for the benefit of the family. The healthcare provider needs to understand clients' and families' world views and how their views and values relate to safety and risk, treatment options, decision making, and informed consent.

Engagement of the family is of utmost importance in working with most ethnocultural communities, and family therapy models also must accommodate the cultural differences in order to be culturally responsive (Campinha-Bacote, 2002).

Working with ethnic communities is a skill seldom taught in professional schools. However, healthcare providers require this kind of skill when they need the assistance of interpreters or cultural consultants, or want to refer to community agencies. It also is an important asset when developing programs for such communities. As in any hospital–community collaboration, the importance of respect and thoughtfulness cannot be overstated.

Program Development

Programs should include systems and processes that provide information about the needs of diverse groups. Developing programs for cultural groups requires thoughtful incorporation of the cultural values of the groups, ideally with input from community members (Lo & Andermann, in press). Healthcare providers need to consider the assumptions on which services are based, and the impact of such assumptions on the accessibility and care that is provided to diverse clients. For example, conventional mental health services that are based on mainstream Western values and assumptions are seldom effective for Aboriginal communities (Kirmayer et al., 2000). Given the evidence that local control by a community contributes to better mental health within such a community (Kirmayer et al., 2000), collaborative program development is vital.

Important questions for program planners to ask on an ongoing basis are:

1. What is the mental health culture and how do the values of this culture compare to values of diverse groups? How are power differentials addressed?
2. How do healthcare providers communicate?
   - Are educational materials provided in various languages?
   - How frequently do healthcare providers work with interpreters?
3. Does the client group reflect the diversity of the general population? Are our program services accessible?
4. Are members from diverse groups involved in, or do they have input into, planning the program?

On the other hand, the cultural mix among clients in the program may lead to certain conflicts. Members of the treatment team often are equally diverse, and the cultural dynamics among them is another important area for team leaders to consider. Any discord will readily lead to disruption in client care.

Clinical Tools

One of the difficulties in developing cultural competence is the lack of concrete tools to bridge the gap between having cultural awareness and incorporating it into everyday practice. Below, the authors describe tools that they have found helpful in clinical practice.

Cultural Formulation

Cultural formulation is a tool included in the *DSM IV* (APA, 1994) as Appendix I, just before the list of contributors; therefore, even those who use the *DSM* daily could easily miss it. However, it represents a hard-won victory for a small group of advocates within the American psychiatric community. The development of the *DSM* itself demonstrates how much a cultural artifact this document is in and of itself, each version reflecting the cultural mores of the generation. The *DSM*'s cultural formulation indicates several areas for inquiry, which would provide a systematic review of all the cultural factors that influence clients and how these potentially affect the working relationship with the clients (Mezzich, 1995). Each area is described briefly, and specific tools are presented that may be helpful in exploring these areas.

Cultural Identity

There are significant connections between mental health and **cultural identity**, which is the sense of belonging to a group or culture based on shared characteristics with other members of the cultural group (see also the discussion of "identity" in Chapter 3). It is important to ascertain the cultural identities of clients, and not base identity solely on appearance (Quastel & Lo, in press). There may be intra-ethnic differences, and for each client with his or her unique life history, the identity could be equally unique (Uba, 1994).

It is helpful to identify the patterns of acculturation, or cultural adaptation (Berry & Sam, 1996), and their implications on mental health. For example, a biracial client with a Black father and a White mother may need to actively explore one or the other side of his or her heritage to arrive at a cohesive sense of self, which is essential to one's mental health.

It also is important to remember that the same identity issues, along with their implications for interactions, apply to healthcare providers and to everyone they encounter in practice, including families, interpreters, and colleagues. Identity is an important aspect of mental health well-being not only for individuals but also for communities.

Cultural Explanations

Cultural explanations are meanings, beliefs, and attitudes that a culture ascribes to a particular phenomenon. Kleinman (1988) formulated the idea that in different cultures, there may be different languages of distress, like somatization, and different explanatory models of illnesses. He proposed a series of questions to clarify the explanatory model of the clients involved (see Chapter 4), and the College of Nurses of Ontario (CNO) has added to that list in its *Culturally Sensitive Care* practice guidelines (College of Nurses of Ontario, 1999). These aim to elicit the client's view of the nature, cause, consequences, and treatment of the problem or situation. To respond to differences between the models of the client and the healthcare provider, Leininger (1995) proposes three paths of action (described in Chapter 4):

1. *Preservation:* respecting and preserving the values where possible
2. *Negotiation*: accommodating and negotiating across preferences and world views where needed
3. *Repatterning*: creating new options and approaches for the client, health-care provider, or system

Cultural Factors Related to Psychosocial Environment and Levels of Functioning

The idea here is to list the many possible social stressors that could contribute to the client's presentation, including those we have discussed in the section above. **Social stressors** are "events or conditions that are linked to individuals' and families' social characteristics, positions, and roles" (Menaghan, n.d.). Supportive factors, such as community and religion, also are considered here. The level of functioning also needs to be interpreted differently in various cultural context; for instance, a single Italian man in his thirties living with his parents may not indicate any dependency issue.

Cultural Elements of Client and Healthcare Provider Relationships

Aside from language and cultural differences having an obvious impact on assessment and treatment, cultural transference and counter-transference occurs in the therapeutic relationship (Cheng & Lo, 1991; Comas-Diaz & Jacobsen, 1991). The therapeutic pairings (which scholars call dyads) are shown in Figure 11-1. Majority (M) and minority (m) refer to power dynamics and do not necessarily

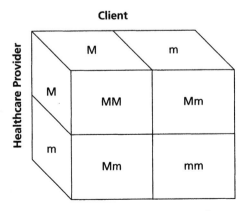

M = majority culture; m = minority culture

FIGURE 11-1 ▪ **Psychodynamics of the Healthcare Provider–Client Relationship**

indicate numbers, so that a White healthcare provider working in a Black neighbourhood would still be considered a member of the majority culture.

With a majority therapist and minority client (Mm), the client may be more trusting of the healthcare provider, feeling that a majority healthcare provider is more educated than a minority one, leading to a positive transference; or the client may feel discriminated against by the majority healthcare provider because of past experience, leading to negative transference. On the other hand, the healthcare provider may feel good to be helping a minority client, contributing to positive counter-transference; or the healthcare provider may harbour preconceived ideas that the client may be lazy and uneducated—negative counter-transference. Different types of dynamics could emerge with different pairings, and it is even more complicated with "mm" because of the many possible variations—the client and healthcare provider may be from the same ethnic group or two different minority groups.

Case Formulation

Case formulation is a tool that allows the healthcare provider to incorporate all the clinical data into an overall assessment of the client. The authors use an expanded version (see Table 11-1) of the holistic bio-psycho-social grid approach (Engel, 1977)—where "bio" refers to the biological and physiological; "psycho," the thinking and feeling aspects; and "social," to social networking—with the following included:

▪ A *spiritual* dimension, to include the spiritual issues often prominent in various ethnocultural groups (Larson, Milano, & Lu, 1998)
▪ A *presenting* column, to summarize the clinical features being presented
▪ A *protective* column, to consider strengths
▪ A *plan* column, to indicate types of interventions

This tool provides a way of capturing, in clinical assessments, all relevant information—cultural included—that will guide intervention planning.

The use of the grid is illustrated in Table 11-1 by the formulation of the hypothetical case of Kyoko, a single Japanese woman of 39 who immigrated to Toronto one year ago. She managed to find work and has done well. However, she is quite shy, and, without her family for the first time, she felt lonely and became depressed. Then her family doctor told her that she had a breast lump, possibly cancer. Her mother died of breast cancer six years earlier, and Kyoko often felt she did not do enough for her. She had to wait for the specialist to give her the diagnosis and prognosis. She could not tell anyone about the possibility of breast cancer and became obsessed with its potential consequence and the associated fear and stigma. She used to pray at a temple, but had not been to one in Toronto. She was referred to a male Caucasian therapist. She had difficulty expressing herself in English, and also was reticent in discussing her negative emotions.

TABLE 11-1

Case Formulation of Kyoko

	PRESENTING	PREDISPOSING	PRECIPITATING	PERPETUATING	PROTECTIVE	PLAN
Biological	Insomnia	Family history of cancer	Breast lump	Cancer diagnosis unclear	Healthy otherwise	Antidepressant
Psychological	Depressed	Shyness Guilt about mother	Manner in which she was given the diagnosis/ prognosis	Difficulty expressing emotion	Lack of trust in therapist	Encouraged to seek therapy and support
Social	Withdrawal	Alone in Canada		Further isolation	Working well	Advocacy with specialist
Spiritual	Confused			Not using religious resource	Prays at home	Seek out temple

Note: Some items can be put in different categories, and some categories can be left blank if information is not available.

Kluckhohn Triangle

Every man is in certain respects like all other men, like some other men, and like no other man. (Kluckhohn & Murray, 1953, p. 388)

The above quotation is wonderfully helpful in conceptualizing the nature of culture. "Like all other men" represents the universal, "like some other men" represents the cultural, and "like no other men" represents the individual. Envisaged as a triangle with three layers, it is a graphic reminder for us to consider the influence that culture has at all levels of our clinical interactions.

For the uninitiated, there are only two layers, the individual and the universal; one would consider the presentation of any clinical data from the individual client by comparing it with ourselves—our own universal view, which is assumed to be applicable to all. Then we intervene in ways that are thought to be universally valid. By introducing the cultural layer, we would have three layers; the information from the client would then be filtered through the cultural layer, and we would interpret it with our cultural knowledge, always remembering to check our interpretations with the client so as not to engage in stereotyping. Only then would we be able to arrive at a position to truly understand the universal, the feelings we all share as humans. From that position, using our professional knowledge, we intervene. However, the intervention again needs to pass through the cultural layer so that it is culturally appropriate and capable of accomplishing the desired goal (see Figure 11-2).

As an example, Mr. Chan, a 65-year-old Chinese man, became depressed with various somatic preoccupations after his retirement and immigration to Canada. The healthcare provider considered him non-compliant when he did not continue his antidepressants. Using the "cultural" layer, one might appreciate that depression has not been a known illness in the Chinese culture. One might also find out that Mr. Chan was scared by the dizziness he was experiencing, which he interpreted as sign of a serious illness. Besides, he could not see how his problem could be helped by medication. At the "universal" level, the healthcare provider could then understand that a client would not take anything that is scary without being convinced of its usefulness. The healthcare provider would proceed to explain Mr. Chan's condition to him, using the concept of neurasthenia, which is well established in Mr. Chan's culture, and present the medication as a "tonic," and reassure him that the dizziness was not serious and would not last long.

Cultural Mindedness

The authors of this chapter believe that people vary in their aptitude for dealing with cross-cultural encounters, and refer to this as **cultural mindedness** (CM).[1] This is what healthcare providers bring to the clinical encounter. Part of that aptitude is derived from nature, but part of it also can be purposefully nourished. We

---

[1]The notion of cultural mindedness described here is similar to the concept of cultural sensitivity discussed in Chapter 3.

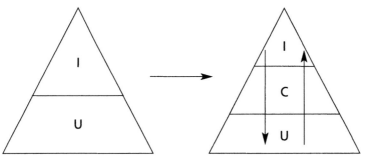

I = Individual   U = Universal   C = Cultural

FIGURE 11-2 ▪ **The Kluckhohn Triangle**
Based on *Personality in nature, society and culture* (p. 53), by C. Kluckhohn and H. A. Murray (Eds.), 1953, New York: Knopf.

consider this aptitude to be the basis of clinical cultural competence, and enhancing our CM will further develop it. A conceptualization of CM, with some of its domains, is as follows:

1. *Attitude*—certain attitudinal attributes contribute to CM:
   - Curiosity—propels us to inquire into the culture of another person (Dyche & Zayas, 1995)
   - Respect—guides our interaction so that the other person does not feel encroached upon or intimidated
   - Desire to connect—we try not just to understand but also to connect with the other person
2. *Awareness*—certain types of awareness also contribute to CM:
   - Awareness of the fact that the other person has his or her own world view
   - Awareness that the healthcare provider also has a distinctive world view
   - Awareness of the power dynamics between client and healthcare provider and their effect on the relationship (Pinderhughes, 1988)
3. *Autobiography* or personal experience—the healthcare provider's unique life experience, which also powerfully contributes to CM:
   - Past (e.g., the healthcare provider may have a bicultural heritage or experience of being a member of a minority group)
   - Present (e.g., current social network, exposure to other cultures through the media)
   - Future (e.g., aspirations and direction in life)

To enhance one's CM, the healthcare provider should ask the following questions on an ongoing basis:
- *Before any encounter, ask:* "Do I want to connect with this person in a respectful manner?"
- *At the encounter, ask:* "Am I aware that we have different world views, and that there also may be a power differential between us?"
- *At all times, ask oneself:* "Am I living a 'culturally conscious' life?"

These questions can be a useful tool in developing cultural competence, and can be used during reflective practice and clinical supervision of healthcare providers involved in mental health care.

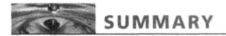

SUMMARY

Culturally competent health care requires a client-centred approach (CNO, 1999), which enables healthcare providers to understand individuals as unique cultural beings. This is true for the mental health practice as much as for any other area of health care. Healthcare providers focus on clients' perspectives and use their wishes and views to guide care and treatment. Even with different clients from a similar cultural background, there is no single approach or intervention that will always work. Culturally competent mental health care also is holistic care, in that all the bio-psycho-social and spiritual spheres are considered.

This chapter identified key issues within mental health care that are influenced by culture and presented specific and generic competencies that are necessary for healthcare providers. Cultural identity and cultural explanations are two important areas that require assessment before appropriate interventions can be determined. Power dynamics between healthcare providers and clients are highlighted through a discussion on the psychodynamics of this relationship and its potential impact on the therapeutic relationship. The chapter ends with a case formulation exercise that illustrates how this tool can be used to incorporate the relevant clinical data into an overall assessment and plan of care.

This chapter focused on the individual healthcare provider involved in mental health care, however, culturally competent individuals can exert little influence if the system in which they work is not culturally competent. Conversely, to develop a culturally competent mental health system, individual healthcare providers also must be trained and supported in their development of cultural competence. This interrelationship cannot be overstated in view of the uneven development in the field.

Although the development of cultural competence may be an ethical responsibility and a practical necessity, tremendous personal rewards can be gained from practising in a culturally competent manner, such as a unique perspective on the full richness of the human experience. Developing cultural competence is an ongoing journey with no specific end point, a journey that the reader is encouraged to embark on.

ONLINE LEARNING RESOURCES

http://sfghdean.ucsf.edu/barnett/DBS/cd.asp
Barnett-Briggs Medical Library (University of California), Cultural Competence and Diversity Collection

www.mentalhealth.samhsa.gov/publications/allpubs/SMA00-3457/default.asp
Cultural Competence Standards in Managed Care Mental Health Services, National Mental Health Information Center

http://www.omhrc.gov
Home page of the Office of Minority Health, US Department of Health and
Human Services; features data on minority populations as well as cultural
competency

www.surgeongeneral.gov/library/mentalhealth/cre/
Mental Health: Culture, Race and Ethnicity, A Supplement to Mental Health: A
Report of the Surgeon General (US Department of Health and Human Services)

REFERENCES

American Psychiatric Association. (1994). *Diagnostic and statistical manual of mental disorders* (4th ed.). Washington, DC: Author.

Andermann, L., & Lo, H. T. (2006) Cultural competence in psychiatric assessment. In D. Goldbloom (Ed.), *Psychiatric Clinical Skills* (pp. 21–28). St. Louis: Mosby.

Beiser, M., & Hyman, I. (1997). Refugees' time perspective and mental health. *American Journal of Psychiatry, 154*, 996–1002.

Berry J. W., & Sam, D. (1996). Acculturation and adaptation. In J. W. Berry, M. H. Segall, & C. Kagitcibasi (Eds.), *Handbook of cross-cultural psychology. Vol 3: Social behavior and applications* (pp. 291–325). Boston: Allyn & Bacon.

Campinha-Bacote, J. (1994). Cultural competence in psychiatric mental health nursing: A conceptual model. *Nursing Clinics of North America, 29*(1), 1–8.

Campinha-Bacote, J. (2002). Cultural competence in psychiatric nursing: Have you asked the right questions? *Journal of American Psychiatric Nurses Association, 8*, 183–187.

Canadian Task Force on Mental Health Issues Affecting Immigrants and Refugees. (1988). *After the door has been opened: Mental health issues affecting immigrants and refugees in Canada*. Ottawa: Health and Welfare Canada.

Cheng, L. Y., & Lo, H. T. (1991). On the advantages of cross-culture psychotherapy: The minority therapist/mainstream patient dyad. *Psychiatry, 54*(4), 386–396.

Cheung F. M. (1987). Conceptualization of psychiatric illness and help-seeking behaviour among Chinese. *Culture, Medicine & Psychiatry, 11*(1), 97–106.

Chiu, L. H. (1988). Locus of control differences between American and Chinese adolescents. *Journal of Social Psychology, 128*, 411–3.

College of Nurses of Ontario. (1999). *Practice guideline: Culturally sensitive care*. Toronto, ON: Author.

Comas-Diaz, L., & Jacobsen, F. M. (1991). Ethnocultural transference and countertransference in the therapeutic dyad. *American Journal of Orthopsychiatry, 61*(3), 392–402.

D'Avanzo, C. E., & Geissler, E. M. (2002). *Pocket guide to cultural assessment* (3rd ed.). St. Louis, MO: Mosby.

Dyche, L., & Zayas, L. (1995). The value of curiosity and naivete for the cross-cultural psychotherapist. *Family Process, 34*(4), 389–399.

Eid, M., & Diener, E. (2001). Norms for experiencing emotions in different cultures: Inter- and intranational differences. *Journal of Personality and Social Psychology, 81*(5), 869–885.

Engel, G. L. (1977). The need for a new medical model: A challenge for biomedicine. *Science, 196*, 129–136.

Fernando, S. (1991). *Mental health, race and culture*. Basingstoke: Macmillan.

Gao, G., Ting-Toomey, S., & Gudykunst, W. B. (1996). Chinese communication process. In M. H. Bond (Ed.), *Handbook of Chinese psychology* (pp. 280–293). New York: Oxford University Press.

Hall, E. T., & Whyte, W. F. (1960). Intercultural communication: A guide to men of action. *Human Organization, 19*, 5–12.

Herrick, C., & Brown H. (1998). Underutilization of mental health services by Asian-Americans residing in the United States. *Issues in Mental Health Nursing, 19*(3), 225–240.

Ho, M. (1987). *Family therapy with ethnic minorities*. Newbury Park: Sage.

Hsieh, T., Shybut, J., & Lotsof, E. (1969). Internal versus external control and ethnic group membership: A cross-cultural comparison. *Journal of Consulting and Clinical Psychology, 33*, 122–124.

Ipsos Reid Survey. (2005). One in six Canadians say they have personally been victims of racism. Retrieved February 12, 2006, from www.ipsos-na.com/news/pressrelease.cfm?id=2602

Jilek, W. G. (1993). Traditional medicine relevant to psychiatry. In N. Sartorius, G. de Girolamo, & G. Andrews (Eds.), *Treatment of mental disorders: A review of effectiveness* (pp. 341–383). Washington, DC: American Psychiatric Press.

Kirmayer, L. J. (1997). Failures of imagination: The refugee's narrative in psychiatry. *Anthropology and Medicine, 10*(2), 167–185.

Kirmayer, L. J., Brass, G., & Tait, C. (2000). The mental health of Aboriginal peoples: Transformations of identity and community. *Canadian Journal of Psychiatry, 45*, 607–616.

Kirmayer, L. J., Dao, T. H. T., & Smith, A. (1998). Somatization and psychologization: Undertaking cultural idioms of distress. In S. Okpaku, (Ed.), *Clinical methods in transcultural psychiatry* (pp. 233–265). Washington: American Psychiatric Press.

Kirmayer, L. J., Galbaud du Fort, G., Young, A., Weinfeld, M., & Lasry, J. C. (1996). Pathways and barriers to mental health care in an urban multicultural milieu: An epidemiological and ethnographic study. *Culture and Mental Health Research Unit Report No. 6*, (Summary, pp. 13–15). Retrieved August 11, 2005, from http://upload.mcgill.ca/tcpsych/Report6.pdf

Kirmayer, L. J., Groleau, D., Guzder, J., Blake, C., & Jarvis, E. (2003). Cultural consultation: A model of mental health service for multicultural societies. *Canadian Journal of Psychiatry, 48*(3), 145–153.

Kleinman, A. (1988). *The illness narratives: Suffering, healing and the human condition*. New York: Basic Books.

Kluckhohn, C. (1951). Values and value orientations. In T. Parsons (Ed.), *Toward a general theory of action* (pp. 388–433). Cambridge, MA: Harvard University Press.

Kluckhohn, C., & Murray, H. A. (Eds.). (1953). *Personality in nature, society and culture*. New York: Knopf.

Larson, D., Milano, M., & Lu, F. (1998). Religion and mental health: The need for cultural sensitivity and synthesis. In: S. Okpaku, (Ed.), *Clinical Methods in Transcultural Psychiatry* (pp. 191–210). Washington, DC: American Psychiatric Press.

Leininger, M. (1995). *Transcultural nursing: Concepts, theories, research & practices*. New York: McGraw-Hill, Inc.

Levine, E., & Gaw, A. (1995). Culture-bound syndromes. *The Psychiatric Clinics of North America, 18*(3), 523–536.

Lo, H. T., & Andermann, L. (in press). Challenges in mental health service delivery to ethnocultural populations: A review of models. In A. Rummens, and M. Beiser, (Eds.), *Immigration, health and ethnicity*. Toronto: University of Toronto Press.

Lo, H. T., & Fung, K. (2003). Culturally competent psychotherapy. *Canadian Journal of Psychiatry, 48*, 161–170.

Lu, F. H., Lim, R. F., & Mezzich, J. E. (1995). Issues in the assessment and diagnosis of culturally diverse individuals. In J. M. Oldham & M. B. Riba (Eds.), *Review of psychiatry* (Vol. 14, pp. 477–510). London: American Psychiatric Press.

Marcos, L. R. (1979). Effects of interpreters on the evaluation of psychopathology in non-English–speaking patients. *American Journal of Psychiatry, 136*, 171–174.

Menaghan, E. (n.d.). Stress. Retrieved December 23, 2005 from http://encyclopedias.families.com/stress-1573-1579-iemf

Mezzich J. (1995). Cultural formulation and comprehensive diagnosis. *Psychiatric Clinics of North America, 18*(3), 649–57.

Noh, S., Beiser, M., Kaspar, V., Hou, F., & Rummens, J. (1999). Perceived racial discrimination, depression, and coping: A study of Southeast Asian refugees in Canada. *Journal of Health and Social Behavior, 40*, 193–207.

Noh, S., & Kaspar, V. (2003). Perceived discrimination and depression: Moderating effects of coping, acculturation, and ethic support. *American Journal of Public Health, 93*(2), 232–238.

Pinderhughes, E. (1988). *Understanding race, ethnicity, and power: The key to efficacy in clinical practice.* New York, NY: Free Press.

Quastel, A., & Lo, H. T. (in press). Cultural considerations in psychiatric assessment. In A. Rummens, & M. Beiser, (Eds.), *Immigration, health and ethnicity.* Toronto: University of Toronto Press.

Ruiz, P. (Ed.). (2000). *Ethnicity and psychopharmacology.* Washington, DC: American Psychiatric Press.

Sue, S. (1998). In search of cultural competence in psychotherapy and counseling. *American Psychologist, April*, 440–444.

Sue, D. W., & Sue, S. (2003). *Counseling the culturally diverse.* New York: John Wiley & Sons, Inc.

Tsang, A., Bogo, M., & George, U. (2003). Critical issues in cross-cultural counseling research: Case example of an ongoing project. *Journal of Multicultural Counseling and Development, 31*, 63–78.

Tseng, W. S., & Streltzer, J. (2001). *Culture and psychotherapy: A guide to clinical practice.* Washington, DC: American Psychiatric Association.

Tsui, P., & Schultz G. L. (1988). Ethnic factors in group process: Cultural dynamics in multi-ethnic therapy groups. *American Journal of Orthopsychiatry, 58*, 136–142.

Uba, L. (1994). *Ethnic identity: Asian Americans.* New York: Guilford Press.

Warren, B. J. (2000). Cultural competence: A best practice process for psychiatric mental health nursing. *Journal of the American Psychiatric Nurses Association, 6*, 135–138.

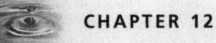

CHAPTER 12

Immigrant Women's Health

ILENE HYMAN AND SEPALI GURUGE

LEARNING OBJECTIVES

At the end of this chapter, the learner will be able to:

- Describe factors that determine health
- Understand how income, education, work, social support, stress, health practices, and health services impact on the health of immigrant women
- Identify ways of responding to the health needs of immigrant women
- Explain the roles of policymakers, health planners, and health practitioners in improving immigrant women's health

KEY TERMS

Determinants of health	Health promotion
Determinants of immigrant women's health	Healthy immigrant effect

Many broad determinants have been found to influence the health of all Canadians. This chapter discusses what they are and begins with an overview of immigrant women in Canada. Some of the specific determinants of immigrant women's health then are examined. Finally, the implications of findings for policymakers, health planners, and practitioners are discussed.

Overview: Immigrant Women in Canada

Cultural diversity is a reality in Canada. Since 1990, the country has accepted approximately 230,000 immigrants a year, or about 0.7 percent of the Canadian population (van Kessel, 1998). Women comprise just over half (51 percent) of the new immigrants each year, and immigrant women represent 18 percent of all women living in Canada (Chard, Badets, & Howtson-Leo, 2000). Immigrant women are not a homogeneous group; there is a great deal of diversity among these women with respect to country of origin, official immigration category under which the women entered Canada, length of stay in Canada, race, culture, age, socio-economic status, education, and knowledge of host country languages.

The ethnic composition of Canada's immigrants has shifted dramatically since the 1960s, changing from largely European to largely non-European countries of origin (van Kessel, 1998). Today, 60 percent of recent immigrants come from Asia and the Middle East (Citizenship and Immigration Canada, 2003). If we study the number of immigrants coming from individual countries, male immigrants generally outnumber females—except in the case of the Philippines and Jamaica (Citizenship and Immigration Canada, 2000). In 1996, 44 percent of immigrant women in Canada belonged to a visible minority group compared with just 4 percent of Canadian-born women who belong to a visible minority group (Chard et al., 2000).

Immigrants to Canada fall into several categories, depending on their reasons for immigrating: economic/business class (56 percent), family class (29 percent), refugees (13 percent), and "others," such as caregivers and retirees (3 percent) (Citizenship and Immigration Canada, 2000). However, who is in which category is sometimes unclear; for example, when family members of refugees reunite, they may come to Canada under the family class. In 1998, 40 percent of female immigrants came as spouses of economic immigrants, and 35 percent came as family class immigrants (Chard et al., 2000). The five leading source countries for refugees to Canada in 1999 were Bosnia Herzegovina (11.1 percent), Sri Lanka (10.7 percent), Afghanistan (7.4 percent), Iran (5.9 percent), and Somalia (5.7 percent). Approximately one-third of these refugees were female (Citizenship and Immigration Canada, 2000).

Immigrants to Canada tend to be highly educated, in part reflecting the fact that the majority of immigrants who come to Canada do so through the independent or business streams. For example, the proportion of men and women holding university degrees is significantly higher among recent immigrants (24 percent and 19 percent, respectively) than among the Canadian-born population (13 percent and 12 percent). Women among the most recent group of immigrants tend to be somewhat less likely than men to be able to carry on a conversation in English or French. In 1996, females accounted for 64 percent of recent immigrants who could not speak English or French. Among older recent immigrants (aged 45 to 64 years), 79 percent of females and 64 percent of males could not speak English or French (Chard et al., 2000).

Immigration and Health

In Canada, as in other countries, notably the United States (Stephen, Foote, Hendershot, & Shoenborn, 1994) and Australia (Donovan, d'Espaignet, Metron, & van Ommeren, 1992), the "healthy immigrant effect" represents a major health concern (Hyman, 2001, 2004). The **healthy immigrant effect** refers to the observation that immigrants (male and female) often are in superior health compared to the native-born population when they first arrive in a new country but lose this health advantage over time (Chen, Ng, & Wilkins, 1996a, 1996b; Pérez, 2002). Similar findings have been reported when immigrant women alone are studied. Based on data from a Canadian Community Health Survey, immigrant women who had been in Canada for less than two years were less likely to report poor health; women who had immigrated to, and resided in, Canada for at least ten years were more likely to report poor health than Canadian-born women (Vissandjée, Desmeules, Cao, Abdool, Kazanjian, 2003). Whether these findings were a result of self-selection or influenced by other determinants of immigrant women's health could not be ascertained.

Determinants of Immigrant Women's Health

It has been suggested that the process of immigration and resettlement may influence immigrant health indirectly through so-called **determinants of health**. According to the "Population Health Approach" (see Table 12-1), many broad determinants influence the health of all Canadians, including gender, income, and social status; employment and working conditions; health practices; social and physical environments; and culture (Health Canada, 2002).

In a review of the important health issues that immigrants and refugees face, Fowler (1998) notes that "of paramount importance are the social determinants of health, including age, social isolation, language barriers, separation from family, changes in family roles and norms, and lack of information about available resources and unemployment" (p. 389). She also proposed that "cross-cultural differences in information-seeking patterns, communication styles, perceptions of health risk, and ideals about prevention of disease have an impact on health" (p. 389). Specific **determinants of immigrant women's health,** which are examined in the pages that follow, include:

- Income, education, and work
- Social support and stress
- Health practices
- Use of health services

TABLE 12-1

Population Health Approach

Key Determinants of Health
1. Income and social status
2. Social support networks
3. Education
4. Employment/working conditions
5. Social environments
6. Physical environments
7. Personal health practices and coping skills
8. Healthy child development
9. Biology and genetic endowment
10. Health services
11. Gender
12. Culture

From *Population health*, 2002, Ottawa: Health Canada. Retrieved November 28, 2004, from http://www.phac-aspc.gc.ca/ph-sp/phdd/determinants/index.html#determinants

Income, Education, and Work

There is strong and growing evidence that high social and economic status is associated with better health. In fact, socio-economic status seems to be the most important determinant of health. High income determines living conditions, such as safe housing and the ability to buy sufficient healthy food. Unemployment, underemployment, and stressful or unsafe work conditions are associated with poorer health (Health Canada, 2002).

Immigrants, especially women, are disproportionately poorer than the Canadian-born population, making poverty a confusing factor in determining any relationship between immigration and health. The lives of many immigrant women are characterized by several factors:

▪ Poverty
▪ Marginalization
▪ Gender inequities
▪ Social processes that reinforce the conditions listed above (e.g., under-employment, discrimination, and the loss of pre-existing support systems) (Oxman-Martinez, Abdool, & Loiselle-Leonard, 2000; Vissandjée, Leduc, Gravel, Bourdeau, & Carigan, 1998)

Among the immigrant population, immigrant women are more likely to be living in low-income situations than their male and Canadian-born counterparts. In 2000, 23 percent of all foreign-born women lived in poverty, compared with 20 percent for immigrant men and just 16 percent for Canadian-born women. Even within the immigrant women group, recent immigrants (those who arrived in Canada within the past decade) are more disadvantaged. In 2000, 35 percent of females who immigrated in the past decade were living in poverty, compared with 21 percent of women who immigrated between 1981 and 1990 (Statistics Canada, 2006).

For immigrant women who work outside the home, occupational health and safety factors constitute other health determinants (Vissandjée, Weinfeld, Dupéré, Abdool, 2001). Exposure to job strain, reduced autonomy, and long working hours are related to the development of chronic illness, particularly heart disease (Kaplan & Keil, 1993; Roxborough, 1996). In the following excerpt, Anderson et al. (1993) describe how a group of Chinese immigrant women managed chronic illness in a way that was influenced by the realities of their daily lives and their often inferior position within the labour market:

> Without job security, many were forced to conceal their chronic illness. This can have dele-terious effects on health. For example, they were reluctant to test their blood sugar at work or to inform co-workers about the signs of low blood sugar. (p. 16)

Education is closely tied to socio-economic status, and effective education for children and lifelong learning for adults are key contributors to health and prosperity for individuals. Although immigrant women, particularly those who are recent immigrants, usually have higher levels of education than Canadian-born females, immigrant women experience more difficulty finding work and their average income is lower than that of their Canadian counterparts. Among women aged 25 to 44 who were employed in Canada in 1995/96, 12 percent of

immigrant women and 17 percent of recent immigrant women were manual workers, compared with 6 percent of Canadian-born females. In the 1996/97 National
Population Health Survey (Hyman, 2002), recent immigrants reported higher
levels of education than their Canadian-born counterparts, but their rates of
poverty were more than double (29.7 percent and 12.6 percent, respectively).

Few empirical studies have examined the effects of poverty and its associated
social processes on immigrant women's health and well-being (Janzen, 1998;
Mulvihill & Mailloux, 2000). In the area of infectious disease, there is strong
evidence that poverty, poor living conditions, substance abuse, and malnutrition
are associated with the reactivation of tuberculosis in North America (Kent, 1993;
McSherry & Connor, 1993).

Social Support and Stress

Support from families, friends, and communities is associated with better health.
Social support networks could be very important in helping people solve problems and deal with adversity, as well as in maintaining a sense of mastery and
control over life circumstances. The caring and respect that occur in social relationships, and the resulting sense of satisfaction and well-being, seem to act as a
buffer against health problems. Furthermore, recent studies show that limited
options and space for dealing with stress increase vulnerability to a range of
diseases, through sequences of reactions that involve the immune and hormonal
systems (Health Canada, 2002).

Many studies attest to the relationship between social support, stress, and
health status in both immigrant and native-born populations. Moving into
Western, industrialized societies is hypothesized to be stressful, and this stress, in
turn, is associated with increases in blood pressure (Kasl & Berkman, 1983).
Findings from the Whitehall I and II studies of British civil servants suggest that
immigrants, whose lives are characterized by underemployment and socio-
economic marginalization, are at particularly high risk of heart disease
(Vissandjée et al., 2001). Re-settlement stress also has been associated with the
development of tuberculosis during the early years of resettlement (Davies, 1995;
Grenville-Mathers & Clark, 1979; Powell, Meador, & Farer, 1981; Proust, 1971),
with diabetes (Greenhalgh, 1997; Williams, Bhopal, & Hunt, 1994), and with
mental health problems (Beiser, Turner, & Ganesan, 1989). However, few studies
have specifically examined the relationship of stress, social support, and health
among immigrant women.

Research suggests there is a need to refocus attention on immigrant women's
resiliency and capacity to maintain health and well-being despite adversity.
Attachment to the culture of one's country of origin is believed to exert a protective effect on health and well-being, as the following examples illustrate:

▪ The classic study by Marmot and Syme (1976) compared rates of heart
disease among Japanese migrants to Hawaii and found that rates were
three to five times higher among the subgroup considered to be the most
adapted to Western culture.

- In a study of low birth weight (LBW) among Latinos of Mexican descent, Scribner and Dwyer (1989) found that factors associated with a traditional Mexican cultural orientation were protective against the risk of LBW.
- Hyman and Dussault (2000) reported similar findings. In their study of acculturation and LBW, the experiences of newly arrived non-English or non-French-speaking pregnant Southeast Asian women in Montreal were compared to their "more acculturated" (i.e., English- or French-speaking, with longer residency) counterparts. The more acculturated study participants were more likely to exhibit conventional risk factors for LBW, such as engaging in intense work during pregnancy, and also reported increased levels of stress and lower levels of social support than their less acculturated counterparts.

Immigrants' retention of cultural identity also has been associated with their maintenance of practices that enhance health, such as eating a lot of fibre; and abstaining from smoking, using alcohol, and taking drugs (Escobar, 1998; Marmot & Syme, 1976; Scribner & Dwyer, 1989). With respect to mental health, there is substantial evidence linking the provision of social support by a like ethnocultural community with positive mental health outcomes (Beiser, 1988; Beiser & Hou, 2001).

According to Carballo, Divino, and Zeric (1998), Canadian resettlement policies stressing the geographic dispersal of immigrants often contribute to immigrant women's isolation. The lack of social support (e.g., the inability to visit family and friends or have a good family environment and support) has been described as a major impediment to personal health care (MacKinnon & Howard, 2000). Many immigrant women prefer the support of family and friends to cope with psychological distress, depression, or other emotional illness rather than, or before, going to a doctor. Without a social connection and a feeling of belonging, these options for self-care are greatly reduced. However, having access to extended family, friends, and members of one's own ethnocultural community can have a downside; for example, Lepore (1992) found that the detrimental effects of social negativity (e.g., criticism, rejection, and conflicts) outweigh the benefits of positive support.

There is currently a debate in healthcare literature about whether violence in immigrant communities is tied to family, social, and religious values that dictate male dominance in gender relationships and condone violence against women, or whether it is connected with post-migration stresses such as poverty, underemployment, minority status, discrimination, isolation, and gender-role reversals that affect the power dynamics between men and women (Bui & Morash, 1999; Narayan, 1995; West, 1998; Yick & Agbayani-Siewert, 1997). Data suggest that, after arriving in the new country, immigrants experience many changes that affect marital relationships (Hyman et al., 2004), including changes in the following areas:

- Household help and support
- Income and status
- Gender roles
- Communication and intimacy

Health Practices

Health practices refer to the positive actions that individuals can take to:

▪ Prevent diseases and promote self-care
▪ Cope with challenges
▪ Develop self-reliance
▪ Solve problems
▪ Make choices that enhance health

There is a growing recognition that personal life "choices" are greatly influenced by the socio-economic environments in which people live, learn, work, and play.

A number of Canadian studies have suggested that immigrant health practices change over time to resemble those of the majority culture. Previous research using data from the National Population Health Survey (NPHS) demonstrated that new immigrants smoked less, used less alcohol, and were less likely to be obese than longer-term immigrants (those having lived here more than ten years) and those born in Canada (Beiser, Devins, Dion, Hyman, & Lin, 1997). Data from Canada's 1996/1997 NPHS examined changes in health practices among immigrant and visible minority women in Ontario, and confirmed that most of the recent immigrant women were less likely to regularly drink alcohol or smoke and less likely to be overweight than were their Canadian-born counterparts. They also were less likely to engage in regular physical activity in the years immediately following immigration.

Several studies have demonstrated a relationship between changes in immigrants' health practices and changes in their health status. For instance, differences in the extent to which immigrants adopt the host country's health practices (e.g., smoking) have been used to explain why cancer rates among immigrants converge with those of the native-born population over time (Kliewer & Smith, 1995). Dietary changes—such as eating more saturated fats and less cereals or grain product, fruits, and vegetables than residents of their countries of origin—have been associated with increases in hypertension, diabetes, coronary heart disease, and some cancers (Huang et al., 1996; Newell, Borrud, McPherson, Nichaman, & Pillow, 1988; Savage & Harrell Bond, 1991). Alcohol and drug abuse have been associated with the following factors in immigrants' lives:

▪ Alienation from traditional supports
▪ Racism and sexism
▪ Internalization of negative host-societal beliefs
▪ Acculturative stress (i.e., stress in adapting to the new country)
  (Rogler, Cortes, & Malgady, 1991)

Use of Health Services

Health services contribute to a population's health, particularly when the services have been designed to achieve the following:

▪ Maintain and promote health
▪ Prevent disease
▪ Restore health and function

Treatment and secondary prevention are also part of the full spectrum of health service care (Health Canada, 2002).

A number of studies have examined the use of health services by immigrants, using data from the National Population Health Survey and provincial health records. For example, Globerman (1998) used data from the 1994/95 NPHS to examine differences in the use of healthcare services among four groups of immigrants to Canada, namely immigrants from the United States or Mexico; South America or Africa; Europe or Australia; and Asia. He found that differences between Canadian-born respondents and respondents from the four groups were quite modest. There was no significant difference in visits to physicians; Canadian-born individuals and European immigrants were marginally more likely to make frequent visits to specialists.

Wen, Goel, and Williams (1996) used data from the 1990 Ontario Health Survey to examine whether in Ontario there was variation between immigrant and Canadian-born clients in terms of contact with physicians and specialists and the use of hospital emergency departments. They found that the use of all forms of health services was similar between the two groups. Recent Asian immigrants, in particular, registered lower rates of usage for all three healthcare services than Asian immigrants who had been in the country for more than ten years, and these differences persisted even after controlling for differences in health status and age.

Chen et al. (1996a) used data from the 1994/95 NPHS to compare age-adjusted rates of physician contacts between male and female immigrants and the Canadian-born population. In both the immigrant and Canadian-born populations, women reported more frequent contacts with physicians. Low household income, female gender, and low education were significantly associated with a higher frequency of physician contacts, but not with length of stay in Canada.

Under-use of health services was more evident for both preventive health services and mental health services. In a study of the help-seeking behaviours of 2246 healthcare clients—comprising Canadian-born anglophones and francophones, as well as Vietnamese, Caribbean, and Filipino immigrants in an ethnically diverse neighbourhood in Montreal—researchers Kirmayer, Galbaud du Fort, Young, Weinfeld, and Lasry (1996) found that rates of healthcare service use for mental health problems were significantly lower among immigrants. The immigrants were less likely to make use of primary-care mental health services and even less likely to be referred to, or seek out, specialty mental health care. These differences could not be accounted for by lower levels of need or by the use of alternative health care.

Data from the 1996/97 NPHS were used to examine the use of women's preventive health services (Pap and mammography screening, and use of a regular source of care) among immigrant and visible minority women in Ontario. The majority of women (more than 90 percent) interviewed had a regular source of care. Approximately 22.3 percent of recent immigrant women and 12 percent of long-term immigrant women had never had a Pap test compared with 5.3 percent of Canadian-born women. With respect to mammography,

26 percent of recent immigrant women had never undergone mammography compared with 18.3 percent of long-term immigrant women and 18.7 percent of Canadian-born women. There was less variation between immigrant and visible minority groups in the proportion of women who engaged in regular screening (i.e., every three years for Pap and every two years for mammography), suggesting that once initial barriers to screening are overcome, immigrant and visible minority women are committed to continuing these preventive health practices (Hyman, 2002).

A number of barriers to immigrant women's use of healthcare services have been identified, including:

- Differences in cultural values belief systems and practices
- Lack of access to culturally appropriate services
- Under-representation of immigrant and racial minority women in the healthcare professions and on boards of directors of hospitals, universities, and other major institutions
- Compromised mental health care due to stigmatization, racism, and general marginalization
- Geographic factors
- Financial factors
  (Hyman & Guruge, 2002; Mulvihill & Mailloux, 2000; Simms, 1999; Vissandjee et al., 1998)

The barriers also include fewer choices in screening and treatment offered to immigrant and refugee women compared with Canadian-born women.

Reports have consistently suggested that immigrant women who experience abuse under-use medical and legal services, shelters, and hotlines, compared with abused women in the majority population (MacLeod & Shin, 1994; Smith, 2004). However, data from the 1999 General Social Survey on Victimization demonstrated that this under-use was more prominent for recent immigrant women in Canada (those who had been here for less than ten years) compared with their non-recent counterparts.

Recent immigrant women were significantly more likely to report violence to police compared with non-recent immigrant women (50.8 percent versus 26 percent) but were significantly less likely to use "any social services" (30.8 percent versus 52 percent) (Hyman et al., 2006). This has been attributed to the following kinds of multiple and intersecting barriers that immigrant women face in accessing help:

- Social isolation
- Linguistic and cultural barriers
- Discrimination
- Dependency on spouse
- Fear (e.g., of isolation/ostracization, financial insecurity, or deportation)
  (Bui, 2003; Smith, 2004)

These context-specific barriers also may explain why immigrant women depend more on family and friends than on more formal sources of support (Abu-Ras, 2003; Bauer, Rodriquez, Flores-Oritz, & Szkupinski Quiroga, 2000).

Implications for Service Delivery

Policymakers

The health of immigrant women is largely shaped by environment and living conditions, and may change in response to real pressures associated with poverty, marginalization, and class inequity. Such considerations have implications for the delivery of services to this group.

The findings reported in this chapter suggest that comprehensive approaches that involve many sectors of public life are needed to promote and sustain the good health of immigrant women, which in Canada requires the co-operation and co-ordination of different levels of government. Federal settlement services, for example, need to broaden their scope to address the determinants of health identified in this review, to co-ordinate and support services provided by provincial and municipal levels of government, and to ensure communication and information sharing between all jurisdictions.

Other findings highlight the critical role of social support in promoting and sustaining the health and well-being of immigrant women, couples, and their families. Policymakers need to re-evaluate policies that limit family reunification and immigrants' choice of where to reside. Current research that links host country attitudes and mental health means that effort needs to be made through public education and social legislation to improve the image and value of immigrant women in Canadian society.

Health Planners

The evidence that immigrant women use health services less than the Canadian-born population—particularly mental and preventive health services—may be viewed as a positive finding. However, rather than reflecting the superior health status of immigrant women, it may reflect the inadequacy of present services to meet their needs.

Removing barriers to services is of particular importance in the area of infectious diseases, such as tuberculosis, because with early intervention and treatment these conditions can be controlled. Improvements in the accessibility, appropriateness, and comprehensiveness of healthcare services would help ensure the continued good health of new immigrant women and reduce the development of long-term chronic diseases such as diabetes, cancer, and heart disease. This could be accomplished by providing more comprehensive services that address immigrant women's health needs, as well as access to services such as job counselling and training, language and literacy training, family and individual counselling, transportation, and child care.

Other evidence suggests that programs that empower immigrant women to develop and maintain their own ethno-specific institutions and health-promoting practices have positive long-term effects. For example, there are numerous benefits to creating community nutrition projects that include activities such as the purchase and distribution of locally grown fruits and vegetables, community gardens in which neighbours plan and grow a garden together, and community kitchens that involve several people meeting to cook food together enhance learning and the sharing of skills; these benefits include:

- Cutting costs (e.g., of seeds and tools)
- Providing mutual assistance
- Reducing isolation
- Improving language skills
- Increasing social support and networking
- In some cases, as has been attempted already, using the activities to generate income (e.g., catering services)
  (Hyman & Guruge, 2002)

Increasing the proportion of immigrant women among the ranks of healthcare service providers also may enhance quality of care, thus indirectly influencing health status.

Health Practitioners

Being culturally safe and relevant is an important quality of effective and accountable health care. At the individual level, healthcare providers require education that exposes them to two important areas:

1. Ways in which immigrant women understand and conceptualize health
2. The unique circumstances of immigrant women's lives

It has been recommended that healthcare providers at all levels and across all disciplines should receive formal, mandatory, and ongoing training on cultural competence, diversity, and equity (Betancourt, Green, & Carrillo, 2002). For example, although recommendations from doctors have consistently been shown to be a major determinant for participation in screening tests, many studies attest to the fact that immigrant women are less likely to be screened for breast and cervical cancers compared with women in the general population (Hyman et al., 2002).

At the institutional level, many of the essential components of becoming a culturally competent organization have been identified, including developing and making systematic use of the following:

- Cultural interpretation programs or personnel
- Educational materials that are in specific languages and that incorporate cultural nuances
- Assessments of the constraints, obligations, priorities, and barriers in immigrant women's lives
  (Guruge, Donner, & Morrison, 2000)

The participation and representation of community members at meetings of the boards of directors of universities and colleges, hospitals, health councils, and provincial and federal government departments also should be actively sought and supported. Plans can be drawn up to incorporate the knowledge and expertise of such people in the development and implementation of educational, therapeutic, preventive, health promotional, and healing activities. Creating linkages with family practitioners, lay practitioners, and community leaders would help to facilitate early interventions and reduce delays in seeking care (Williams, 1999).

Finally, it cannot be assumed that theoretical models and **health promotion** ideas that are grounded in research based on the majority culture will apply equally to subgroups of immigrant women whose choices may be influenced by barriers of an cultural, linguistic, economic, or informational nature. For some immigrant women, health promotion activities include avoiding shifts between heat and cold or dryness and moisture; avoiding wind and drafts; and staying warm and eating and resting well. Others may not actively seek or participate in health promotion activities because activities of this kind are unconsciously integrated into their everyday lives.

Even though immigrant women in Canada may readily make use of access to home heating, appliances, and indoor plumbing, some may not consider fitness classes or jogging to be essential or appropriate for the maintenance of fitness. While there is a definite need for health promotion materials to be developed in different languages, cultural nuances also must be considered, along with culturally specific patterns of learning (e.g., the use of songs, stories, or drama, as appropriate), to disseminate health information.

An example of an exemplary health promotion program is the Pathways project in the San Francisco Bay area, which obtained impressive increases in cervical and breast screening among different racial and ethnic groups (Haitt et al., 1996). Unique to this intervention was the involvement of each cultural community in the development, planning, and delivery of the screening programs and in the adoption of outreach strategies (e.g., the use of culturally and linguistically appropriate educational materials and program delivery at multiple settings). Other innovative approaches include the use of community "link leaders" and the media (Hyman & Guruge, 2002).

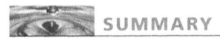 SUMMARY

Health issues and concerns of immigrant women must be located "within the complex socio-economic, historical, political, and institutional structures and dynamics in the pre- and post-migration context" (Guruge & Khanlou, 2004, p. 33). Effective and improved care to immigrant women requires an understanding of the determinants of health for such women and how these interact and intersect to influence health.

The chapter began with a general discussion of immigrant women in Canada. The relationship between immigration and health was examined in general terms and specifically in relation to women. When caring for immigrant women, cultural competence requires an understanding of these broad determinants and how they affect immigrant women and their ability to use healthcare services. Many factors contribute to the challenges faced by immigrant women, especially those who are recent immigrants. These factors are examined under the headings of income, education, and work; social support and stress; and health practices and use of health services. The discussion highlights the relationship between these factors and health. Healthcare literature indicates that while immigrant women have frequent contact with healthcare providers, they tend to under-use preventive services. Healthcare providers must take advantage of the contacts to use a broad and holistic approach to care that fosters healthcare promotion and prevention.

The chapter concluded with a discussion of the roles of policymakers, health planners, and health practitioners in improving immigrant women's health. In particular, approaches that include the community perspective and plan *with* (not just *for*) the diverse communities are recommended. With respect to immigrant women, cultural competence means that healthcare providers understand the unique circumstances of immigrant women's lives and work with the strengths and barriers that arise.

ONLINE LEARNING RESOURCES

www.acewh.dal.ca/e/info/reports.asp
The Atlantic Centre of Excellence for Women's Health

www.bccewh.bc.ca/Pages/publications.htm
The British Columbia Centre of Excellence for Women's Health

http://secure.cihi.ca/cihiweb/dispPage.jsp?cw_page=AR_342_E&cw_topic=342
Canadian Institute for Health Information (Women's Health Surveillance Report)

www.cwhn.ca/search/byTerm.html
The Canadian Women's Health Network

www.cewh-cesf.ca/en/index.shtml
Centres of Excellence for Women's Health

www.pwhce.ca/ptsd-immigrant.htm
The Prairie Women's Health Centre of Excellence (Immigrant/Refugee Women's Health: Post Traumatic Stress Disorder)

REFERENCES

Abu-Ras, W. M. (2003). Barriers to services for Arab immigrant battered women in a Detroit suburb. *Journal of Social Work Research and Evaluation, 4*(1), 49–66.

Anderson, J., Moeschberger, M., Chen, M. S., Jr., Kunn, P., Wewers, M. E., & Guthrie, R. (1993). An acculturation scale for Southeast Asians. *Social Psychiatry and Psychiatric Epidemiology, 28*(3), 134–141.

Bauer, H., Rodriguez, M., Flores-Ortiz, Y., & Szkupinski Quiroga, S. (2000). Barriers to health care for abused Latina and Asian Immigrant Women. *Journal of Health Care for the Poor and Underserved, 11*(1), 33–44.

Beiser, M. (1988). Influences of time, ethnicity, and attachment on depression in Southeast Asian refugees. *American Journal of Psychiatry, 145*, 46–51.

Beiser, M., Devins, G., Dion, R., Hyman, I, & Lin, E. (1997). *Immigration, acculturation and health: Final report*. Ottawa: National Health Research and Development Program.

Beiser, M., & Hou, F. (2001). Language acquisition, unemployment and depressive disorder among Southeast Asian refugees: A 10-year study. *Social Science & Medicine, 53*(10), 1321–1334.

Beiser, M., Turner, R. J., & Ganesan, S. (1989). Catastrophic stress and factors affecting its consequences among Southeast Asian refugees. *Social Science and Medicine, 28*, 183–195.

Betancourt, J. R., Green, A. R., & Carrilo, J. E. (2002). *Cultural competence in health care: Emerging frameworks and practical approaches.* New York: Commonwealth Fund. Retrieved November 28, 2004 from http://www.cmwf.org/publications/publications_show.htm?doc_id=221320

Bui, H. N. (2003). Help-seeking behavior among abused immigrant women: A case of Vietnamese American women. *Violence Against Women, 9*(2), 207–239.

Bui, H. N., & Morash, M. (1999). Domestic violence in the Vietnamese immigrant community. An exploratory study. *Violence Against Women, 5*(7), 769–795.

Carballo, M., Divino J. J., & Zeric, D. (1998). Migration and health in the European Union. *Tropical Medicine and International Health, 3*(12), 936–944.

Chard, J., Badets, J., & Howtson-Leo, L. (2000). Immigrant Women. *Women in Canada 2000.* Cat. No. 89-503-XPE. Ottawa: Statistics Canada.

Chen, J., Ng. E., & Wilkins, R. (1996a). The health of Canada's immigrants in 1994–95. *Health Reports, 7*(4), 33–45.

Chen, J., Ng. E., & Wilkins, R. (1996b). Health expectancy by immigrant status. *Health Reports, 8*(3), 29–37.

Citizenship and Immigration Canada. (2000). *Facts and figures 2002: Immigration overview.* Ottawa: Minister of Public Works and Government Services Canada.

Citizenship and Immigration Canada. (2003). *Facts and figures 1999: Immigration overview.* Ottawa: Minister of Public Works and Government Services Canada.

Davies, P. D. (1995). Tuberculosis and migration. The Mitchell Lecture 1994. *Journal of the Royal College of Physicians of London, 29*(2), 113–118.

Donovan, J., d'Espaignet, E., Metron, C., & van Ommeren, M. (Eds.). (1992). *Immigrants in Australia: A health profile.* Canberra: Australian Government Publishing Service.

Escobar, J. I. (1998). Immigrant and mental health: Why are the immigrants better off? *Archives of General Psychiatry, 55*(9), 781–782.

Fowler, N. (1998). Providing primary health care to immigrants and refugees: The North Hamilton experience. *Canadian Medical Association Journal, 159*, 388–391.

Globerman, S. (1998). *Immigration and health care utilization patterns in Canada.* Vancouver: Research on Immigration and Integration in the Metropolis.

Greenhalgh, P. (1997). Diabetes in British South Asians: Nature, nurture and culture. *Diabetic Medicine, 14*(1), 10–18.

Grenville-Mathers, R., & Clark, J. B. (1979). The development of tuberculosis in Afro-Asian immigrants. *Tubercle, 60*(1), 25–29.

Guruge, S., Donner, G., & Morrison, L. (2000). The impact of Canadian health care reform on recent women immigrants and refugees. In D. Gustafson (Ed.), *Care and consequences* (pp. 222–242). Halifax: Fernwood.

Guruge, S., & Khanlou, N. (2004). Intersectionalities of influence: Research health of immigrant and refugee women. *Canadian Journal of Nursing Research, 36*(3), 32–47.

Haitt, R. A., Pasick, R. J., Perez-Stable, E. J., McPhee, S. J., Engelstad, L., Lee, M., Sabogal, F., D'Onofrio, C. N., & Stewart, S. (1996). Pathways to early cancer detection in the multiethnic population of the San Francisco Bay area. *Health Education Quarterly* 23(Suppl.), S10-S27.

Health Canada. (2002). *Population Health.* Retrieved November 28, 2004 from http://www.phac-aspc.gc.ca/ph-sp/phdd/

Huang, B., Rodriguez, B. L., Burchfiel, C. M., Chyou, P. H., Curb, J. D., & Yano, K. (1996). Acculturation and prevalence of diabetes among Japanese-American men in Hawaii. *American Journal of Epidemiology, 144*, 674–681.

Hyman, I. (2001). *Immigration and health.* Health Canada Working Paper Series, 01–05. Ottawa: Health Canada.

Hyman, I. (2002). Immigrant and visible minority women. In D. E. Stewart, A. Cheung, L. E. Ferris, I. Hyman, M. M. Cohen, & L. J. Williams (Eds.), *Ontario women's health: Status report* (pp. 338–358). Toronto: Ontario Women's Health Council.

Hyman, I., Forte, T., Du Mont, J., Romans, S., & Cohen, M. M. (2006). Help-seeking rates for intimate partner violence (IPV) among Canadian immigrant women. *Health Care for Women International, 27*(8), 682–694.

Hyman, I. (2004). Setting the stage: Reviewing current knowledge on the health of Canadian immigrants: What is the evidence and where are the gaps? *Canadian Journal of Public Health, 95*(3), 15–17.

Hyman, I., & Dussault, G. (2000). Negative consequences of acculturation: Low birth-weight in a population of pregnant immigrant women. *Canadian Journal of Public Health, 91*(5), 357–361.

Hyman, I., & Guruge, S. (2002). A review of theory and health promotion strategies for new immigrant women. *Canadian Journal of Public Health, 93*(3), 183–187.

Hyman, I., Guruge, S., Mason, R., Gould, J., Tang, T., Stuckless, N., Teffera, H., & Mekonnen, G. (2004). Post-migration changes in gender relations among Ethiopian immigrant couples in Toronto. *Canadian Journal of Nursing Research, 36*(4), 74–89.

Hyman, I., Singh, M., Meana, M., George, U., Wells, L., & Stewart, D. E. (2002). Physician-related determinants of cancer screening among Caribbean women in Toronto. *Ethnicity and Disease, 12*(2), 268–275.

Janzen, B. L. (1998) *Women, gender and health: A review of the recent literature.* Prairie Women's Health Centre of Excellence. Retrieved November 28, 2004, from http://www.pwhce.ca/pdf/janzen.pdf

Kaplan, G. A., & Keil, J. F. (1993). Socioeconomic factors and cardiovascular disease: A review of the literature. *Circulation, 88*, 1973–1998.

Kasl, S. V., & Berkman, L. (1983). Health consequences of the experience of migration. *Annual Review of Public Health, 4*, 69–90.

Kent, J. H. (1993). The epidemiology of multidrug-resistant tuberculosis in the United States. *Medical Clinics of North America, 77*(6), 1391–1409.

Kirmayer, L., Galbaud du Fort, G., Young, A., Weinfeld, M., & Lasry, J. C. (1996). *Pathways and barriers to mental health care in an urban multicultural milieu: An epidemiological and ethnographic study.* Report No. 6 (Part 1). Montreal: Sir Mortimer B. Davis, Jewish General Hospital.

Kliewer, E. V., & Smith, K. R. (1995). Ovarian cancer mortality among immigrants in Australia and Canada. *Cancer Epidemiology, Biomarkers and Prevention, 4*(5), 453–458.

Lepore, S. J. (1992). Social conflict, social support, and psychological distress: Evidence of cross-domain buffering effects. *Journal of Personality and Social Psychology, 63*(5), 857–67.

MacKinnon, M., & Howard, L. L. (2000, May). *Affirming immigrant women's health: Building inclusive health policy. Final report.* Halifax, NS: The Maritime Centre of Excellence for Women's Health.

MacLeod, L., & Shin, M. Y. (1994). *Like a wingless bird: A tribute to the survival and courage of women who are abused and who speak neither English nor French.* Ottawa: National Clearinghouse on Family Violence.

Marmot, M. G., & Syme, S. L. (1976). Acculturation and coronary heart disease in Japanese Americans. *American Journal of Epidemiology, 104*(3), 225–247.

McSherry, G., & Connor, E. (1993). Current epidemiology of tuberculosis. *Pediatric Annals, 22*(10), 600–604.

Mulvihill, M. A., & Mailloux, L. (2000). *Canadian research on immigrant and refugee women's health: Linking research and policy. First Draft.* Ottawa: Health Canada.

Narayan, U. (1995). "Male-order" brides: Immigrant women, domestic violence and immigration law. *Hypatia, 10*(1), 104–119.

Newell, G. R., Borrud, L. G., McPherson, R. S., Nichaman, M. Z., & Pillow, P. C. (1988). Nutrient intakes of Whites, Blacks and Mexican Americans in Southeast Texas. *Preventive Medicine, 17*, 622–633.

Oxman-Martinez, J., Abdool, S. N., & Loiselle-Leonard, M. (2000). Immigration, women and health in Canada. *Canadian Journal of Public Health, 91*(5), 394–395.

Pérez, C. E. (2002). Health status and health behaviour among immigrants. *Health Reports, 13* (Suppl.). Ottawa: Statistics Canada.

Powell, K. E., Meador, M. P., & Farer, L. S. (1981). Foreign-born persons with tuberculosis in the United States. *American Journal of Public Health, 71*, 1223–1227.

Proust, A. J. (1971). The Australian screening programme for tuberculosis in prospective migrants. *Medical Journal of Australia, 2*, 35–37.

Rogler, L. H., Cortes, D. E., & Malgady, R. G. (1991). Acculturation and mental health states among Hispanics: Convergence and new directions for research. *American Psychologist, 46*, 585–597.

Roxborough, S. (1996). Gender differences in work and well-being: Effects of exposure and vulnerability. *Journal of Health and Social Behavior, 37*, 265–277.

Savage, P. J., & Harrell Bond, B. E. (1991). Racial and ethnic diversity in obesity and other risk factors for cardiovascular disease: Implications for studies and treatment. *Ethnicity and Disease, 1*, 200–211.

Scribner, R., & Dwyer, J. H. (1989). Acculturation and low birthweight among Latinos in the Hispanic HANES. *American Journal of Public Health, 79*(9), 1263–1267.

Simms, G. (1999). *Aspects of Women's Health from a Minority/Diversity Perspective.* Paper prepared for the Canada-USA Forum on Women's Health. Ottawa: Health Canada.

Smith, E. (2004). *Nowhere to turn? Responding to partner violence against immigrant and visible minority women.* Ottawa: Canadian Council on Social Development.

Statistics Canada. (1998). *National population health survey, 1996–97.* Ottawa: Statistics Canada, Health Statistics Division.

Statistics Canada. (1995). *Women in Canada: A statistical report,* (3rd ed.). Cat. No. 89-503E. Ottawa: Statistics Canada.

Statistics Canada (2006). *Women in Canada: A gender based statistical report,* (5th ed.). Cat. No. 89-503-XIE. Ottawa: Statistics Canada. Retrieved on July 9, 2006 from http://dsp-psd.pwgsc.gc.ca/Collection-R/Statcan/89-503-X/0010589-503-XIE.pdf

Stephen, E. H., Foote, K., Hendershot, G. E., & Shoenborn, C. A. (1994). Health of the foreign-born population. *Advance Data from Vital and Health Statistics, 241*, 1–10.

Van Kessel, G. C. J. (1998). *The Canadian Immigration System.* Ottawa: Department of Citizenship and Immigration Canada.

Vissandjée, B., Leduc, N., Gravel, S., Bourdeau, M., & Carignan, P. (1998). Promotion de la santé en faveur des femmes immigrant au Québec. *Revue Epidemiologique et Santé Public, 43*, 124–133.

Vissandjée, B., Desmeules, M., Cao, Z., Abdool, S., & Kazanjian, A. (2003). Integrating ethnicity and migration as determinants of Canadian women's health. In M. Desmeules, D. Stewart, A. Kazanjian, H. Maclean, J. Payne, & B. Vissandjée (Eds.), Women's health surveillance report: Supplementary chapters. Ottawa: Canadian Institute for Health Information. Retrieved November 28, 2004, from http://secure.cihi.ca/cihiweb/dispPage.jsp?cw_page=PG_336_E&cw_topic=336&cw_rel=AR_342_E

Vissandjée, B., Weinfeld, M., Dupéré, S., & Abdool, S. (2001). Sex, gender, ethnicity and access to health care services: Research and policy challenges for immigrant women in Canada. *Journal of International Migration and Integration, 2*(1), 55–75.

Wen, S. W., Goel, V., & Williams, J. E. (1996). Utilization of health care services by immigrants and other ethnic/cultural groups in Ontario. *Ethnicity and Health, 1*(1), 99–109.

West, C. M. (1998). Lifting the "political gag order." Breaking the silence around partner violence in ethnic minority families. In J. L. Jasinski, & L. M. Williams (Eds.), *Partner violence: A comprehensive review of 20 years of research* (pp. 184–209). Thousand Oaks, CA: Sage.

Williams, C. C. (1999). *Ethnoracial services task force report to the Joint General Psychiatry Program Planning Committee.* Toronto: The Clarke Institute of Psychiatry.

Williams, R., Bhopal, R., & Hunt, K. (1994). Coronary risk in a British Punjabi population: Comparative profile of non-biochemical factors. *International Journal of Epidemiology, 23*(1), 29–37.

Yick, A. G., & Agbayani-Siewart, P. (1997). Perceptions of domestic violence in a Chinese- American community. *Journal of Interpersonal Violence, 12*(6), 832–846.

CHAPTER 13

Pain Management

MONA SAWHNEY

LEARNING OBJECTIVES

At the end of this chapter, the learner will be able to:

- Discuss the definition of pain
- Understand how history impacts the current environment of pain and addiction
- Explain the concept of pain threshold and the differences between cultural groups
- Discuss variations in the affective responses to pain among cultural groups
- Understand how to provide culturally sensitive pain care

KEY TERMS

Chronic pain	Pain threshold
Pain	Pain tolerance level
Pain assessment tools	Stoic

Pain is a sensation that is experienced by all people from all cultures, regardless of age, sex, and socio-economic status. It is a "universal experience of human existence" (Davidhizar & Giger, 2004, p. 49); however, there are variations in the way that pain is perceived, interpreted, and responded to. Pain also is one of the most common reasons why clients seek health care (Goldstein et al., 2004).

The International Association for the Study of Pain (IASP, 1994) says **pain** can be described as "an unpleasant sensory and emotional experience associated with actual or potential tissue damage, or described in terms of such damage." This definition allows pain to be described as a phenomenon that affects a client's physical and psychosocial well-being.

Pain is a subjective experience that cannot be determined by tissue damage alone. The emotional experience associated with a client's pain needs to be considered just as carefully as the physical experience. A definition of pain that highlights its subjective and personal nature comes from McCaffery and Pasero (1999). They state that "pain is whatever the experiencing person says it is, existing whenever he says it does" (McCaffery & Pasero, 1999, p. 17). This definition is clinically oriented and helps us to remember that each client is an expert when it comes to his or her own pain. Healthcare providers need to use the client's self-report of pain as the most reliable indicator of pain (McCaffery & Pasero, 1999).

As countries become more culturally diverse, greater attention is being placed on understanding how culture influences the experience of pain. Unless psychosocial factors, such as culture, are taken into account, the assessment and management of pain is limited. Mark Zoborowski (1952) was one of the earliest researchers to examine these cultural differences. Zoborowski recognized that pain acquires specific social and cultural significances, and that certain reactions to pain should be examined in this light. Understanding group attitudes toward pain can aid in the understanding of individual reactions (Zoborowski, 1952) and can help healthcare providers in providing culturally focused pain management.

Traditionally, healthcare providers have not incorporated culturally sensitive practices into their pain management. This chapter reviews historical concepts of pain management among cultural groups, as well as the differences in how various cultural groups experience and express pain. It also provides information on how to incorporate culturally sensitive pain management into practice.

Historical Concepts of Pain Management

The history of the meaning of pain can and does shape our current understanding of the term. History demonstrates the philosophical, religious, and political meanings of pain that prevailed before the medical profession began to study this phenomenon.

Pain has been depicted in theatre and religion as being "a part of life" for centuries. Sophocles and Aristotle both wrote about pain and incorporated meanings of pain into their dramatic works (Jackson, 2002). In the religious context, pain is a common image in Judeo-Christian teaching; two examples of this are the test of faith in the story of Job and the sacrificial redemption of the crucifixion (Meldrum, 2003). An understanding of, or belief about, pain and its management in the general population still is influenced by these early views. For example, many people hold the view that pain is just a part of life, or that pain has been inflicted upon them to atone for previous wrongdoings.

In addition to religious teachings, the political climate of today's world has an influence on our current beliefs about pain. The use of opioids in pain management is one example of treatment that has been affected by historical and political events. Western society, which used to use opioids to manage pain effectively, now lives in a state of fear about creating opioid addicts. Until the late 1800s, opioids were unregulated and readily available in the local pharmacy. They were the standard treatment for the management of acute, recurrent, and cancer or palliative pain. However, in the 1870s, physicians began to be concerned about the misuse of opioids (Meldrum, 2003; Bloodworth, 2005). This introduced the ongoing fear of addiction to opioids that many healthcare providers have today. One of the major reasons why pain continues to be under-treated in Canada is healthcare providers' fear of creating addiction (Kohr & Sawhney, 2005; Morley-Forster, Clark, Speechley, & Moulin, 2003).

The events of the First and Second World Wars, Prohibition, and the ongoing fight against street drugs continue to shape our current attitudes about pain and its management. For example, in nineteenth-century China, as a result of the Opium Wars, there were roughly twenty million opium addicts before the founding of the People's Republic in 1949. Although drug abuse was essentially eradicated in the early 1950s, fear of addiction became part of Chinese culture. As a result, the Chinese government has adopted very strict measures to control the movement and use of opioids (World Health Organization, n.d.).

Differences in Pain Threshold Among Various Cultural Groups

Why do different people or different groups of people experience and express pain in different ways? Are there differences in the pain thresholds of various cultural groups? In pain research, the **pain threshold** is defined as the level at which 50 percent of stimuli would be recognized as painful, and **pain tolerance level** is the greatest level of pain that a subject is prepared to endure. It is important to note that both pain threshold and pain tolerance level are the subjective experiences of the individual (IASP, 1994).

Research studies comparing pain thresholds in different cultural groups have reported varying results, with no study clearly identifying differences between different groups. Edwards and Fillingim (1999) examined the effects of African American ethnicity versus non-Hispanic Caucasian ethnicity on experimental thermal pain (contact heat stimuli) in healthy volunteers. They found that African American subjects, compared with non-Hispanic Caucasian subjects, had lower thermal pain tolerance and rated thermal stimuli as more unpleasant; however, the two groups did not differ in thermal pain thresholds or ratings of thermal intensity. Yosipovitch, Meredith, Chan, and Goh (2004) examined pain threshold using thermal sensory testing in healthy volunteers in three distinct East Asian populations— Chinese, Malaysian, and Indian. They found no significant differences in pain thresholds between the three populations.

Studies examining the tolerance level of people within various cultural groups have found that African American subjects rated cutaneous heat and tourniquet pain as more unpleasant and more intense than did non-Hispanic Caucasians; therefore, African Americans had a lower pain tolerance (Edwards, Doleys, Fillingim, & Lowery, 2001; Sheffield, Biles, Orom, Maixner, & Sheps, 2000). The studies also found that women rated the stimuli as more painful than men did (Sheffield et al., 2000).

These studies indicate that different people experience variations in pain tolerance, but they do not show a difference in pain threshold based on culture or ethnicity. It is important to note that all of these studies had a small sample size, thereby limiting a broad application of the findings to the general public. The identification that a specific stimulus is painful (e.g., a thermal probe at 30°C), also known as pain threshold, does not indicate how long that painful stimulus will be tolerated, or the severity of the pain an individual will experience. There is no strong evidence that pain threshold varies among cultural groups (Lee, Gin, & Oh, 1997), yet stereotypes continue to influence the practice of healthcare providers. Each individual has personal beliefs and preconceptions about pain that are based on cultural, sociological, and ethnic factors. Social and cultural norms within an ethnic group often dictate how and to what degree pain behaviour is expressed (Yosipovitch et al., 2004). We can learn more about these norms in response to pain from clinically based, observational studies that focus on affective responses to pain.

Differences in Affective Responses to Pain from Around the World

Mark Zoborowski (1952), one of the first researchers to examine the influence of cultural norms on pain experience and pain management, concluded that differences exist among varying cultural groups.

In a landmark study, he examined the pain experience of three cultural groups in a hospital in New York City: Jewish, Italian, and "Old American" (Caucasians of Protestant religion, whose grandparents were born in the United States). He reported that Jewish and Italian cultures allow for free expression of feelings and emotions using words, sounds, and gestures. Both groups feel free to talk or complain about their pain, and vocalize by, for example, moaning and crying. The difference between the groups lies in the meaning they ascribe to their pain. Italian clients were concerned about the actual pain they experienced and how it affected their immediate ability to perform their roles. Jewish clients were concerned about the meaning of the pain and whether the pain was a threat to their health. In contrast, Old Americans tried to minimize pain and avoided complaining so they would not be a "nuisance." However, if the pain became severe, there was a tendency to express pain and vocalize through, for example, moaning. This group of clients saw pain as a warning sign, indicating that something is wrong. Pain was considered as bad and unnecessary, and as something that should be immediately addressed (Zoborowski, 1952). Two conclusions from this study are:

1. Similar reactions to pain by members of different cultural groups do not necessarily reflect similar attitudes toward pain
2. Similar reactions toward pain may have different functions or meanings in various cultures (Zoborowski, 1952)

Zoborowski's early study has been important to further studies that explore cultural influence on pain:

▪ *Old American versus Jewish, Italian clients.* Greenwald (1991) examined inter-ethnic differences in pain perception in clients with cancer pain, in regions of the United States where ethnic groups had assimilated with the American culture. He found that those who identified as Old Americans (whose original heritage was from Britain, Germany, and Scandinavia) expressed pain less rapidly than Jewish or Italian clients did. He also found that Jewish and Italian clients did not differ in their expression of pain from the clients in the Old American group. Greenwald felt that this lack of difference could be due to acculturation.

▪ *Intra-ethnic clients.* Bates, Edwards, and Anderson (1993), in a study of intra-ethnic group variations of clients in the United States with chronic pain, found that clients who identified themselves as coming from the Hispanic and Italian culture indicated a belief that emotional expression of pain was an appropriate response to pain, whereas members of the Polish and Old American cultural groups indicated that non-expression of pain was ideal (Bates et al., 1993).

▪ *Mexican American, Anglo-American clients.* Calvillo and Flaskerud (1993) examined the differences in Mexican American and Anglo-American women's response to cholecystectomy pain. They found no significant differences between the two groups in their description of the pain, the amount of pain experienced, and the amount of pain medication administered. In Hispanic culture, when an individual is in pain, stoicism (indifference or lack of affective response to pain) is valued, and signs and symptoms of pain often are not acknowledged. It is believed that a lack of stamina is considered a sign of weakness. Many Hispanics value the religious concepts of pain and believe that one's fate is to suffer in this world (Calvillo & Flaskerud, 1993; McNeill, Sherwood, Starch, & Nieto, 2001). When defining what pain meant to them, a population of Hispanic clients with cancer pain described pain as physical and or emotional suffering. They also waited until the pain was severe before calling their doctor or nurse for assistance (Anderson et al., 2002). However, Mexican American clients, especially women, moan when uncomfortable. In Mexican culture, crying out in response to pain is an acceptable expression and does not necessarily indicate that the pain is severe or the person is experiencing a loss of self-control. This pattern of moaning and crying may be used to help relieve pain, rather than being a way of communicating a request for an intervention (Calvillo & Flaskerud, 1993).

▪ *African American clients.* African Americans are reported to express a greater severity of pain than Caucasians, as evidenced by both experimental and clinical pain studies (Edwards, Fillingim, & Keefe, 2001; White, Asher, Lai, & Burton, 1999). A study of African Americans and Caucasians with rheumatoid arthritis found that distraction, praying, and hoping were strategies to manage pain that were used more frequently by clients of African American descent (Jordan, Lumley, & Leisen, 1998). A study of a population of African American cancer clients showed that prayer was the most frequently used alternative or complementary technique of managing pain (Anderson et al., 2002). When defining what pain meant to them, they described pain as a sensory experience or "hurt." They, like Hispanic cancer clients, waited until the pain was severe before calling their doctor or nurse for assistance (Anderson et al., 2002).

▪ *Clients of Arabic culture.* Reizian and Meleis (1986) examined Arab Americans' perception and response to pain. They defined Arab Americans as Arabic-speaking people of Semitic origin who had migrated to the United States. Reizian and Meleis report that people of Arab culture do not respond favourably to painful experiences. They have a present-time orientation to pain as they are concerned about the current pain experience and how to control or avoid the pain. In private, among trusted family members, there is free expression of pain and suffering through crying, groaning, moaning, and complaining. In the presence of healthcare providers, their response to pain is more constrained. However, during labour and delivery, women of Middle Eastern descent may express pain with loud moans, groans, and screams. Callister, Khalaf, Semenic, Kartchner, and Vehvilainen-Julkunen (2003) report that Muslim women of Middle Eastern descent are verbally expressive during labour, often crying and screaming. However, these women gain comfort and support from their faith in God and other female members of their family (Callister et al., 2003).

◦ *Australian study.* A study of the effects of culture on back pain in Australian Aboriginals found that Aboriginals have a high tolerance for pain and displayed no public pain or illness behaviours, even after acknowledging the presence of back pain. Most Aboriginals preferred ointments and traditional methods of healing, and back pain did not interfere with their activities of daily living. Without direct inquiry regarding pain, healthcare providers would not be aware of the pain that this population experiences (Honeyman & Jacobs, 1996).

◦ *Chinese ties.* Clients of Chinese descent also tend to be more reluctant to express pain. Pain is seen as something that should be accepted as fate, and endured. This pain endurance belief is influenced by Confucian thought, which does not value expressing physical or emotional distress to others (Callister et al., 2003; Chung, Thomas, & Yang, 2000; Lai et al., 2003; Lee et al., 1997). When in labour, women of Chinese descent tend to have soft voices and a quiet demeanour. It is thought to be shameful to scream, and that screaming and crying expends energy that can be used to give birth (Callister et al., 2003).

◦ *Taiwanese men and women.* In their testing of the Pain and Opioid Analgesics Beliefs Scale with cancer clients in Taiwan, Lai and colleagues (2003) found that men believe in the value of enduring pain more than women. They also found that the majority of clients studied had negative beliefs about opioids and their related side effects (Lai et al., 2003).

In summary, these studies show us that people with different cultural backgrounds express pain in various ways and attach different meanings to the pain they experience. Healthcare providers should recognize that some people adapt or assimilate to the culture into which they migrate. Healthcare providers should not assume that every client affiliated with a specific cultural group will display the pain behaviours of that cultural group. For example, clients who live in Canada, but whose grandparents moved here from Italy may not be expressive when experiencing post-operative pain. They may display a more stoic response to their pain, as learned in Western culture.

Understanding how a cultural group may express or perceive pain should not limit our ability to identify pain as an individual, subjective experience. An understanding of these affective responses to pain should help us to recognize the variations in the way pain is expressed and be amenable to these variations. Effective pain management requires that each client be viewed as an individual with many characteristics, including a particular cultural background.

Using Non-Western or Complementary and Alternative Pain-Management Treatments

Some healthcare clients in Canada incorporate traditional Chinese medicine (TCM), traditional Ayurvedic medicine, or so-called complementary and alternative medicine (CAM) into their pain-management regimes. (These forms of healing are also discussed in Chapter 8.)

TCM has existed for more than 5000 years and involves an understanding of the human body based on the circulation of the universe (a person and heaven are one entity) (Ho, 2001). It involves balancing the energy within and around the individual. It includes treatments such as acupuncture, moxibustion (in which the mugwort herb moxa is burned near the skin), massage, and diet. There is evidence that acupuncture is effective in relieving dental pain, chronic back pain, and migraines (Ho, 2001; MacPherson, Thorpe, Thomas, & Campbell, 2003). It is important to be aware that clients may be using traditional therapies to help manage their pain, and to be open to evaluating the usefulness of these therapies.

TCM bears similarities to Ayurvedic medicine, which has also provided a traditional perspective on the management of pain. Ayurvedic medicine is a comprehensive medical system that has been part of the traditional system of health care in India for more than 5000 years. It is similar to TCM in that it focuses on establishing and maintaining balance of the life energies within an individual, rather than focusing on individual symptoms. Ayurvedic treatments include meditation, yoga, massage, herbs, and diet. Herbal treatment can include the application of ointments, including "pain ointments." A study investigating pain and disability in rural India found that rheumatic disease was the most common pain-causing disability (18 percent of the adult population). Moderate pain greater than two years' duration was reported by almost 60 percent of those with rheumatic diseases (Chopra, Saluja, Patil, & Tandale, 2002). This incidence of painful rheumatoid arthritis highlights the importance of investigating a pain treatment that has been a part of traditional healing for many years. Studies have investigated the effectiveness of topical Ayurvedic pain ointments in the management of pain and swelling in clients with rheumatoid arthritis and osteoarthritis. The studies found that ointments were safe to use but had variable outcomes in relation to pain management (Chopra, Lavin, Patwardham, & Chitre, 2000; Singh et al., 2003).

Acknowledging that clients may be using traditional medicine or complementary and alternative medicine as part of their pain management plan is important. Approximately 12 percent of Canadians use CAM (Andrews & Boon, 2005). For pain management, this includes, but is not limited to, treatments such as acupuncture, reiki, massage, and topical or herbal remedies. The body of evidence for CAM in pain management is increasing and as its use increases, healthcare providers may be expected to answer clients' questions about the potential value of these treatments in the management of pain.

Access to Pain Care and Analgesics in North America

Persistent/Chronic pain—pain that has persisted for at least six months, or occurs for longer than the time of expected tissue healing—carries an estimated annual price tag of more than $10 billion in Canada (Chronic Pain Association of Canada, 2004; Jovey et al., 2003). This figure is based on direct care costs and does not include less quantifiable costs, such as quality of life.

A survey conducted by Moulin, Clark, Speechley, and Morley-Forster (2002) reports the prevalence of chronic pain in Canada to be approximately 30 percent of the population, with the majority of chronic pain sufferers reporting moderate to severe pain. They also found, from a sample of 340 people who live with chronic pain, that only 22 percent were treated with opioids and of those, only 7 percent were treated with a major opioid such as morphine (Moulin et al., 2002). This may be due to the fear of addiction and the related prescribing practices as identified by Morley-Forster et al. (2003). A survey of 100 Canadian physicians, all with a defined interest in palliative care for non-cancer pain, found that up to 35 percent would never use opioids for non-cancer pain, even if the pain were severe. These statistics are similar to prescribing practices for the treatment of cancer and non-cancer pain throughout North America (Morley-Forster et al., 2003).

To understand how this problem can affect people of different cultural backgrounds, we need to review the American literature because the Canadian literature has not differentiated among cultural groups in relation to prescription of medications to manage pain:

- *Unrelieved pain.* Studies of culturally diverse populations have found that there is a high prevalence of unrelieved pain among minority groups. Cleeland, Gonin, Baez, Loehrer, and Pandya (1997) found that outpatients with cancer who received treatment from clinics that mainly treated people of African American and Hispanic descent were more likely to receive inadequate analgesia than those who received treatment in non-minority treatment settings; 59 percent to 74 percent of African American and Hispanic outpatients received inadequate analgesic prescriptions. There was also a discrepancy between client report and healthcare provider estimates of pain, with pain being underestimated by the healthcare providers (Cleeland et al., 1997).

- *Discrepancies in surgery rates.* A study of ethnic differences in a chronic pain population found that there were no differences in the number of pain locations or percentage of clients taking opioids, benzodiazepines, or antidepressants (Edwards, Doleys, et al., 2001). The researchers did find a significant difference in the number of pain-related surgeries, with Caucasian clients having more surgery than African Americans. They also found that African American clients were more likely to be taking muscle relaxants to manage pain before admission to the chronic pain program (Edwards, Daniels, et al., 2001).

- *Hospital setting.* This shortfall in pain management also is observed for clients in a hospital setting. Studies of Hispanic clients found that even when analgesics were prescribed, they were not administered to Hispanic clients experiencing pain (McNeill et al., 2001). A study of Mexican American clients found that there were differences between the clients' and the nurses' assessment of clients' pain, with the clients assessing pain as being more severe than the nurses' assessment of pain (Calvillo & Flaskerud, 1993). Ng, Dimsdale, Rollnick, and Shapiro (1996) studied the effect of ethnicity on the use of patient-controlled analgesia for post-operative pain management. They found that there was no difference in the amount of opioid self-administered using the patient-controlled analgesia, but there were differences in the amount of opioid prescribed based on ethnicity. Clients of Hispanic and Asian descent were prescribed less opioid than African Americans and Caucasians (Ng et al., 1996).

▪ *Doctors' versus clients' assessments of pain.* Todd, Lee, and Hoffman (1994) examined the influence of ethnicity on the estimates that doctors made of pain severity in Caucasian and Hispanic clients with extremity trauma in an emergency setting. They found that client pain assessment was higher than physician pain assessment in both groups (Todd et al., 1994). Another study used clinical vignettes to examine the prescribing practice of emergency physicians as influenced by race or ethnicity. The three conditions studied were migraine headache, non-traumatic back pain, and ankle fracture. The race of clients was stated in the vignette, and the clients were given racially identifiable names. The study found that clients' race or ethnicity was not related to rates of opioid prescription at discharge in any of the vignettes (Tamayo-Sarver et al., 2003). However, a vignette cannot replace a clinical interaction with clients and their families, where a healthcare provider is immersed in the immediacy of the pain experience.

▪ *Access to opioids.* Once a client receives a prescription for an opioid to manage pain, will he or she have access to the drug? A study of the availability of commonly prescribed opioids in New York City pharmacies found that only 25 percent of pharmacies in "non-White" neighbourhoods (where less than 40 percent of residents had a white skin colour) had opioid supplies that were insufficient to treat clients in severe pain. In contrast, 72 percent of the pharmacies in predominantly White neighbourhoods (where at least 80 percent of residents had a white skin colour) had opioid supplies that were sufficient to treat clients in severe pain (Morrison, Wallenstein, Natale, Senzel, & Huang, 2000). African American and Hispanic cancer clients have reported difficulties in obtaining pain medications. These barriers included cost, limited availability, and physician reluctance to prescribe opioids (Anderson et al., 2002).

▪ *Addiction fears.* Pain care that is delivered to clients is greatly affected by the healthcare providers' knowledge and attitudes regarding pain and pain management. Surveys of healthcare providers have documented knowledge deficits and attitudinal barriers related to the control of pain (Clarke, et al., 1996; Watt-Watson, Stevens, Garfinkel, Streiner, & Gallop, 2001). Healthcare providers still fear the possibility of addiction when clients in pain take opioids, and they warn clients about addiction (Morley-Forster et al., 2003; Watt-Watson et al., 2001). This can create reluctance on the part of the client to take opioids to manage pain when appropriate, and reluctance on the part of the healthcare provider to incorporate culturally identified meanings of pain into the management of pain.

It is important to recognize that clients view physicians and nurses as trusted sources of pain-management information and expect them to "know" they are experiencing pain and to treat it (Anderson et al., 2002).

Providing Culturally Sensitive Pain Care

To enhance cultural sensitivity, healthcare providers need to work with clients and their families so that mutual goals are identified and the clients' understanding and beliefs about pain are taken into account (McCaffery & Pasero, 1999). The following approaches can be used to help provide culturally sensitive pain care.

Be Aware of Personal Values and Knowledge That May Affect Responses to Pain

It is important for healthcare providers to explore their personal values regarding pain management so they can differentiate their own values from the values of those for whom they provide care. The client's ethnic background may unconsciously influence healthcare providers' decisions regarding pain management. Studies of healthcare providers' views of clients' experience of pain have found that medical and nursing personnel underestimate clients' pain and limit analgesics (Anderson et al., 2002; Calvillo & Flaskerud, 1993; Cleeland et al., 1997; Todd et al., 1994; Ng et al., 1996; Watt-Watson et al., 2001).

When the healthcare provider and the client who is experiencing pain share common values regarding the expression and meaning of pain, there may be little conflict regarding pain management. However, when the values regarding the expression and meaning of pain are different, conflict can arise when determining the most effective pain-management plan (Calvillo & Flaskerud, 1993).

Western society values a stoic response to pain. When clients are expressive regarding their pain, they may be seen as unable to cope and may be identified as "bad" or "unco-operative" clients. Healthcare providers must be aware of these biases and should avoid labelling clients. One way to assist in the elimination of negative client labels is to avoid using the phrase "complaints of pain." A more objective way to communicate a client's pain, either verbally or in writing, would be to cite "the client's report of pain" (McCaffery & Pasero, 1999).

Be Conscious of Variations in Affective Responses and the Meaning of Pain Among Cultures

A **stoic** is defined as "one apparently or professedly indifferent to pleasure or pain" (Merriam-Webster Online Dictionary, 2005). Stoic behaviour on the part of a client does not necessarily mean that within the client's culture there is a high tolerance to pain. However, there may be cultural norms that determine how pain should be expressed. Conversely, an emotional response to pain does not mean the client is seeking analgesics. Avoid cultural stereotyping. It is important to individually assess each client who is experiencing pain (Lasch, 2000).

Use Established Pain Assessment Tools to Assist in Measuring Pain

Clients from many different cultures may be assessed using similar pain assessment tools, and the findings will have similar meanings across cultures. Behavioural expression of pain may differ among cultural groups; however, pain ratings and tools to assess pain can be applied across cultures with success (McCaffery & Pasero, 1999). Self-report of the intensity of pain should be measured using valid and reliable tools. Examples of **pain assessment tools** include, but are not limited to, the Numeric Rating Scale (NRS), faces scales, and simple descriptors of pain, as well as behavioural and observational tools to assess pain in infants and non-verbal adults (American Pain Society, [n.d.]; Herr, Spratt, Mobily, & Richardson, 2004; Hicks, von Baeyer, Spafford, van Korlaar, & Goodenough, 2001; McCaffery & Pasero, 1999; Paice & Cohen, 1997).

Numeric Rating Scale (NRS)

A numeric rating scale of pain intensity consists of a range of numbers from 0 to 10 (see Figure 13-1). Individuals are informed that 0 represents "no pain," and 10 represents "worst pain imaginable." The NRS may be used either verbally or visually. A client with pain would state or record the number that best represents his or her level of pain intensity.

The Faces Pain Scale—Revised (FPS-R)

Faces pain scales present the client with drawings of facial expressions, representing increasing levels of pain intensity. The client is asked to select the face that best represents his or her pain intensity (or level), and the resulting score is the corresponding number (rank order) of the expression chosen. Clients do not see the numbers; these are shown in Figure 13-2 only for reference purposes. The FPS-R is available in 22 languages (www.painsourcebook.ca). It was developed to assess pain intensity in children but can also be used with adults, even when a language barrier exists.

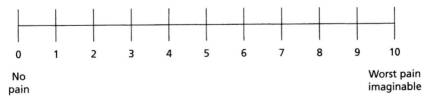

FIGURE 13-1 ▪ A Numeric Rating Scale for Pain

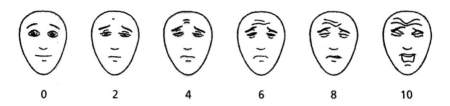

0   2   4   6   8   10

FIGURE 13-2 ▪ **The Faces Pain Scale—Revised (FPS-R)**
From "Faces of pain scale—revised," Copyright 2001 International Association
for the Study of Pain (IASP), Web site: http://www.painsourcebook.ca

Additional Pain Assessment Tools

A multi-dimensional tool can be used when a more comprehensive pain assessment
is necessary. The "McGill Pain Questionnaire" and the "Brief Pain Inventory" are
two examples of comprehensive pain assessment tools. Both tools are available
online and have been used with clients from a variety of cultural backgrounds
(Cleeland, Nakamura, & Mendosa, 1996; Greenwald, 1991; Lasch, 2002; Melzak,
1975; Saxena, Mendoza, & Cleeland, 1999). There may be other pain type-specific
or discipline-specific tools that can be used to assess aspects of pain, including
tools related to function and quality of life (American Pain Society, n.d.).

Remember that a client's self-report of pain is the most reliable indicator of
the presence and intensity of pain and its impact on quality of life. In addition to
the established pain assessment tools indicated above, Table 13-1 presents questions that may assist the healthcare provider in obtaining a culturally sensitive
pain assessment.

Learn About Biological Differences in the Metabolism of Medications

Clients' genetic makeup, as influenced by their ethnic background, can have an
impact on how medication is metabolized. For example, codeine, a weak opioid
analgesic, is metabolized in the liver to morphine, its active analgesic form. It
is converted from codeine into morphine using a cytochrome P-450 enzyme,
CYP 2D6. However, some people produce only a small amount of CYP 2D6
and are therefore unable to metabolize codeine into morphine, making it ineffective as an opioid analgesic (Williams, Patel, & Howard, 2002). Approximately 5 to 10 percent of Caucasians, up to 20 percent of African Americans, and
1 percent of Asians are poor metabolizers of drugs handled by CYP 2D6 (Rogers,
Nafziger, & Bertino, 2002).

Due to the ineffectiveness of the drug, poor and rapid metabolizers may be
mistakenly labelled as drug seeking. Switching to an opioid that is not activated
by CYP 2D6 may provide more effective pain relief (Rogers, Nafziger, & Bertino,
2002). Examples of such opioids include morphine, hydromorphone, oxycodone,
and fentanyl.

TABLE 13-1

Questions You Can Ask to Assess an Individual's Beliefs About Pain

- What do you call your pain? What name do you give it?
- Why do you think you have this pain?
- What does your pain mean for your body?
- How severe is it? Will it last a long or short time?
- Do you have any fears about your pain? If so, what do you fear most about your pain?
- What are the chief problems that your pain causes for you?
- What kind of treatment do you think you should receive? What are the most important results you hope to receive from the treatment?
- What cultural remedies have you tried to help you with your pain?
- Have you seen a traditional healer for your pain? Do you want to?
- Who, if anyone, in your family do you talk to about your pain? What do they know? What do you want them to know?
- Do you have family and friends that help you because of your pain? If so, who helps you?

From "Culture, pain, and culturally sensitive pain care," by K. E. Lasch, 2000, *Pain Management Nursing*, *1*(3) Suppl. I, p. 19.

Incorporate Culturally Specific Practices, Desired by the Client, into the Pain Management Plan

The healthcare team can discuss, with both the client and the family, how culturally specific practices can be incorporated into the plan of care. Although it may not be possible to incorporate all culturally specific practices into the plan of care, this type of discussion can help to clarify which methods of treatment the client would find helpful or unhelpful in managing his or her pain.

Understanding the common beliefs about pain in various cultures is helpful for providing culturally sensitive pain management. It may not be realistic to try to learn every culture's common beliefs about pain; however, healthcare providers can become informed about the beliefs of the populations they regularly see in their practice (Crawley, Marshall, Lo, & Koenig, 2002).

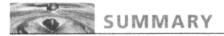 SUMMARY

As cultural diversity increases, healthcare providers will be required to care for individuals from many backgrounds that are different from their own, with pain management being an important aspect of the care provided. It is important to recognize that different cultural groups express pain in a variety of ways: some groups allow for free expression of pain, while others value stoicism. Different cultural groups also ascribe different meanings to their pain. The concept of acculturation also is important; individuals who have immigrated may adopt their new homeland's common expression and meaning of pain, leaving behind their traditional cultural values.

CULTURAL COMPETENCE IN ACTION

Client Won't Budge on Ointment Preference

Clients may have treatment preferences that healthcare providers need to understand, as is the case with a 62-year-old woman of East Indian descent who has been admitted to hospital for the treatment of community-acquired pneumonia.

She also has painful rheumatoid arthritis in her right knee. At home, she managed the pain in her knee with a topical "pain ointment" that her younger brother sent from India. She has experienced decreased mobility since being admitted into hospital, which she attributes to the pain in her knee. However, she refuses to take the oral analgesic that was prescribed as she feels it would be unnecessary if she were able to use her own pain ointment.

Although based on your personal beliefs, you think she should use oral analgesics as the first-line treatment for her pain, you understand that the topical treatment is her preference. After researching the literature regarding this topical treatment for the management of arthritis pain, you find limited but positive evidence to support this practice. You then advocate on behalf of the client that she be allowed to continue her topical treatment for her painful rheumatoid arthritis while in the hospital. The client's family is happy to bring the pain ointment to the hospital for her to use as necessary.

This example highlights how personal beliefs regarding the treatment of pain may differ, but how discussion and research can help healthcare providers to incorporate personal and cultural preference into the plan of care for their clients.

Concepts of culture may be useful for making generalizations about populations; however, these generalizations should not be used to predict individual behaviour (Crawley et al., 2002). One way to help avoid making these generalizations in pain assessment and management is to remember the definition of pain: pain is an individual, subjective experience, with both emotional and sensory components. Only the individual who is experiencing the pain can describe it and indicate when it occurs. Non-verbal cues to determine the presence and intensity of pain may not always be present. Using valid and reliable pain assessment tools, and asking questions that can assist in obtaining a culturally sensitive pain assessment, will aid healthcare providers in determining the presence and intensity of the pain, and the best treatment plan.

ONLINE LEARNING RESOURCES

www.ama-cmeonline.com/pain_mgmt/module01/02intro/index.htm#
American Medical Association (Pain Management)

www.ampainsoc.org
American Pain Society

http://ccmadoctors.ca
Canadian Complementary Medical Association

www.curepain.ca
Canadian Consortium on Pain Mechanisms, Diagnosis and Management

www.canadianpainsociety.ca
The Canadian Pain Society

www.chronicpaincanada.com
Chronic Pain Association of Canada

www.iasp-pain.org
International Association for the Study of Pain

www.painhurtscanada.ca
Pain Hurts Canada, an initiative of the Canadian Pain Coalition

www.postoppain.org
Procedure Specific Postoperative Pain Management

www.paincare.ca
Purdue Pharma's painCare.ca (Canadian resource for pain management)

http://www.rnao.org/Storage/11/543_BPG_assessment_of_pain.pdf
Registered Nurses Association of Ontario (Best Practice Guidelines)

REFERENCES

American Pain Society (n.d.). http://www.ampainsoc.org/ce/npc/II/b_measurement.htm

Anderson, K. O., Richman, S. P., Hurley, J., Palos, G., Valero, V., Mendoza, T., Gning, I., & Cleeland, C. (2002). Cancer pain management among underserved minority outpatients. *Cancer, 94*(8), 2295–2304.

Andrews, G., & Boon, H. (2005). CAM in Canada: Places, practices, research. *Complementary Therapies in Clinical Practice, 11*, 21–27.

Bates, M., Edwards, W. T., & Anderson, K. O., (1993). Ethnocultural influences on variation in chronic pain perception. *Pain, 52*(1), 101–112.

Bloodworth, D. (2005). Issues in opioid use. *American Journal of Physical Medicine and Rehabilitation, 84* (S), S42–S55.

Callister, L. C., Khalaf, I., Semenic, S., Kartchner, R., & Vehvilainen-Julkunen, K. (2003). The pain of childbirth: Perceptions of culturally diverse women. *Pain Management Nursing, 4*(4), 145–154.

Calvillo, E. R. & Flaskerud, J. H. (1993). Evaluation of the pain response by Mexican American and Anglo American women and their nurses. *Journal of Advanced Nursing, 18*, 451–459.

Chopra, A., Lavin, P., Patwardhan, B., & Chitre, D. (2000). Randomized double-blind trial of an Ayurvedic plant-derived formulation for treatment of rheumatoid arthritis. *Journal of Rheumatology, 27*(6), 1365–1372.

Chopra, A., Saluja, M., Patil, J., & Tandale, H. S. (2002). Pain and disability, perceptions and beliefs of a rural Indian population: A WHO-ILAR COPCORD study. *Journal of Rheumatology, 29*(3), 614–21.

Chronic Pain Association of Canada. (2004). *Pain Facts.* Retrieved February 5, 2005, from http://www.chronicpaincanada.com/

Chung, J. W. Y., Thomas, W. K. S., & Yang, J. C. S. (2000). The lens model: Assessment of cancer pain in a Chinese context. *Cancer Nursing, 23*(6), 454–461.

Chung, T. K., French, P., & Chan, S. (1999). Patient-related barriers to cancer pain management in a palliative care setting in Hong-Kong. *Cancer Nursing, 22*(3), 196–203.

Clarke, E. B., French, B., Bilodeau, M. L., Capasso, V. C., Edwards, A., & Empoliti, J. (1996). Pain management knowledge, attitudes and clinical practice: The impact of nurses' characteristics and education. *Journal of Pain and Symptom Management, 11*(1), 18–31.

Cleeland, C. S., Gonin, R., Baez, L., Loehrer, P., & Pandya, K. J. (1997). Pain and treatment of pain in minority outpatient pain study: The eastern cooperative oncology group minority outpatient pain study. *Annals of Internal Medicine, 127*(9), 813–816.

Cleeland, C. S., Nakamura, Y., & Mendoza, T. R. (1996). Dimensions of the impact of cancer in a four-country sample: New information from multidimensional scaling. *Pain, 67,* 267–273.

Crawley, L. M., Marshall, P. A., Lo, B., & Koenig, B. (2002). Strategies for culturally effective end-of-life care. *Annals of Internal Medicine, 1*(9), 673–679.

Davidhizar, R., & Giger, J. N. (2004). A review of the literature on care of clients in pain who are culturally diverse. *International Nursing Review, 51,* 47–55.

Edwards, C. L., Fillingim, R. B., & Keefe, F. (2001). Race, ethnicity and pain. *Pain, 94*(2), 133–137.

Edwards, R. R., Doleys, D. M., Fillingim, R. B., & Lowery, D. (2001). Ethnic differences in pain tolerance: Clinical implications in a chronic pain population. *Psychosomatic Medicine 63,* 316–323.

Edwards, R. R., & Fillingim, R. B. (1999). Ethnic differences in thermal pain responses. *Psychosomatic Medicine, 61,* 346–354.

Greenwald, H. (1991). Interethnic differences in pain perception. *Pain, 44*(2): 157–164.

Goldstein, D., Ellis, J., Brown, R., Wilson, R., Penning, J., Chisom, K., VanDenKerkhof, E., (with members of the Canadian Collaborative Acute Pain Initiative). (2004). Meeting proceedings: Recommendations for improved acute pain services: Canadian collaborative acute pain initiative. *Pain Research and Management, 9*(3), 123–130.

Herr, K. A., Spratt, K., Mobily, P. R., & Richardson, G. (2004). Pain intensity assessment in older adults: Use of experimental pain to compare psychometric properties and usability of selected pain scales with younger adults. *Clinical Journal of Pain, 20*(4), 207–219.

Hicks, C. L., von Baeyer, C. L., Spafford, P. A., van Korlaar, I., & Goodenough, B. (2001). The Faces Pain Scale—Revised: Toward a common metric in pediatric pain measurement. *Pain 93*(2), 173–83.

Honeyman, P. T., & Jacobs, E. (1996). Effects of culture on back pain in Australian Aboriginals. *Spine, 21*(7), 841–843.

Ho, N. K. (2001). Understanding traditional Chinese medicine—A doctor's viewpoint. *Singapore Medical Journal, 42*(10), 487–492.

International Association for the Study of Pain. (1994). Retrieved December 22, 2005 from www.iasp-pain.org/terms-p.html

Jackson, M. (2002). *Pain the fifth vital sign.* Toronto: Random House Canada

Jordan, M. S., Lumley, M. A., & Leisen, J. C. (1998). The relationships of cognitive coping and pain control beliefs to pain and adjustment among African-American and Caucasian women with rheumatoid arthritis. *Arthritis Care and Research, 11*(2), 80–88.

Jovey, R. D., Ennis, J., Gardner-Nix, J., Goldman, B., Hays, H., & Lynch, M. (2003). Use of opioid analgesics for the treatment of chronic non-cancer pain—A consensus statement and guidelines from the Canadian Pain Society, 2002. *Pain Research and Management, 8*(Suppl. A), 3A–14A.

Kohr, R. & Sawhney, M. (2005). Advanced practice nurses' role in the treatment of pain. *Canadian Nurse, 101*(3), 30–34.

Lai, Y. H., Dalton, J. A., Belyea, M., Chen, M. L., Tsai, L. Y., & Chen, S. C. (2003). Development and testing of the pain opioid analgesics beliefs scale in Taiwanese cancer patients. *Journal of Pain and Symptom Management, 25*(4), 376–385.

Lasch, K. E. (2000). Culture, pain and sensitive pain care. *Pain Management Nursing 1*(3 Suppl. I), 16–22.

Lasch, K. E. (2002). Culture and pain. *Pain Clinical Updates, 10*(5), Retrieved December 22, 2005, from http://www.iasp-pain.org/PCU02-5.html

Lasch, K. E., Wilkes, G., Montuori, L. M., Chew, P., Leonard, C., & Hilton, S. (2000). Using focus group methods to develop multicultural cancer pain education materials. *Pain Management Nursing, 1*(4), 129–139.

Lee, A., Gin, T., & Oh, E. (1997). Opioid requirement and responses in Asians. *Anaesthesia and Intensive Care, 25*, 665–670.

MacPherson, H., Thorpe, L., Thomas, K., & Campbell, M. (2003). Acupuncture for low back pain: Traditional diagnosis and treatment of 148 clients in a clinical trial. *Complementary Therapies in Medicine, 12*, 38–44.

McCaffery, M. & Pasero, C. (1999). *Pain Clinical Manual* (2nd ed.). St. Louis, MO: Mosby.

McNeill, J. A., Sherwood, G. D., Starch, P. L., & Nieto, B. (2001). Pain management outcomes for hospitalized Hispanic patients. *Pain Management Nursing, 2*(1), 25–36.

Meldrum, M. (2003). A capsule history of pain management. *Journal of the American Medical Association, 290*(18), 2470–2475.

Melzak, R. (1975). The McGill pain questionnaire: Major properties and scoring methods. *Pain, 1*, 277–299.

Merriam-Webster Online Dictionary. (2005). *Stoic.* Retrieved December 22, 2005 from http://www.m-w.com/dictionary/stoic

Morley-Forster, P. K., Clark, A. J., Speechley, M., & Moulin, D. E. (2003). Attitudes toward opioid use for chronic pain: A Canadian physician survey. *Pain Research and Management, 8*(4), 189–194.

Morrison, R. S., Wallenstein, S., Natale, D. K., Senzel, R. S., & Huang, L. (2000). "We don't carry that"—Failure of pharmacies in predominantly nonwhite neighborhoods to stock opioid analgesics. *The New England Journal of Medicine, 342*(14), 1023–1026.

Moulin, D. E., Clark, A. J., Speechley, M., & Morley-Forster, P. K. (2002). Chronic pain in Canada: Prevalence, treatment and the role of opioid analgesia. *Pain Research and Management, 7*(4), 179–184.

Ng, B., Dimsdale, J. E., Rollnick, J. D., & Shapiro, H. (1996). The effect of ethnicity on prescriptions for patient-controlled analgesia for post-operative pain. *Pain, 66(1)*: 9–12.

Paice, J. A., & Cohen, F. L. (1997). Validity of a verbally administered pain rating scale to measure cancer pain intensity. *Cancer Nursing, 20*, 88–93.

Reizian, A., & Meleis, A.I. (1986). Arab-Americans' perceptions of and responses to pain. *Critical Care Nurse, 6*(6), 30–36.

Rogers, J. F., Nafziger, A. N., & Bertino, J. S. (2002). Pharmacogentics affects dosing, efficacy, and toxicity of cytochrome P450-metabolized drugs. *American Journal of Medicine, 113*, 746–750.

Saxena, A., Mendoza, T., & Cleeland, C. (1999). The assessment of cancer pain in North India: Validation of the Hindi Brief Pain Inventory–BPI-H. *Journal of Pain and Symptom Management, 17*(1), 27–41.

Sheffield, D., Biles, P. L., Orom, H., Maixner, W., & Sheps, D. (2000). Race and sex differences in cutaneous pain perception. *Psychosomatic Medicine, 62*(4), 517–523.

Singh, B. B., Mishra, L. C., Vinjamury, S. P., Aquilina, N., Singh, V. J., & Shepard, N. (2003). The effectiveness of Commiphora mukul for osteoarthritis of the knee: An outcomes study. *Alternative Therapies in Health & Medicine, 9*(3), 74–9.

Tamayo-Sarver, J. H., Dawson, N. V., Hinze, S., W., Cydulka, R. K., Wigton, R. S., Albert, J. M., Ibrahim, S. A., & Baker, D. W. (2003). The effect of race/ethnicity and desirable social characteristics on physicians' decisions to prescribe opioid analgesics. *Academic Emergency Medicine, 10*(11), 1239–1248.

Todd, K. H., Lee, T., & Hoffman, J. R. (1994). The effect of ethnicity on physician estimates of pain severity in patients with isolated extremity trauma. *Journal of the American Medical Association, 271*(12), 925–928.

Watt-Watson, J., Stevens, B., Garfinkel, P., Streiner, D., & Gallop, R. (2001). Relationship between nurses' pain knowledge and pain management outcomes for their postoperative cardiac patients. *Journal of Advanced Nursing, 36*(4), 535–545.

Williams, D. G., Patel, A., & Howard, R. F. (2002). Pharmacogentics of codeine metabolism in an urban population of children and its implications for analgesic reliability. *British Journal of Anesthesia, 89*(6), 839–845.

White, S. F., Asher, M., Lai, S. M., & Burton, D. C. (1999). Patients' perceptions of overall function, pain and appearance after primary posterior instrumentation and fusion for idiopathic scoliosis. *Spine, 24*(16), 1693.

World Health Organization. (n.d.). Cancer Pain Release. 1995. Vol 8(3) Retrieved December 22, 2005. http://www.whocancerpain.wisc.edu/eng/8_3/chinese.html

Yosipovitch, G., Meredith, G., Chan, Y. H., & Goh, C. L. (2004). Do ethnicity and gender have an impact on pain thresholds in minor dermatologic procedures? A study on thermal pain perception thresholds in Asian ethnic groups. *Skin Research and Technology, 10*, 38–42.

Zoborowski, M. (1952). Cultural components in responses to pain. *Journal of Social Issues, 8*, 15–30.

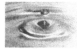

CHAPTER 14

Caring–Healing and Complementary Therapies

SHEILA M. LEWIS

LEARNING OBJECTIVES

At the end of this chapter, the learner will be able to:

- Understand the major classifications and definitions of complementary therapies
- Explain what human science means as it relates to complementary therapies in Canada
- Describe the evolving relationship between caring–healing healthcare practice and culturally congruent care
- Explore the cultural considerations in caring–healing healthcare practice in relation to complementary therapies

KEY TERMS

Caring–healing

Complementary and alternative health care (CAHC)

Complementary and alternative medicine (CAM)

Culturally congruent care

Human science

Integrative health care

What do consumers need for their health and healing journey? What role should healthcare providers play in facilitating the healthcare needs of consumers? How can this care be provided in a way that incorporates major values and beliefs of the client (i.e., is **culturally congruent care**)? What role do alternative and complementary therapies play in health and healing? What are the results when the healthcare provider–client relationships are based on a foundation of compassionate caring healing practices? How can healthcare providers gain knowledge, competence, and skill in the provision of culturally congruent complementary therapies? These are some of the questions that this chapter will reflect upon. These issues will be addressed through an exploration of the following:

- The definitions and classifications of complementary therapies
- The human science context for complementary therapies

▪ The evolving connection between caring–healing healthcare practice and culturally congruent care
▪ Cultural considerations in caring–healing healthcare practice in relation to complementary therapies

Major Classifications and Definitions of Complementary Therapies

The National Center for Complementary and Alternative Medicine (NCCAM) in the United States provides basic definitions to assist with understanding the difference between conventional, alternative, complementary, and integrative health care (see Table 14-1). These definitions focus on the differences between therapies that have been accepted by mainstream medicine (i.e., conventional, allopathic, and traditional Western therapies) versus those that are considered alternative or unconventional approaches (i.e, are non-traditional in the West); complementary (i.e., used together with conventional medicine); and integrative (i.e., are evidence-based therapies).

Complementary and alternative medicine also is known more commonly as **CAM,** a "group of diverse medical and healthcare systems, practices, and products that are not presently considered to be part of conventional medicine—that is, medicine as practiced by holders of MD (medical doctor) or DO (doctor of osteopathy) degrees and their allied health professional, such as physical therapists, psychologists, and registered nurses" (NCCAM, 2002, p. 1). In Canada, Health Canada's health systems division has gone beyond the medical term CAM, broadening the terminology to **complementary and alternative health care** (CAHC) to include non-medical practices and practitioners and to reflect a more holistic perspective that is consistent with consumer demands. Another term, **integrative health care**, is used to describe approaches that blend complementary and conventional practices to provide holistic care (also see Chapter 8). These terms will be used for the remainder of this chapter.

Classifying Common Complementary and Alternative Healthcare Practices

Now that definitions of CAHC have been clarified, attention should be turned to understanding the fluid boundaries within these practices and what implications this may have for cultural competence in health care.

What at first appears to be a simple matter of categorizing practices into either conventional or CAHC actually is a complex process. Many alternative or complementary practices also may be delivered by conventional healthcare providers, and "clearly, the boundaries between conventional medicine and CAHC can not be delineated through the training or orientation of the providers" (Achilles, 2001, p. I.3). Achilles goes on to suggest that many of these therapies can be classified as healthcare promotion activities in relation to the "health care

TABLE 14-1

Definitions for Major Complementary Therapy Classifications

Alternative medicine	Used *in place of* conventional medicine (e.g., special diet to treat cancer instead of undergoing surgery, radiation, or chemotherapy, that has been recommended by a conventional doctor) (NCCAM, 2002, p. 2)
Complementary medicine	Used *together with* conventional medicine (e.g., aromatherapy to help lessen a client's discomfort following surgery) (NCCAM, 2002, p. 4)
Integrative medicine	Combines mainstream medical therapies and CAM [complementary and alternative medicine] for which there is some high-quality scientific evidence of safety and effectiveness (NCCAM, 2002, p. 5)
Conventional medicine or biomedicine	Western medical practices, modern, allopathic, orthodox, scientific (Fontaine, 2005, p. 4)
Complementary and alternative health care (CAHC)	Eastern, ancient, homeopathic, traditional, indigenous healing methods (Fontaine, 2005, p. 4)

From *What is complementary and alternative medicine (CAM)?* by National Center for Complementary and Alternative Medicine (NCCAM), May 2002. Retrieved October 30, 2004, from http://nccam.nih.gov/health/whatiscam/
Also from *Complementary and alternative therapies for nursing practice* (2nd ed., p. 4), by K. L. Fontaine, 2005. Upper Saddle River, NJ: Pearson/Prentice Hall.

organization, the environment, lifestyle, and human biology" (p. I.3). This means that many CAHC practices clearly are holistic, personal health practices, and preventive care practices, which reflect the values and beliefs of the individual, family, and community. This is in contrast to the "continuing monopoly of the medical model in definitions of CAHC" (Achilles, 2001, p. I.4). Such a client-centred approach suggests that the CAHC practices would be supported within a model of health promotion and disease prevention, instead of a conventional medical model.

Ultimately, a client-centred health promotion approach would help healthcare providers to accept and promote world views, or outlooks, other than the traditional world view that the Western medical model represents. This shift toward a more client-centred approach also recognizes the importance of cultural competence.

Complementary and alternative healthcare practices are not always classified using those names. Canadian academic Douglas Tataryn (2002), for example, has developed a classification system that is based on the following four perspectives of health and illness (see also Table 14-2):

1. Health of body
2. Body–mind
3. Body–energy
4. Body–spirit

TABLE 14-2

Four Paradigms of Health and Disease

Classifying Common Alternatives and Complementary Therapies

BODY	BODY–MIND	BODY–ENERGY	BODY–SPIRIT
1) Physical substances	Affirmations/suggestion	Acupressure	Ceremonies and rituals
a) *Diets and supplements*	Counselling	Acupuncture	Dervish dancing
(Natural or synthetic)	Dream interpretation	Ayurvedic medicine	Exorcism
Aromatherapy	Expressive art therapies	Chinese medicine	Faith healing
Gerson diet	Hypnosis	Crystal therapy	First Nations traditions
Herbal remedies	Imagery/visualization	Healing touch	Laying-on-of-hands
Macrobiotic diet	Meditation	Homeopathy	Magic/occult practices
Vitamin and mineral therapies	Psychotherapy	Magnetic therapy	Prayer
b) *Extracts and concentrates*	Stress reduction	Polarity therapy	Psychic diagnosis
Antineoplastons	Support groups	Qigong	Psychic interventions
Laetrile		Reflexology	Sacraments/rites
Live cell therapies		Reiki	Shamanic healing
Ozone therapy		Therapeutic touch	
Shark cartilage		Tai chi	
c) *Chemicals/ synthetics*		Yoga	
714-X			
Chemotherapy			
Chelation therapy			
2) Physical manipulation			
(Natural or invasive)			
Chiropractic			
Colonic irrigation			
Enemas			
Hypo-/hyperthermic therapy			
Massage			
Physiotherapy			
Surgery			

From "Paradigms of health and disease: A framework for classifying and understanding alternative medicine," by D. Tataryn, 2002, *The Journal of Alternative and Complementary Medicine, 8*(6), 881.

Each perspective, or paradigm, reflects the assumptions of health and disease with which it is associated. For example, the body paradigm reflects the assumptions that are associated with biological factors being seen as the primary determinants of health; the body–mind paradigm considers factors such as psychological coping, stress, and social supports as primary determinants of health; the body–energy paradigm reflects health and illness in relation to the harmony and flow of life energies; and the body–spirit paradigm considers factors such as transcendence and aspects of health and illness outside of the material universe as we know it.

Tataryn (2002) assumes a hierarchical relationship among these four paradigms, with each incorporating the assumptions of the previous one and adding other assumptions to qualify previous paradigms. Again, this model depicts a more holistic approach that considers the varying cultural and belief systems of people. As such, it is a suitable framework from which to begin to understand multiple perspectives. In addition, as Tataryn (2002) points out, "Many Western families of European descent now fully embrace vegetarian diets and non-Judeo-Christian belief systems, such as Buddhism, Taoism, and different forms of yoga. Conversely, many North American First Nations people and people of Japanese and Chinese descent are second- and third-generation Christians who now live what was once the 'typical' North American philosophy and lifestyle" (p. 878). Thus, these four paradigms of health reduce the potential for labelling people based on their distinctive culture.

Critics of this model point to its continuing use of the word "body" in each paradigm, which they say serves the continued domination of the body in Western culture. But, as Tataryn clearly states (2002, p. 880), "other cultures might have different dispositions and might perceive the 'person' or 'spirit' as being healthy or becoming sick" and prefer those terms instead of "body." Future research should investigate the development of a cross-cultural paradigm of health that would classify common CAHC practices.

One final example of a classification system for CAHC is seen in Table 14-3. It clearly identifies those therapies that are considered alternative within our dominant Western culture. Many of these practices are considered to be mainstream or integrative within other cultures. This example, once again, emphasizes the need for healthcare providers to move beyond their own etic (outsider or provider) world view, to one that considers the emic (lay, indigenous, or folk) practices of each person (Leininger, 2002).

A Human Science Context for Complementary Therapies in Health Care

Having looked at some of the common classification systems within complementary and alternative health care, we can turn our attention to what these various therapies mean with respect to cultural competence in clinical care.

To provide care that "focuses on people of diverse cultures in many different living contexts and environments" (Leininger, 2003, p. 283), we must first ask

TABLE 14-3

Classification of Complementary and Alternative Medicine Therapies
As Defined by the US National Center for Complementary and Alternative Medicine (NCCAM)

ALTERNATIVE MEDICAL SYSTEMS

These therapies are built upon complete systems of theory and practice. They often have evolved earlier and apart from conventional medical approaches used in Canada and elsewhere.

Examples of systems that have developed in Western cultures include homeopathic medicine and naturopathic medicine. Examples of systems that have developed in non-Western cultures include environmental medicine, traditional Chinese medicine, and Ayurveda.

Examples of specific therapies include:
- Acupuncture
- Environmental medicine (e.g., air quality, ergonomics)
- Aboriginal practices (e.g., drumming, herbs, sweat lodge)
- Natural products
- Past-life therapy
- Shamanism
- Tibetan therapies (e.g., herbs, meditation)

MIND–BODY INTERVENTIONS

Mind–body medicine uses a variety of techniques designed to enhance the mind's capacity to affect bodily function and symptoms. Some techniques that were considered CAM in the past have become mainstream (e.g., client support groups and cognitive-behavioural therapy). Other mind–body techniques are still considered CAM, including meditation, prayer, mental healing, and therapies that use creative outlet (e.g., art, music, or dance).

Specific examples include:
- Yoga
- Counselling
- Humour therapy
- Relaxation techniques
- Tai chi
- Dance therapy
- Support groups
- Guided imagery
- Biofeedback
- Hypnotherapy

BIOLOGICALLY BASED THERAPIES

Biologically based therapies in CAM use substances found in nature, such as herbs, foods, and vitamins. Examples include dietary supplements, herbal products, and the use of other so-called "natural" but as yet scientifically unproven therapies (e.g., using shark cartilage to treat cancer).

Specific examples include:
- Anti-oxidizing agents
- Botanical medicines
- Cell treatment
- Chelation therapy
- Metabolic therapy
- Oxidizing agents (ozone, hydrogen peroxide)
- Gerson therapy
- Macrobiotics and other therapeutic diet programs
- Megavitamins
- Nutritional supplements

MANIPULATIVE AND BODY-BASED METHODS

Manipulative and body-based methods in CAM are based on manipulation and/or movement of one or more parts of the body. Examples include chiropractic or osteopathic manipulation and massage.

Other examples include:
- Acupressure
- Alexander technique
- Biofield therapies
- Feldenkrais method
- Reflexology
- Trager method
- Zone therapy

ENERGY THERAPIES

Energy therapies involve the use of energy fields. They are of two types:

Biofield therapies are intended to affect energy fields that purportedly surround and penetrate the human body. Some forms of energy therapy manipulate biofields by applying pressure and/or manipulating the body by placing the hands in or through these fields.

Examples include:
- Qigong
- Healing touch
- Therapeutic touch
- Reiki

Bioelectromagnetic-based therapies involve the unconventional use of electromagnetic fields, such as pulsed fields, magnetic fields, or alternating current or direct current fields.

Examples include:
- Electroacupuncture
- Electromagnetic fields
- Electrostimulation and neuromagnetic stimulation devices
- Magnetoresonance spectroscopy
- Magnets/magnetic fields

From *What is complementary and alternative medicine (CAM)?* by National Center for Complementary and Alternative Medicine (NCCAM), May 2002 [NCCAM Publication No. D156]. Retrieved October 30, 2004, from http://www.nccam.nih.gov/health/whatiscam Also from *Holistic nursing: A handbook for practice* (pp. 18–19), by B. Dossey, L. Keegan, and C. Guzzetta, 2005. Boston: Jones & Bartlett Publishers.

ourselves what our own values, beliefs, and assumptions are in relation to our thinking or knowing, being, and doing in health care. This reflection encourages each of us to remember who we are and to relate to others as "pan-dimensional" beings (Rogers, 1992). To understand more fully what we cherish in our own clinical practice, education, research, and/or teaching, it may be helpful to consider three basic paradigms or perspectives in health care, and then reflect upon which one best "fits" with our own values and beliefs and those of the clients we serve.

Three perspectives dominate the field of health care and healing (see also Table 14-4):
1. Particulate–deterministic perspective (Paradigm I)
2. Interactive–integrative perspective (Paradigm II)
3. The emerging unitary–transformative perspective (Paradigm III)
   (Newman, 1997; Parse, 1995; Rogers, 1992; Watson, 1999)

As Newman (1992) explains, "The idea here is that the first of the paired words describes the view of the entity being studied and the second describes the notion of how change occurs" (p. 10). These paradigms have also been categorized respectively as Era I, Era II, and Era III by Dossey (1999).

TABLE 14-4

Paradigms of Health

PARADIGM	VIEW OF HUMAN BEING	ROLE OF HEALTH CARE
I Particulate–deterministic (biophysical science)	▪ Reducible into parts ▪ Relationships and reality linear and causal ▪ Separate and dualistic	▪ Healthcare provider as expert ▪ Objectivity and "doing-to" versus "being with" ▪ Distant and not interactive ▪ Emphasis on functional tasks and skills ▪ Cultural needs secondary to treatment plan
II Interactive–integrative (bio-psycho-social science)	▪ Reality multidimensional and contextual ▪ Acknowledge local effect of mind on the body	▪ Objectivity and subjectivity ▪ Control and predictability ▪ Consider client's experience, psychosocial and emotional needs ▪ Cultural context of client considered
III Unitary–transformative (human science)	▪ Unitary (human field) "is an irreducible, indivisible, pan-dimensional energy field identified by pattern and manifesting characteristics that are specific to the whole and which cannot be predicted from knowledge of the parts" (Rogers, 1992, p. 29)	▪ Client as expert ▪ Transpersonal relational, ethical caring–healing ▪ Mutuality, relatedness, and connectedness ▪ Creative unfolding including but not limited to "caring–healing modalities: ethical, relational, and energetic through caring consciousness, intentionality, presence, authenticity; non-invasive, non-intrusive, natural-environmental healing modalities; those modalities that help to connect with universal field to access inner healer; intentional use of form, colour, light, energy, sound, touch, visual, consciousness, etc." (Watson, 2005, p. 225). ▪ Cultural context of client embedded in healthcare provider–client relationship

Based on Newman, et al., 1991; Newman, 1992, 1997; Parse, 1995; Rogers, 1992; Watson, 1995, 2005.

Paradigm/Era I

The particulate–deterministic perspective (Paradigm/Era I) is based on a view of humans as reducible into parts, with a focus on the physical causes of illness, along with mechanical techniques, technology, and objectivity. Practitioners using complementary therapies within this frame of reference would focus on "doing to" versus "being with." The cultural needs and wishes of each client would be secondary to the primacy of the "treatment" and the mechanical curative aspects of each treatment.

Of course, this world view isn't very compatible with client-focused approaches to care—embraced by the various health disciplines—that call for the kind of compassionate caring–healing processes that support each client's quality of life. In the words of Madeleine Leininger (2002), "Care is the essence of nursing and a distinct, dominant, central and unifying focus" (p. 192). Cody (2000) explored the literature regarding existing guiding frameworks for science, society, and health care, and noted that Paradigm I generally has been dominated by men and "at best serve[s] women only poorly and at worst oppress[es] and harm[s] women, and [has] little relevance for nurses in learning about women" (p. 191). He goes on to state that this results in a perpetuation of "unequal, harmful, and unjust relationships between men and women, rich and poor, light-skinned and dark-skinned people, and straight and gay people" (p. 191). He suggests that one answer to this oppression is through an ongoing critique of the power relationships that exist among people. This may result in heightened social consciousness.

Another theoretical approach to consider is the adoption of a healthcare framework that serves as the foundation for thinking, speaking, writing, and practice for both the individual healthcare practitioner as well as the healthcare system (Cody, 2000). If human health–life experiences are the central focus for health care within a caring, culturally sensitive framework, then we must look to the underpinnings of Paradigms II and III for guidance in order to determine which healthcare theory best speaks to each of us.

Paradigm/Era II

Within the interactive–integrative paradigm or world view (Paradigm/Era II), the healthcare provider's frame of reference becomes that of a bio-psycho-social science perspective, in which she or he now extends the values of Paradigm II to consider the experience and context of the client. However, this approach generally is taken from the healthcare provider's own expert perspective.

Complementary therapies would be used within this frame of reference as *tools* that could enable healthcare providers and clients to understand their lived experiences more clearly. Within Paradigm II, the cultural context of the client is of some importance to health and healing. This perspective is reflective of the Florence Nightingale call to "put the patient in the best condition" for self-healing to take place. This may include holistic approaches to health and healing, but as Rogers (1992) notes, the term "holistic" often refers to summation of parts, rather than irreducible wholeness.

Healthcare providers practising from this paradigm may be led to use their knowledge of complementary therapies and culture with the best intentions as a partner in care. However, this world view may not necessarily support the belief that clients "know 'the way' somewhere within self" (Parse, 1990, p. 139). Likewise, Engebretson (2002) warns those who practise CAHC:

> Many of these modalities with origins in other cultures or historical periods have been popularized through New Age or Holistic Health movements. As these techniques have been taken out of the cultural context of their historical and geographical or ethnic setting, these techniques are often used without a full understanding of cultural or philosophical underpinnings, beliefs and values. (p. 178)

Engebretson (2002) cautions us against a blending of the values and beliefs of Western biomedicine when trying to apply more ancient healing systems. When we interpret only fragments of a healing system from another culture, we face the results of reductionism and mechanism.

Paradigm/Era III

This third paradigm calls for an ongoing process of relational–transformative connectedness, which now is emerging as a unitary–transformative perspective (Paradigm/Era III). This world view requires a deep respect for the healing traditions of all clients.

As Newman (2002) notes, "Each succeeding level transcends and includes the previous ones. So having reached the unitary perspective, we do not discard the physical, interpersonal and integrative knowledge. All are vital to the greater whole" (p. 3). Within this postmodern world view, concepts that were not fully understood in either Paradigm I or Paradigm II could now be explored more fully. This includes a fuller understanding of concepts, such as energy, non-contact touch, time and space relativity, non-local or collective consciousness, and transcendence. While Paradigm II perspectives acknowledged the local effect of the mind on the body or "psychosomatic" perspectives, it was unable to transform our thinking regarding broader meanings of health and healing (Watson, 1999). Phenomena such as healing are viewed from a self-organizing unitary field that is embedded in a larger self-organizing field. As Gerber (2001) tells us:

> The more advanced quantum and particle physicists are now coming to the same conclusions about the underlying unity of humanity and nature the ancient Chinese and Indian philosophers described in their writings depicting subtle human relationships with the cosmos. The only difference in approach between the ancient and modern viewpoints is that the old Oriental and Vedic teachers came to their insights through meditation and inner psychic probing of the universe, while modern scientists have arrived at their conclusions through a more mechanistic, electronic, and empirical approach. (pp. 416–417)

The use of complementary therapies that often are ancient methods of caring–healing, focus on "body–mind–spirit integration through auditory, visual, olfactory, sensory, tactile, and cognitive modalities that potentiate wholeness, comfort, relaxation, pain control, symptom management, self-care, and sense of well-being" (Watson, 1995, p. 68). Integration of mind–body–spirit cannot occur without cultural sensitivity, awareness, knowledge, and skills that go beyond simply acknowledging diversity. This includes a process of "becoming aware of personal cultural values and beliefs and then developing an awareness of the cultural beliefs of the healthcare system, and finally growing to be aware of the cultural belief systems of patients" (Engebretson, 2003, p. 217).

Human science is embedded in the understanding of important contexts, such as culture, history, and gender. In healthcare practice, **human science** means a focus on clients as unitary wholes—a focus on clients' values and beliefs and the meanings they gain from their lived experience.[1] Each client's circumstances reflect his or her past and present, everyday, lived experiences. Multiple perspectives are honoured and respected. Thus, it is within the unitary–transformative paradigm that healthcare professionals can most fully actualize these complementary caring–healing practices and respect the wholeness of each person.

Cultural competence embraces these concepts because they reflect an ethical caring and connectedness that is vital to preserving the dignity, wholeness, and humanity of those clients we are privileged to serve. Within this holographic,[2] non-linear model of health, healing, and the universe, both the seen and the unseen interconnections between everything show us more clearly that we are "all constructed from the same subatomic building blocks. At a microcosmic level, we are each complex yet uniquely arranged aggregates of the same particularized universal energy" (Gerber, 2001, p. 417).

This view holds great promise for the future of health care. It implies that culturally congruent complementary therapies are practised with reference to the subjectivity of each client. Within this model of health and caring–healing, our primary concern is to take the time to listen, understand, and respect the world view, ethical values, concerns, hopes, and wishes of each individual, family, and community.

Putting Paradigm/ERA III to Work

> Sources of knowing in nursing are unbounded; that is to say that as unitary beings in relation, nurses draw on multiple sources of knowing including rational, empirical, theoretical, philosophical, personal, moral and ethical, intuitive and transcendent. Caring nurses utilize these multiple sources of knowing to be with, witness and co-create quality of life with clients, their families and the community they serve. (York University School of Nursing, 2003, p. 2)

There are a number of human science nursing theories that reflect a unitary–transformative Paradigm/Era III perspective as the foundation for a caring–healing, culturally congruent healthcare practice. Four such nursing theories are:

1. Martha Rogers Science of Unitary Human Beings (1986, 1990, 1992)

---

[1]A more formal definition for human science calls it a "knowledge-acquiring enterprise that uses an approach and method that is faithful to the unique qualities of human beings. That is, radically nonreductionistic" (Giorgi, 2005, p. 78).

[2]The term "holographic" refers to the notion that the whole is reflected in each part.

2. Jean Watson's Theory of Human Caring (1999, 2005)
3. Rosemarie Rizzo Parse's Theory of Human Becoming (1995, 1998, 2001)
4. Margaret Newman's Theory of Expanding Consciousness (1992, 1994, 1997)

An application of Jean Watson's (1999, 2005) philosophy of caring science as sacred science in relation to cultural considerations in caring–healing and complementary therapies is presented below. The term "caring–healing" is used extensively by Watson in the context of bringing the sacred to healing work. **Caring–healing** relates to a way of being and belonging, as well as to caring–healing practices that help the healthcare providers remember who they are and that they belong to that which is greater than any one individual person or individual culture. Watson's theory offers the opportunity for healthcare providers to unite their energy with their caring–healing consciousness, in any given moment in space and time.

Watson (2002) advocates a renewed understanding of the importance of intentionality, and suggests that caring–healing consciousness "also renews some of the esoteric core of religions of all worlds, as well as the perennial wisdom traditions of the ages" (p. 15). This understanding offers deeper possibilities for a movement away from the traditional goal-oriented healthcare practice of Paradigm/Era I, to a transcultural, transpersonal caring–healing practice that "invites spirit-energy to enter into one's life and work, and into the caring–healing processes and outcomes" (Watson, 2002, p. 14).

From this perspective, health care plays a witnessing, facilitative role in assisting all people to "maintain their ability to cultivate and manifest deep values, beliefs, and meaningfulness in the midst of suffering and disease" (Watson, 2002, p. 15). Inner healing is possible when healthcare providers practise from such an ethical, humanitarian, transpersonal awareness. In fact, Watson (2005), Rogers (1992), Newman (2002), and Parse (1997) might all agree that "the predominant belief is that the human uniquely co-creates a personal health in mutual process with the universe; thus, the theory is not specific to any one culture, nor is there any effort to categorize people according to their culture" (Parse, 1997, p. 34).

Clients are honoured for their deeply embedded values and longings. It is within this sacred act of communion with another that "we are remembering our own and others' humanity and our shared belonging to the infinity of [the] universal field of love that embraces spirit. We are remembering we are touching the life force, the very soul of another person, hence ourselves" (Watson, 2005, p. 61).

Readers are encouraged to explore these theories further, because doing so provides the greatest opportunity for self-understanding and a guide to transpersonal, transcultural healthcare practice, education, research, and administration.

CULTURAL COMPETENCE IN ACTION

A Healing Touch Case Study

Introduction

The following case study is a reflection based on my* experience as a volunteer healing touch practitioner (HTP-A) at an inner-city agency in Ontario that has a mission to support underhoused and low-income women in the community. The agency staff are guided by feminist principles of anti-racism or anti-oppression, which enable clients to take greater control of their lives.

The women who participate in the various day programs requested my services after one of my students was nearing completion of her clinical placement at the agency. One woman participant acted as the co-ordinator and encouraged other women to consider seeing me at some point during my experience. One requirement for my final healing touch certification process (Level 5) was to document 100 client assessments and healing touch processes. During the previous summer, I had volunteered at an independent nurse-run counselling program and had completed almost half of my client assessments there; clients had been very willing to answer my assessment questions and to have me document my healing touch sessions with them.

My orientation to the policies and procedures at the agency emphasized client confidentiality and respect for the dignity and wholeness of each woman. During my allotted time, I met with five to eight women over a period of six weeks. This case study reflects the integration of these shared times, with all names having being changed.

Each client signed up for a one-hour healing touch session (see Table 14-5 for an overview of healing touch). At the completion of each session, each client decided whether or not she would like to return for another session the following week. Everyone returned for at least five sessions. At the beginning and end of each day and before each caring–healing session, I centred myself and meditated briefly in order to be truly present with each client with whom I spent time. Sometimes, this centring was done with the client as we began the mutual process of engaging in healing touch. The women collectively helped with the preparation of the room, including putting a poster on the window of each door to provide additional privacy; ensuring that there were few interruptions during each session; and deciding on the times that each of them would visit me (schedules changed based on activities, etc.).

They commented on my attempts to create a sacred healing space.** For example, I played some soothing music during each session. Finally, after two sessions Lori*** said to me, "That music is pretty blah. Haven't you got anything a little more upbeat?" On another occasion, someone was playing the piano outside our healing space, and Chris felt that it was not conducive to our session together. She went out and asked the pianist to either stop playing or else change the tune (the tune changed!). I quickly learned that being client-centred meant that they would guide the caring–healing dance and I would follow their lead.

---

*This case study represents a personal account by the chapter author, Sheila M. Lewis.

**Sacred healing space is a safe, protective environment characterized by trust created through caring, honesty, integrity, gentleness; intentionality and caring consciousness; honouring the wholeness; and listening.

***Names of the women have been changed to protect confidentiality.

The nurse co-ordinator had warned me that my formal documentation might not be accepted by many of the clients since often they mistrusted the traditional healthcare system as a result of their negative experiences with healthcare personnel. The first day, I dutifully brought my forms out and learned that this was the quickest way to shut down the development of a transpersonal caring–healing relationship with each woman. After consultation with a few of the clients, it was agreed that I would document essentials very briefly on a pad of blank paper.

The Process

I began each session by exchanging hellos and asking each woman what would be helpful for our time together. This proved to be an excellent way to begin to listen to clients' experiences and respond to their needs for that particular day.

Rhonda, for example, sat with me during our first visit and told me about her animals and how she was having problems healing the cat bites on her arms. She had finished her antibiotic treatment but still had considerable drainage and inflammation at the site of each bite. She asked me to do some healing touch on her cuts, after I explained the options. We spent the next 30 minutes talking while I slowly entered her energy field and began to complete an assessment, followed by two techniques called energetic ultrasound and energetic laser. Later, she decided that she wanted to lie on the table for the remainder of the healing touch treatment. She spoke about her relationship with her animals and her long-time experience at the agency. She also asked me many questions about my work and my life, as did a number of the clients. We were co-participants in the healing process. This meant that I also experienced healing in this mutual process of caring. Through the sharing of their lives, these women showed me their resilience and the impact that social and economic inequalities have on the lives of all women.

Many of the clients that I had the privilege of being with were recent immigrants to Canada. They had experienced isolation, poverty, and a high incidence of abuse. Each of them showed courage and determination to meet their own goals for quality of life and for harmony of mind–body–soul. In addition, some of them had been isolated by their own cultural communities since they had broken a code of silence in relation to their abuse by husbands/uncles/partners. They spoke of how important their friendship with other women was to their own healing. Through this friendship, they formed communities of caring and healing, within the sacred hoop of one circle. I joined this circle for a brief time and was sheltered in turn by their caring. Through this process, I did not see myself alone as the healing environment but saw the women collectively enfolded together. We moved from listening to talking and sharing, from crying to laughing, and from strangers to souls in search of peace.

Within this caring–healing space and time, specifics such as ethnicity, religion, sexual preference, and so on were not essential to understanding their healing process. Instead, what unfolds is a mutual process that goes beyond language and requires authentic caring–healing consciousness and intentionality. This resulted in multiple meanings and caring–healing experiences for each client.

I was given a thank-you card from the women that said: "You have been a bright light in the darkness . . . thank you very much for helping me to be me." This card came from a woman who told me during our first visit that she had "trouble trusting anyone" as a result of abuse over a long period of time. She told me that she wasn't "between the cracks" but "in" the cracks, "and it is a long way out." During our third visit, she told me that "people are more open with me and I feel more grounded." At another visit she said, "I feel like my heart has been closed a long time." This is a small part of her lived experience and the meaning she gained from our transpersonal caring–healing relationship.

In reflecting upon my precious time with each woman, I feel that I have been given a number of lessons to continue my own healing process and lessons as a healer. Here are a few of these lessons:

Lesson 1
Control is an illusion since people "knowingly participate in creating their reality by being aware, making choices, feeling free to act on their intentions, and involving themselves in creating changes" (Barrett, 2000, p. 4). Each of the clients that I worked with struggled with her own past, present, and future. We had moments of synchronized rhythms, and we had moments of despair and non-engagement. For example, on my final day, Jin met me outside and told me that she just couldn't see me that day, and that she needed to be somewhere else. In her eyes, I saw fear and loneliness. Later that day, the card they gave me included a note from Jin thanking me for my gentle touch and signing it "your challenge."

Lesson 2
Energy fields are open and pan-dimensional. They do not differentiate based on ethnicity, race, gender, sexuality, or any other label that we place on people. The patterns that are expressed in our energy fields reflect our infinite past, present, and future, unbounded by time and space. In many of our healing touch sessions, we had non-linear experiences that had no spatial or temporal attributes. These experiences fostered "a sense of oneness with the universe. This same notion of oneness is present in non-Western cultures as well as the notion of respect for life and stewardship of the resources provided to us" (Cox, 2003, p. 31). For example, in one session, I sensed that Jin had experienced a great loss and that someone else was with us in spirit, during this healing session. Jin responded, "It might have been the loss of myself you were sensing." She went on later to talk at length about the loss of herself "with no way out sometimes." She expressed that life was a real struggle for her. In those brief moments, Jin was able to access her own inner healer and invite creative emergence within herself.

Lesson 3
Telling a woman's story "preserves her traditions, values, and way of life. The woman is the interpreter of her own lived experiences. The woman is the Keeper of the Wisdom, the Knower" (Lambert Colomeda, 1996, p. xx). Each client expressed her story in her wholeness, dignity, and integrity. Feeling listened to and understood offered opportunities for mutual meaning and for paradoxical expressions of hope/hopelessness, grieving/joy, humour/sadness, loss of self/finding self, control/no control, content/

discontent, isolation/togetherness, vulnerability/resilience, fear/courage, clarity/lack of clarity, holding/sharing, aloneness/togetherness, weakness/strength, and silence/voice. I cherished my time with each client, in the knowing and in the unknowing that we shared together. From this witnessing of each other's humanness, we often are able to transcend the ego level and create new possibilities for each of us, while at the same time living the suffering and loss associated with lived experience.

Lesson 4
Complementary therapies such as healing touch are simply a doorway or pathway to self-healing. There are many pathways to remembering ourselves and what we are called to in this lifetime. The opening of the doorway to our centre includes, but is not limited to, caring–healing consciousness, intentionality, presence, authenticity, caring–healing ontologies such as healing touch, mutual support, an ethic of deep caring as a way of being and belonging, along with respect for the dignity and wholeness of each person. It also is closely aligned to each person's cultural values, beliefs, and practices that support her in her wholeness.

Lesson 5
Each of us carries light that resonates in varying, concentric circles. A healthcare provider's caring consciousness and heart/mindfulness and intentionality carry a higher frequency energy than non-caring consciousness. I learned to take time to begin and end my day with meditation/breathwork and gratitude, to let go of those things that I could not control, and to ask for divine spirit and love as I lived day to day. This practice enabled me to see more fully and to be more fully present with the spirit-filled clients that I had the privilege to meet.

Lesson 6
There are still barriers to the availability of caring–healing complementary therapies, which recognize and integrate unitary ways of being, knowing, and doing (praxis). They include:
- Attitudes and values of healthcare providers
- Cost of treatment
- The ongoing need for education

If I hadn't offered my services voluntarily, most of these clients wouldn't have been able to afford to pay. Some of them made a strong point of telling me that they thought I should be remunerated for my services. As research and education in complementary therapies advances and practitioners take risks to challenge the status-quo Era I paradigm, we will begin to see increased application of Era II and Era III paradigms. At the present time, nurses and other healthcare providers continually serve as humanizing connections between this mechanistic system and the lived experience of clients and their families. As one nurse said to me recently, "We are overdue for change to a more humanistic, client-centred healthcare system." Caring–healing is needed for both the practitioners and for the clients we serve. This is our call.

TABLE 14-5

Healing Touch (Biofield Therapy)

DEFINITION, GOALS, BENEFITS, AND PRINCIPLES

What Is Healing Touch?

- "An energy based therapeutic approach to health and healing. It uses touch to influence the Energy System, specifically the Energy Field that surrounds the body and the Energy Centers which control the energy flow from the Energy Field to the physical body, thus affecting all physical, mental, emotional and spiritual health and healing" (Mentgen & Trapp Bulbrook, 2000, p. 125)
- "Based on a heart-centered caring relationship in which both healer and client come together energetically to facilitate client's health and healing" (Mentgen & Trapp Bulbrook, 2000, p. 124)

Goal of Healing Touch

- To restore harmony and balance in the energy system, placing the client in a condition to self-heal (Mentgen & Trapp Bulbrook, 2000, p. 125)

Benefits of Healing Touch

- Acceleration of wound healing
- Relief of pain and increased relaxation
- Reduction of anxiety and stress
- Energizing the field
- Prevention of illness
- Enhancement of spiritual development
- Aid in preparation for and follow-up after medical treatments and procedures
- Support for the dying process
  (Mentgen & Trapp Bulbrook, 1996 , p. 13)

PRINCIPLES OF HEALING TOUCH

- Center (become clear in the self)
- Open (be available to receive without judgment)
- Observe verbal, non-verbal, energetic, and intuitive information throughout the whole process
- Be accurate
- Be truthful at your level of understanding in reporting what you find before, during, and post treatment
  (Mentgen & Bulbrook, 2000, p. 19)

Other Principles and Ideas in Healing Touch

- The healing act is a sacred process
- The world and everything in it are interdependent
- A person's health and quality of life are affected by the health and quality of life of the energy system (Mentgen & Trapp Bulbrook, 1996, 2000)

From *Healing touch level I notebook*, by J. Mentgen and M. J. Trapp Bulbrook, 1996, Carrboro, NC: Colorado Center for Healing Touch.
Also from *Healing touch level II notebook*, by J. Mentgen and M. J. Trapp Bulbrook, 2000, Carrboro, NC: Colorado Center for Healing Touch. Retrieved from http://www.healingtouch.net/ccht.shtml

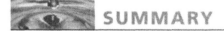

SUMMARY

This chapter has provided an overview of the major classifications and definitions of complementary therapies, with the intent of understanding the complexity and ongoing development of complementary and alternative health care (CAHC) in relation to cultural considerations in caring–healing.

It also has sought to consider what consumers are asking from healthcare providers in relation to their health and healing journey. This has been approached through an analysis of three paradigms for health: particulate–deterministic, interactive–integrative, unitary–transformative. The unitary–transformative paradigm has been further elucidated through consideration of human science nursing theories and their meaning in relation to health care.

The author shared her experience as a healer in order to provide a brief image of how Watson's (2005) philosophy of caring science can be used as a framework for living the values and beliefs of this philosophy. As with complementary therapies and transcultural nursing, "the concepts and frames of reference point toward a Caring Science, but are not *It*" (Watson, 2005, p. ix). Instead, this chapter has represented reminders of our shared soulful path and what it might mean to approach the sacred in all, while deeply respecting and honouring each client's culture and circumstance. The short poem below attempts to capture the essence of the healing path.

THE HEALING PATH
All are sacred
As is the Earth and the Sun and the Sky and the Stars above
Sun spirit, Rain spirit, Wind spirit, Moon spirit
Light my path forward
Light my way home
Help me listen
Listen gently
Remember who I am ~ bless me
Remember who you are ~ bless you
Together
Walking proudly in balance
Upon Mother Earth
Finding our healing path home

—Sheila M. Lewis

ONLINE LEARNING RESOURCES

www.ahna.org/home/home.html
The American Holistic Nurses Association

www.ccnm.edu/
The Canadian College of Naturopathic Medicine

http://www.canadian-health-network.ca
The Canadian Health Care Network (select language and see Complementary and Alternative Health under topics)

http://mypage.direct.ca/h/hutchings/chna.html
Canadian Holistic Nurses Association

www.can-nurses.ca/cna/
Canadian Nurses Association

www.shamanism.org
Foundation for Shamanic Studies

www.thefacts.org/
Friends of Alternative and Complementary Therapies Society

www.healingtouchcanada.net/
Healing Touch Canada

www.healingtouch.net
Healing Touch International

www.noetic/org/
Institute of Noetic Sciences

www.humancaring.org
International Association for Human Caring

www.issseem.org
The International Society for the Study of Subtle Energies and Energy Medicine

www.nccam.nih.gov/
National Center for Complementary and Alternative Medicine (NCCAM)

www.therapeutic-touch.org
Nurse Healers—Professional Associates International

www.herbalists.on.ca/
Ontario Herbalists Association

www.phac-aspc.gc.ca/publicat/pcahc-pacps
Public Health Agency of Canada: Perspectives on Complementary and
Alternative Health

www.therapeutictouchnetwk.com
Therapeutic Touch Network of Ontario

REFERENCES

Achilles, R. (2001). *Defining complementary and alternative health care.* Retrieved August 12, 2004, from http://www.phac-aspc.gc.ca/publicat/pcahc-pacps/pdf/comp_define.pdf

Baker, M., Jones, G., & Schuman, M. (1998). *The healing blanket. Stories, values and poetry from Ojibwe elders and teachers.* Salt Lake City, UT: Commune-A-Key Publishing.

Barrett, E. A. M. (2000). The theoretical matrix for a Rogerian nursing practice. *Theoria: Journal of Nursing Theory, 9*(4), 3–7.

Cody, W. K. (2000). Nursing Science Frameworks for practice and research as means of knowing self. *Nursing Science Quarterly, 13*(3), 188–195.

Cox, T. (2003). Theory and exemplars of advanced practice spiritual intervention. *Complementary Therapies in Nursing and Midwifery, 9*, 30–34.

Dossey, L. (1999). *Reinventing medicine: Beyond mind-body to a new era of healing.* San Francisco: HarperCollins.

Dossey, B., Keegan, L., & Guzzetta, C. (2005). *Holistic nursing: A handbook for practice.* Boston: Jones & Bartlett Publishers.

Engebretson, J. (2002). Culture and complementary therapies. *Complementary Therapies in Nursing and Midwifery, 8*, 177–184.

Engebretson, J. (2003, Sept.). Cultural constructions of health and illness. Recent cultural changes toward a holistic approach. *Journal of Holistic Nursing, 21*(3), 203–227.

Fontaine, K. L. (2005). *Complementary and alternative therapies for nursing practice* (2nd ed.). Upper Saddle River, NJ: Pearson/Prentice Hall.

Gerber, R. (2001). *Vibrational medicine* (3rd ed.). Rochester, VT: Bear and Company.

Giorgi, A. (2005, Jan.). The phenomenological movement and research in the human sciences. *Nursing Science Quarterly, 18*(1), 75–82.

Kavanaugh, K., & Kennedy, P. H. (1992). *Promoting cultural diversity: Strategies for health care professionals*. Newbury Park, CA: Sage.

Krippner, S. (1995). A cross-cultural comparison of four healing models. *Alternative Therapies in Health and Medicine, 1*, 21–29.

Lambert Colomeda, L. A. (1996). *Through the northern looking glass. Breast cancer stories told by northern native women*. New York: National League for Nursing.

Leininger, M. (2002). Culture care theory: A major contribution to advance transcultural nursing knowledge and practices. *Journal of Transcultural Nursing, 13*(3), 189–192.

Leininger, M. (2003). Founder's focus: Some key last challenges. *Journal of Transcultural Nursing, 14*(3), 283.

Mentgen, J., & Trapp Bulbrook, M. J. (1996). *Healing touch level I notebook*. Carrboro, NC: Colorado Center for Healing Touch.

Mentgen, J., & Trapp Bulbrook, M. J. (2000). *Healing touch level II notebook*. Carrboro, NC: Colorado Center for Healing Touch.

National Center for Complementary and Alternative Medicine. (n.d.). *The use of complementary and alternative medicine in the United States*. Retrieved October 20, 2004, from http://nccam.nih.gov/news/camsurvey_fs1.htm

National Center for Complementary and Alternative Medicine. (2002, May). *What is complementary and alternative medicine (CAM)?* Retrieved October 30, 2004, from http://nccam.nih.gov/health/whatiscam/ Publication No. D156).

Newman, M. A. (1992). Prevailing paradigms in nursing. *Nursing Outlook, 40*(1), 10–14.

Newman, M. A. (1994). *Health as expanding consciousness,* (2nd ed.). Sudbury, MA: Jones & Bartlett.

Newman, M. A. (1997). Evolution of theory of health as expanding consciousness, *Nursing Science Quarterly, 7*, 153–157.

Newman, M. A. (2002). The pattern that connects. *Advances in Nursing Science, 24*(3), 1–7.

Newman, M. A., Sime, A. M., & Corcoran-Perry, S. A. (1991). The focus of the discipline of nursing. *Advances in Nursing Science, 14*(1), 1–6.

Parse, R. R. (1990). Health: A personal commitment. *Nursing Science Quarterly, 3*, 136–40.

Parse, R. R. (Ed.). (1995). *Illuminations: The human becoming theory in practice and research*. New York: National League for Nursing.

Parse, R. R. (1997). The human becoming theory: The was, is, and will be. *Nursing Science Quarterly, 10*(1), 32–38.

Parse, R. R. (1998). *The human becoming school of thought: A perspective for nurses and other health professionals*. Thousand Oaks, CA: Sage.

Parse, R. R. (2001). *Qualitative inquiry: The path of sciencing*. New York: National League for Nursing.

Rogers, M. E. (1986). Science of unitary human beings. In V. Malinski (Ed.), *Explorations on Martha Rogers' science of unitary human beings* (pp. 3–8). Norwalk, CT: Appleton-Century-Crofts.

Rogers, M. E. (1990). Nursing: Science of unitary, irreducible, human beings: Update 1990. In E. Barrett (Ed.), *Visions of Rogers' science-based nursing* (pp. 5–11). New York: National League for Nursing.

Rogers, M. E. (1992). Nursing science and the space age. *Nursing Science Quarterly, 5*(1), 27–34.

Tataryn, D. (2002). Paradigms of health and disease: A framework for classifying and understanding alternative medicine. *The Journal of Alternative and Complementary Medicine, 8*(6), 877–892.

Watson, J. (1995, July). Nursing's caring–healing paradigm as exemplar for alternative medicine? *Alternative Therapies in Health and Medicine, 1*(3), 64–69.

Watson, J. (1999). *Postmodern nursing and beyond.* Edinburgh: Churchill Livingstone.

Watson, J. (2002). Intentionality and caring–healing consciousness: A practice of transpersonal nursing. *Holistic Nursing Practice, 16*(4), 12–19.

Watson, J. (2005). *Caring science as sacred science.* Philadelphia: FA Davis.

York University School of Nursing. (2002). *Philosophy of the BScN program.* Toronto, ON: Author.

Glossary

Aboriginal medicine [Ch. 8]: A highly complex group of systems that draws on and develops the physical, mental, and spiritual talents and powers of individuals. It includes intervention by elders and, in some cases, by healers. Practices include, but are not limited to, ceremonies and the use of herbals and medicinal substances.

Acculturation [Chs. 7 and 8]: The process by which members of a cultural group learn and adopt behaviours of a different culture as a result of close, often continuous, contact.

Acupuncture [Ch. 8]: The practice of inserting very fine needles into the skin to stimulate specific anatomic points in the body (called acupoints or acupuncture points) for therapeutic purposes. Acupuncture literally means "needle piercing."

Ad hoc interpreters [Ch. 6]: People serving as interpreters who have not received any training in interpretation, also known as informal interpreters. The individuals are frequently family and friends but also may be untrained volunteers, or professional or non-professional staff.

Advance directive [Ch. 10]: A document that expresses a person's wishes about critical care or life-sustaining medical treatments in the event that the person is unable to make his or her own decisions.

Allopathic medicine [Ch. 8]: Medicine as practised by holders of doctor of medicine (MD) or doctor of osteopathy (DO) degrees and by their allied healthcare providers, such as physical therapists, psychologists, and registered nurses. Other terms include conventional medicine, Western medicine, mainstream medicine, orthodox medicine, biomedicine, and regular medicine.

Assimilation [Chs. 2 and 8]: The process by which different cultural groups come to have a common culture; the term often is used in reference to the process by which a minority group is gradually absorbed into another dominant group and adopts its customs and attitudes while losing its own distinctive features over time.

Awareness [Ch. 10]: The awareness aspect of competency that refers to an understanding of how culture shapes the issues that are of concern to particular populations.

Ayurveda and MAV [Ch. 8]: India's traditional, natural system of medicine that has been practised for more than 5000 years. Ayurveda provides an integrated approach to preventing and treating illness through lifestyle interventions and natural therapies. Ayurvedic theory states that all disease begins with an imbalance or stress in the individual's consciousness. **Maharishi Ayurveda (MAV)** is a revival of Ayurveda brought about by Maharishi Mahesh Yogi and uses meditation techniques to develop a more integrated and coherent functioning of the nervous system and human physiology.

Back translation [Ch. 6]: The process of taking a document that has already been translated into a foreign language and translating it back into the original language—preferably using an independent translator.

Bearing witness [Ch. 10]: The skill of being present with clients and families to share and understand the cultural as well as health- and illness-related issues being experienced in the situation.

Becoming [Ch. 8]: The dimension of the bio-psycho-social-spiritual framework that highlights how an individual's behaviours are connected with purposeful activities undertaken to achieve his or her goals.

Being [Ch. 8]: The dimension of the bio-psycho-social-spiritual framework that refers to the bio-psycho-spiritual foundation reflecting the holistic nature of a person.

Belonging [Ch. 8]: The dimension of the bio-psycho-social-spiritual framework that refers to how one fits in with the surrounding environment.

Bicultural staff [Chs. 2 and 6]: Belonging to or knowledgeable about two cultures. Bicultural individuals have some legitimacy in both cultures and can serve as brokers between the cultures to bridge the cultural gap and negotiate across cultural misunderstandings.

Bi-directional conversations [Ch. 5]: Conversations where information flows from and to both parties and both parties (healthcare providers and clients) give as much time to listening as to talking.

Bilingual [Ch. 6]: Proficiency in two languages. In Canada, bilingualism refers to the ability to speak the two official languages, English and French.

Biomedical [Ch. 1]: The view of medical science that focuses on the application of principles of the natural sciences, especially biology and physiology, to clinical medicine; also referred to as Western medicine.

Bio-psycho-social-spiritual framework of health [Ch. 8]: This is a short way of referring to a holistic perspective where "bio" refers to the biological and physiological aspects; "psycho" refers to the thinking and feeling aspects; "social" refers to the social network, including friends and family; and "spiritual" refers to one's beliefs and relationship with the broader universe.

Birth plan [Ch. 9]: A written plan of preferences and desires for the labour and birthing experience.

Birth stories [Ch. 9]: Memories of women's birthing experiences that are shared with others.

Bonding/infant attachment [Ch. 9]: Bonding, or infant attachment, is defined as the sensitive period and process after birth when parents have close contact with infants, to assist in the development of emotional relationships.

Caring–healing [Ch. 14]: An approach to health care that focuses on the conscious compassion skills of the healthcare provider. It also relates to practices that help healthcare providers remember who they are and that they belong to that which is greater than any one individual person or individual culture. Caring–healing therapies focus on instilling hope and promote body–mind–spirit integration.

Chiropractic [Ch. 8]: A system of diagnosis and treatment based on the concept that the nervous system co-ordinates all of the body's functions and that disease results from a lack of normal nerve function. Chiropractic employs manipulation and adjustment of body structures, such as the spinal column, so that pressure on nerves coming from the spinal cord due to displacement of a vertebral body may be relieved.

Chronic pain [Ch. 13]: Pain that has persisted for at least six months longer than the time of expected tissue healing.

Clinical cultural competence [Ch. 1]: The ability to provide client-centred care that reflects the client's cultural values and beliefs and also reflects a recognition of the impact of marginalization in healthcare interactions and responses.

Collectivism [Chs. 5 and 7]: Social pattern where individuals see themselves as parts of one or more collectives and are primarily motivated by the norms of the group (versus individual pleasures) and duties imposed by the collective (versus individual preferences and desires).

Comfort [Ch. 10]: Comfort is both a process and an outcome. It involves promoting well-being within the physical, interpersonal, social, and spiritual domains.

Common-law family [Ch. 7]: The common-law family consists of two people living together as spouses without the formality of marriage. The family may or may not include children.

Complementary and alternative health care (CAHC) [Ch. 14]: A health- and consumer-driven term that is broader and more holistic in scope than "complementary and alternative medicine." CAHC includes therapies and practitioners outside the scope of medical care.

Complementary and alternative medicine (CAM) [Ch. 14]: The common medical term for diverse medical and healthcare systems, practices, and products that are not presently considered to be part of conventional medicine.

Consecutive interpreting [Ch. 6]: Interpreter session during which the interpreter is present with the healthcare provider and the client, and uses pauses between each one's speech to transform the message into a language understood by the other. Also known as face-to-face interpretation.

Cultural bias [Ch. 1]: A preference for a particular culture's values, beliefs, and norms, often with an accompanying belief that it is the correct perspective and must guide the situation or decisions.

Cultural blindness [Ch. 1]: Unwillingness or inability to recognize the existence of cultural differences, frequently due to a desire to be unbiased and treat everyone the same way.

Cultural care accommodation/negotiation [Ch. 4]: (Originally termed culture care accommodation/negotiation by Leininger.) Refers to actions and decisions that help clients adapt to, or negotiate with, others for beneficial and meaningful healthcare outcomes.

Cultural care reframing/repatterning [Ch. 4]: (Originally termed culture care repatterning/restructuring by Leininger.) Refers to actions and decisions that help clients change, re-order, or modify their lifeways for new and different approaches and outcomes by assisting them to see alternative interpretations of particular events or actions.

Cultural care validation/preservation [Ch. 4]: (Originally termed culture care preservation/maintenance by Leininger.) Refers to actions and decisions that help clients acknowledge and retain their meaningful healthcare values and lifestyles for their health and well-being.

Cultural competence [Ch. 1]: Refers to the ability of healthcare providers to apply knowledge and skill appropriately in interactions with clients in cross-cultural situations.

Cultural destructiveness [Ch. 1]: Refers to attitudes, practices, and organizational policies that focus on the superiority of one culture to the extent that other cultures are dehumanized and destroyed.

Cultural explanations [Ch. 11]: Meanings, beliefs, and attitudes that members of a specific culture ascribe to a particular phenomenon.

Cultural formulation [Ch. 11]: A tool included in the *Diagnostic and Statistical Manual of Mental Disorders* (*DSM*) *IV* that indicates areas for inquiry, which together would provide a systematic review of all the cultural factors that influence clients and the way in which these factors could affect the working relationship between the client and the healthcare provider.

Cultural identity [Ch. 11]: A sense of belonging to a group or culture, based on characteristics that are shared with other members of the cultural group.

Cultural interpretation [Ch. 6]: Interpretation where, in addition to the spoken word, the interpreter uses his or her cultural knowledge to offer additional information regarding potential cultural values and meanings of verbal and non-verbal communication.

Cultural knowledge [Chs. 3 and 4]: As an element of the Culture Care Framework, it identifies that cultural competence is knowledge-based care. Cultural knowledge has two components: see the definitions for "generic cultural knowledge" and "specific cultural knowledge."

Cultural literacy [Ch. 2]: Knowledge of a culture and associated languages, including idioms, slang, and other aspects of communication, leading to an ability to understand and converse in and with the culture.

Cultural mindedness [Ch. 11]: The aptitude for dealing with cross-cultural interactions and situations.

Cultural mosaic [Ch. 2]: Term used to describe the wide array of ethnic groups, languages, and cultures that co-exist within Canadian society with each group retaining its distinct heritage.

Cultural pre-competence [Ch. 1]: Part of the cultural competence continuum. This stage refers to the recognition of needs based on culture and some movement toward meeting those needs (e.g., a commitment to civil rights).

Cultural proficiency [Ch. 1]: Part of the cultural competence continuum. The stage where practitioners and organizations value diversity and seek out the positive role that culture can play in health and health care.

Cultural racism [Ch. 1]: Prejudice and exclusionary practices, by those in power, against another racial, religious, or social group, demeaning the other culture and at times attempting to change its values and ways of being, impose their own values over the other, or eradicate the minority culture.

Cultural reciprocity [Ch. 9]: Occurs when clients or their families feel able to share cultural needs, concerns, and feelings with healthcare providers, and sense that respect and sensitivity characterize the relationship.

Cultural relativism [Ch. 2]: Judging and interpreting the behaviour of others in terms of their traditions and experiences as opposed to one's own experiences and traditions.

Cultural resources [Chs. 3 and 4]: As an element of the Culture Care Framework, it recognizes that what happens in a particular clinical interaction depends not only on the competence of the healthcare provider but also on the resources available in the practice environment. Cultural resources are sources of cultural knowledge and may take the form of expressed information (e.g., in printed, electronic, or art form); policies or guidelines that provide direction; or individuals and groups that assist with information and understanding about cultures.

Cultural sensitivity [Ch. 3]: As an element of the Culture Care Framework, this refers to a complex set of understanding about the concept of culture, about self and one's culture, and about the dynamics associated with issues of difference. Cultural sensitivity focuses on self-awareness and insight versus understanding the other.

Culturally congruent care [Chs. 3 and 14]: Care that incorporates key values and beliefs of the client in a given situation.

Culture [Ch. 1]: Commonly understood, learned traditions and unconscious rules of engagement that people use to interpret experience and to generate social behaviour.

Culture broker [Ch. 2]: One who serves as a bridge between the client's culture and the culture of health care by sharing information and understanding, linking, or mediating between groups or persons of differing cultural backgrounds for the purpose of reducing conflict or producing change.

Culture care [Ch. 3]: Reflects the goal of integrating cultural issues into all aspects of health care.

Curanderismo [Ch. 8]: A healing tradition, common in Hispanic communities, where the healers recognize three levels (*niveles*)—the material, the spiritual, and the mental. It commonly uses herbs as well as objects and religious symbols with healing powers.

Decoding [Ch. 5]: Processes of perceiving and interpreting incoming messages in verbal and non-verbal communication.

Determinants of health [Ch. 12]: Factors that work together in a complex system to influence the extent to which a person is healthy or unhealthy. These factors include individual characteristics (e.g., gender), as well as social and economic characteristics (e.g., income, social status, employment, health practices), and the physical environment—including living and working conditions.

Determinants of immigrant women's health [Ch. 12]: Specific determinants of immigrant women's health include income, education and work, social support and stress, health practices, and use of health services.

Diversity [Ch. 1]: A term used to describe variation between people with respect to a range of characteristics such as ethnicity, national origin, gender, social class, sexual orientation, age, religion, physical abilities, values, and life experiences.

Encoding [Ch. 5]: Processes used to put thoughts, emotions, feelings, or attitudes into verbal and non-verbal communication forms that are recognizable by others.

Energy medicine [Ch. 8]: Energy medicine is a collection of techniques and systems based on the central tenet that human beings are energy systems that manifest the universal life force. The energy may be of the type that can be measured (e.g., magnetism or electromagnetic fields) or biofields that have defied measurement and are based on the concept that humans are infused with a subtle form of energy. This vital energy or life force is known under different names in different cultures, such as *qi* in traditional Chinese medicine (TCM) and *doshas* in Ayurvedic medicine.

Epidemiology [Ch. 8]: The scientific study of the determinants and distributions of health-related outcomes and events in specific populations.

Equity [Chs. 2 and 3]: Equality of opportunity, access, and outcome. Equity is different from equal or same treatment for all, and implies differential treatment to achieve equality in access and outcome.

Ethnic matching [Ch. 2]: Pairing healthcare provider and client of the same ethnic group together.

Ethnicity [Ch. 1]: A group identity based on culture, language, or a common attachment to a place or kin ties.

Ethnocentrism [Ch. 1]: A belief that one's own cultural values, beliefs, and behaviours are the best, preferred, and most superior ways.

Ethno-specific [Ch. 2]: Belonging or referring to a particular ethnic group.

Everyday racism [Ch. 1]: Characterized by routine encounters with discriminatory behaviour from the dominant group that pervade people's daily social interactions. Everyday racism can include mundane hassles as well as overt, severe racist experiences.

Explanatory model of illness [Chs. 2 and 4]: Perceptions and beliefs about the meanings and expectations associated with the illness and the illness experience, including the cause of illness, the severity of illness, the expected treatment, and the prognosis.

Face [Ch. 5]: Refers to the projected image of oneself in a situation involving two or more parties. Face is associated with honour and related concepts such as respect, shame, pride, dignity, and guilt.

Faith [Ch. 10]: An agreed-upon set of beliefs that often are sought by people for comfort and direction during difficult times such as illness.

Familism [Ch. 7]: A social pattern in which family solidarity and tradition have greater value than individual rights and interests.

Family diversity [Ch. 7]: The characteristics associated with the composition of a family, such as structure, membership, world view, race, ethnicity, religion, class, and acculturation stage, that influence how members of the family respond to issues of health and illness.

Family roles [Ch. 7]: Assigned or acquired responsibilities for individuals within a family unit that define what each member does within the family and allows the family unit to maintain equilibrium within the family. Family member roles are influenced by a variety of factors and can change over time and in response to specific events.

Family structure [Ch. 7]: An outline of the composition of a family, with respect to members and their relationship to each other and the family unit.

Family system [Ch. 7]: A recognition of the interdependencies of the family members within the family unit and of the family unit within the broader community and society.

Family Systems Theory [Ch. 7]: Encourages us to consider issues in terms of a multi-generational family system.

Feelings [Ch. 10]: A key area for cultural exploration. Feelings refer to emotions that may be evoked during difficult times across a range of issues that are affected by the situation.

Female circumcision [Ch. 9]: Refers to a number of procedures performed for cultural, rather than medical, reasons on the female genitalia. Also known as female genital cutting or female genital mutilation, the procedures involve tissue removal ranging from clitoridectomy or clitoridotomy (the removal or splitting of the clitoral hood) to infibulation (in which the labia majora is sutured).

Finality [Ch. 10]: Process that focuses on the closure of life as known and lived by a client and his or her family. This is a key area for consideration during culturally competent end-of-life care.

Generational conflict [Ch. 7]: Conflict that arises between family members as a result of differences in acculturation that challenge the pre-existing roles and norms within the family.

Generic cultural competencies [Ch. 10]: A broad set of knowledge, skills, and attitudes that enable the healthcare provider to work cross-culturally with clients from any ethnocultural group.

Generic cultural knowledge [Chs. 3 and 4]: Fundamental knowledge of cultural issues that can be applied across cultural and clinical populations.

Health [Ch. 8]: A state of complete physical, mental, and social well-being, not merely the absence of disease or infirmity.

Health disparities [Ch. 1]: Can exist with respect to either of the following, or both: *Disparities in health outcomes* refer to the differential burden of diseases, death, and morbidity in ethnic and racial minority groups compared with that of non-minorities. *Disparities in health care* refer to the lower-quality care provided to minority populations, even when access-related factors are controlled.

Health inequity [Ch. 1]: The presence of systematic disparities in health (or in the major social determinants of health) between social groups who have different levels of underlying social advantage/disadvantage.

Health promotion [Ch. 12]: Activities undertaken by individuals to optimize their health. These activities may be undertaken consciously or unconsciously as part of everyday life.

Healthy immigrant effect [Ch. 12]: Refers to the observation that immigrants (male and female) often are in superior health compared with the native-born population when they first arrive in a new country, but lose this health advantage over time.

High-context communication [Ch. 5]: Style of communication in which the intent and the meaning of the message are highly dependent on context and less on the words used. The meaning is embedded in how something is said, including what is not said.

Holding knowledge [Ch. 4]: A term coined by Leininger to describe specific knowledge of cultures or cultural patterns that is held by the healthcare provider and is used to reflect on ideas and experiences and determine areas for further inquiry. Holding knowledge allows for hypothesis generation and is not used to make stereotypical judgements.

Homeopathy [Ch. 8]: A system of therapy based on the concept that disease can be treated with drugs (in minute doses) thought capable of producing the same symptoms in healthy people as the disease itself.

Human science [Ch. 14]: In healthcare practice, this means a focus on clients as unitary wholes—a focus on clients' values and beliefs and the meanings they gain from their lived experience.

Identity [Ch. 3]: A concept emphasizing the sharing of a degree of sameness with others of a particular characteristic, which leads to a sense of belonging with the others.

Idioms [Ch. 5]: Phrases or expressions in which meaning is based on cultural understanding rather than the sum of the meanings of each individual word.

Immigrant and refugee experience [Ch. 11]: Includes events and experiences leading up to, involved in, and following the actual physical move that shapes the individual's world views.

Individualism [Chs. 5 and 7]: A social pattern in which individuals are primarily motivated by their own preferences, needs, rights, and desires, and view themselves largely as being independent of the larger collective.

Inquiring responses [Ch. 5]: Responses that inquire into the client's perspectives and invite further conversation.

Integrative health care [Chs. 8 and 14]: An integrated approach to health care that combines knowledge of conventional and complementary healing methods with the belief that the combination is ultimately superior to a single-model approach to health and wellness. Integrative health deals with the whole person, uses a variety of therapies, and is considered both a person-centred and a person-empowering approach to health and healing.

Interpretation [Ch. 6]: Refers to the process of mediating a verbal interaction between people who speak two different languages, without omission, addition, editorializing, or any distortion in meaning.

Joint family [Ch. 7]: In some cultures, the term for a family where parents and adult children and their families live under a single roof.

Layers [Ch. 3]: Dimensions of a person (e.g., race, ethnicity) that contribute to the person's identity and influence his or her viewpoints. Layers are dynamically intertwined with legacies and contribute to the ideas, beliefs, and perceptions about a variety of situations and issues.

Legacies [Ch. 3]: Powerful historical events, such as colonization, slavery, capture and redistribution of land, and religious conflict, experienced by our ancestors, family, and community of origin that continue to have ripple effects in our lives today. While these events may have happened decades ago, the impact has been so powerful that the influence extends across time and generations.

Lifeways [Chs. 1, 2, 3, 4, and 7]: A term used to describe a cultural group's way of life with respect to customs and practices.

Linguistic interpretation [Ch. 6]: Interpretation of the spoken word without the addition of cultural context or meanings.

Low-context communication [Ch. 5]: Style of communication in which information and meaning are made explicit in the language used. What is said is more important than how it is said.

Marginalization [Ch. 1]: To relegate or confine to a lower or outer limit or edge, as of social standing. The social process of marginalization refers to a lack of equitable access to social, political, and economic benefits, including health, on the basis of one's membership in an identifiable group.

Meritocracy [Ch. 3]: A belief that success and positive outcomes are based on merit, hard work, ability, and accomplishment rather than systemic or social factors.

Minority [Ch. 1]: Existing in proportionally smaller numbers. Within social contexts it is a misleading term to describe non-dominant ethnic identities.

Monochronic time (M-time) [Ch. 5]: View of time that is linear and emphasizes schedules, appointments, and promptness.

Multiculturalism [Ch. 2]: A condition in which many cultures co-exist in society and maintain their cultural differences. Multiculturalism also refers to the public policy of managing cultural diversity in a multi-ethnic society, emphasizing tolerance and respect for cultural diversity. Multiculturalism is regarded as a fundamental characteristic of Canadian society.

Naturopathic medicine [Ch. 8]: A system of primary health care based on the belief that given the proper opportunity, the body can heal itself with the healing power of nature. Naturopathic medicine uses natural methods and substances to stimulate the body's inherent self-healing processes. It includes botanical medicine, clinical nutrition, homeopathic approaches, lifestyle counselling, stress management, manipulation, Asian medicine, and physical therapies including hydrotherapy, light therapy, and massage.

Nuclear family [Ch. 7]: Traditionally, the nuclear family was a household consisting of two married, heterosexual parents and their legal children. In recent years, the "nuclear" family has come to be viewed as the immediate or the smallest family unit, and may include same-sex couples.

Osteopathy [Ch. 8]: A system of therapy based on the concept that the body can formulate its own remedies against diseases when the body is in a normal structural relationship, has a normal environment, and enjoys good nutrition. Osteopathy is particularly concerned with maintaining correct relationships between bones, muscles, and connective tissues.

Pain [Ch. 13]: An unpleasant sensory and emotional experience associated with actual or potential damage to a person's physical and psychosocial well-being.

Pain assessment tools [Ch. 13]: These include the Numeric Rating Scale (NRS), faces scales, and simple descriptors of pain, as well as behavioural and observational tools to assess pain in infants and non-verbal adults.

Pain threshold [Ch. 13]: The level at which 50 percent of stimuli would be recognized as painful.

Pain tolerance level [Ch. 13]: Greatest level of pain that an individual is prepared to endure.

Perinatal loss [Ch. 9]: An unwanted end of pregnancy during 40 weeks of gestation (through miscarriage or stillbirth) or during the first 28 days of life (the neonatal period). Perinatal loss is estimated to occur in 20 to 25 percent of all conceptions.

Perinatal period [Ch. 9]: The perinatal period is defined differently by different authors but generally extends over the period of time before and up to 28 days after birth.

Perspectives [Ch. 2]: Conceptual landscapes or sets of ideas that form the overall picture on a given topic.

Polychronic time (P-time) [Ch. 5]: A view of time that is circular, prompting people to do several things at once and value involvement with others over schedules and appointments. As a result, members of P-time cultures may come to appointments late or change schedules frequently.

Power [Ch. 3]: The ability to produce intended effects on oneself, on other people, and on things or situations. Within the healthcare provider–client relationship, power refers to the healthcare provider's sense of authority in the healthcare system that comes with the position, specialized knowledge, ability to influence and access other healthcare providers and other parts of the system, and access to privileged information.

Prejudice [Ch. 2]: A set of attitudes held by one person or group about another person or group, which casts the other in an inferior light despite the absence of legitimate or sufficient evidence.

Pre-session [Ch. 6]: A brief meeting between the healthcare provider and interpreter before the interpreted session in order to provide the interpreter with basic client information, clarify the purpose and objectives of the encounter, establish necessary ground rules and boundaries for the upcoming session, and reinforce the role of the interpreter on the team.

Privilege [Ch. 3]: Unearned resources or advantages associated with being a member of a particular (generally dominant) social or cultural group.

Race [Ch. 1]: Grouping of individuals based on genetically transmitted physical characteristics, such as skin colour, hair type, and body proportions. Race may be regarded either as a biological or social category and has been used to denote superiority and inferiority between groups.

Racism [Ch. 1]: An attitude as well as specific actions through which one group exercises power over others on the basis of skin colour and/or racial heritage. The effect is to marginalize and oppress some people and to sustain advantages for people of certain social groups.

Remote interpreting [Ch. 6]: Refers to situations when the interpreter is not in the presence of the speakers; it is usually done via a telephone (telephonic interpreting) but may be done using other technologies (e.g., video conferencing).

Self-reflexivity [Ch. 3]: Process of critical self-examination that challenges the stance of neutrality and instead examines own reality and the assumptions on which it is based.

Skip-generation family [Ch. 7]: An example is a family in which a grandparent takes on the dual role of parent and grandparent.

Social stressors [Ch. 11]: Events or conditions that are linked to individuals' and families' social characteristics, positions, and roles.

Somatization [Ch. 11]: A phenomenon where emotional or mental distress is expressed as a physical complaint.

Specific cultural competencies [Ch. 10]: Intimate knowledge of the culture, community, and culturally appropriate treatment approaches and skills, such as language fluency, that enable the healthcare provider to practise effectively with clients who identify with a particular cultural group.

Specific cultural knowledge [Chs. 3 and 4]: In-depth cultural knowledge that is pertinent to specific clinical or cultural populations.

Spirituality [Ch. 10]: Concerned with matters related to the spirit. Spirituality may or may not encompass faith or religion, and is manifested by what gives meaning to one's life.

Stereotype [Ch. 2]: A generalized conception of a group of people that results in the unconscious or conscious categorization of each member of that group, without regard for individual differences.

Stoic [Ch. 13]: Seemingly indifferent to, or unaffected by, joy, grief, pleasure, or pain.

Strategy [Ch. 2]: A guiding method that allows healthcare providers to move forward with an approach that can be modified as the situation unfolds.

Suffering [Ch. 10]: The bearing of pain or distress.

Telephonic interpreting [Ch. 6]: Refers to situations when the interpreter is not in the presence of the speakers but is available via a telephone. A form of remote interpreting.

Traditional Chinese medicine (TCM) [Ch. 8]: A health system that is said to be between 3000 and 7000 years old that sees diseases, disorders, and dysfunctions as imbalances in the body's energy. It includes nutritional therapy, massage, herbal therapy, acupuncture, and exercise regimes for relaxation and balancing of the body's energies.

Translation [Ch. 6]: Refers to the process of transcribing written documents from one language to another.

Triadic communication [Ch. 6]: Communication requiring three people, such as the healthcare provider, patient, and interpreter.

Trust [Ch. 3]: A valued and critical concept in all relationships, particularly client–healthcare provider relationships. Client trust is based on expectations that the healthcare provider will be knowledgeable, will take responsibility for the care that is needed, and will make the client's welfare a high priority.

Truth telling [Ch. 10]: The process of full disclosure (versus selective disclosure), in which healthcare providers feel obligated to share all information regarding diagnosis and prognosis with the client.

Visible minorities [Ch. 1]: In North America, persons, other than Aboriginal peoples, who are non-Caucasian in race or non-White in colour.

Western cultures [Ch. 1]: Refers to those cultures that value and use modern technologies, are industrialized, emphasize efficiency, use scientific approaches and equipment that make them "progressive" or "modern," and are dependent upon high technologies. Western cultures tend to be younger and generally include Canada, the United States, Europe, Russia, and related areas. Non-Western cultures refer to those cultures that have existed for thousands of years and have a long history of surviving and living with different philosophies of life. Non-Western cultures tend to have traditional values and lifestyles and rely less on modern technologies. Non-Western cultures include China, Japan, India, Vietnam, Indonesia, Egypt, Borneo, and the Caribbean.

World view [Ch. 3]: A perspective about values, life, and the surrounding world that serves as a reference point to make sense of the world.

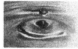

About the Contributors

SALMA DEBS-IVALL, RN, BSCN, MSCN, is corporate associate co-ordinator in nursing education at The Ottawa Hospital. She also works as a cultural care consultant, and as a part-time professor at the University of Ottawa in the Faculty of Health Sciences. She holds a BScN from the American University of Beirut in Lebanon and an MScN from the University of Ottawa. She has given multiple poster and oral presentations, as well as workshops and seminars, at regional, provincial, national, and international conferences. At press time, she was involved with the collaborative initiative of the Registered Nurses Association of Ontario, the Ontario Ministry of Health and Long-Term Care, and Health Canada's Healthy Work Environment Best Practice Guidelines project, working on the guideline titled "Embracing Cultural Diversity: Developing Cultural Competence."

SEPALI GURUGE, BSCN, MSC, is an associate professor at the School of Nursing at Ryerson University. She holds both a BScN and an MSc from the University of Toronto, and is currently completing her PhD in Nursing there, on intimate partner violence in immigrant communities. She is a co-investigator on a number of the Canadian Institutes of Health Research–funded research projects on intimate partner violence in various immigrant communities to Canada. She is also co-investigator on a study examining perceptions and experiences of immigrant and refugee women using an urban mobile health unit. She has published a number of articles and book chapters, and presented at many conferences nationally and internationally. She is also the co-editor of a book titled *Working with Women and Girls in the Context of Immigration and Settlement: Issues and Strategies for Mental Health Professionals* on immigrant and refugee girls and women's mental health, being published by the Centre for Addiction and Mental Health in 2007.

RAJU HAJELA, MD, MPH, CCSAM, FASAM, FCFP, is the clinical medical director, Addiction Network, Calgary Health Region, and a clinical associate professor, Faculty of Medicine, University of Calgary. He is a retired major (Canadian Forces) and former assistant professor at Queen's University in the Faculty of Medicine, Departments of Family Medicine and Psychiatry. He grew up and received his early education in India. He completed his MD at Dalhousie University in Halifax (1982), and his Master of Public Health (MPH) at Harvard School of Public Health (1988). He completed training in Maharishi Ayurveda at the Maharishi University of Management in Fairfield, Iowa (1994). His long-standing interests include physics, philosophy, religion, spirituality, behavioural sciences, and international health. He has held leadership positions in the Canadian Society of Addiction Medicine, the American Society of Addiction Medicine, the International Society of Addiction Medicine, the Ontario Medical

Association, and the Canadian Medical Association since the early 1990s. He is frequently invited to address professional and public audiences, and has conducted numerous workshops in the areas of pain and addiction, psychiatric disorders and addiction, and models of health and disease. He is a member of the editorial advisory board of *Crosscurrents,* the journal of addiction and mental health published by the Centre for Addiction and Mental Health in Toronto.

DAVID HOWES, Rev., BA, M.Div., is an ordained Presbyterian minister (University of Toronto, 1982) by training. He served for ten years in Quebec, first in a predominantly francophone area and then for seven years in the heart of Montreal. During those latter years, he was the director of an inner-city community centre that worked with refugees from all over the world and with the local Black community. In 1992, he returned to Ontario and worked in a suburban parish and then a village setting. In 2000, he went to Sunnybrook Hospital and began to study for chaplaincy. He was a part of the burn unit and also served on the emergency ward. At the present time, David is the director for spiritual care at Bridgepoint Health Hospital, a multicultural rehabilitation hospital in Toronto, with 29 languages spoken on staff, and people from all over the world as patients in "slow stream rehab and complex care." Over the past year, he has worked to take what was a Christian-based religious program and open it up to become a spiritually based program that responds to the needs of both the religious and non-religious.

ILENE HYMAN, BSc(PT), MHSc, PhD (Community Health/Epidemiology), is a research scientist in the Violence and Health Research Program at the Centre for Research in Women's Health, and an assistant professor in the Department of Public Health Sciences at the University of Toronto. Her expertise is in the areas of immigrant health, women's health, intimate partner violence (IPV), and cross-cultural issues in health care. Prior research experience includes studies of perinatal health, mental health, cancer screening, and determinants of health in immigrant and cultural communities. Much of this research has focused on acculturation, the process through which immigrants incorporate new values, attitudes, and behaviours, and on exploring the mechanisms through which this process affects health and health behaviour. She has most recently completed research on the prevalence of IPV and IPV help-seeking behaviour among recent and non-recent Canadian immigrants. She is currently conducting research on post-migration changes in marital relationships among Ethiopian immigrants in Toronto and on perceptions of, and responses to, IPV among Tamil women in Toronto. She has written extensively on immigration and health, and women's health, including policy reports for government agencies and scientific publications.

SHEILA M. LEWIS, BSCN, MHSc, is an associate lecturer in nursing at York University, Atkinson Faculty of Liberal and Professional Studies, in Toronto. In addition to full-time teaching, she is a healing touch practitioner (HTP) with a strong interest in complementary therapies, women's health, Aboriginal health, and human science nursing theories as a guide to nursing praxis. Her extensive clinical background includes roles in senior nursing leadership, education, and primary and secondary clinical nursing practices. Sheila recently completed a research study to explore the lived experience of residents, families, and nurses in long-term care in relation to implementation of the Registered Nurses Association of Ontario Client Centred Care Best Practice Guideline.

HUNG-TAT (TED) LO, MBBS, MRCPsych, FRCPC, is an assistant professor in the Faculty of Medicine, University of Toronto, consulting to the Culture, Community and Health Studies Program at the Centre for Addiction and Mental Health. He is a community psychiatrist who has been actively involved in ethno-cultural mental health over the past twenty years. He established the Hong Fook Mental Health Association in Toronto in 1982 and also started the Friends of Alternative and Complementary Therapies Society in Toronto in 1998. Recently, he has been engaged in cultural competence training for physicians and mental health professionals, and research toward its measurement.

CLAIRE McDONALD, RN, BScN, received a diploma in nursing from the Hamilton and District School of Nursing, a BScN from the University of Windsor, and certificates in midwifery and perinatal intensive care nursing from the State of Victoria, Australia. Claire worked as a staff nurse in neonatal intensive care nurseries in Canada for many years. She is currently the perinatal nurse educator/neonatal at St. Joseph's Hospital in London, Ontario.

ATHINA PERIVOLARIS, RN, BScN, MN, is an advanced practice nurse at the Centre for Addiction and Mental Health in Toronto. She obtained her BScN and a master of nursing degree from the University of Toronto. She has extensive experience in both mental health and gerontological nursing practices across a range of healthcare settings. In her role as an advanced practice nurse over the years, Athina has focused her scholarship and practice on enabling older persons with irreversible dementias, and on enhancing the quality of their living experience. She is an expert at designing interventions for maximizing older persons' abilities and for minimizing the occurrence of challenging behavioural patterns of patients.

ANN POTTINGER, RN, BASc, BScN, MN, is an advanced practice nurse at the Centre for Addiction and Mental Health, Toronto. She has extensive experience in providing nursing care, in both hospital and community settings, to diverse clients and families who have mental health and addiction issues. Throughout her career, Ann has focused on care strategies and approaches that honour the values and preferences of persons from diverse groups.

MONAKSHI SAWHNEY, RN, MN, ACNP, is a clinical nurse specialist, acute care nurse practitioner for pain management at North York General Hospital in Toronto. She has a clinical appointment to the University of Toronto, Faculty of

Nursing, and is involved in teaching in the undergraduate program. Mona has published and presented in the area of pain management, both nationally and internationally. She is currently involved in a national project that focuses on the hospital accreditation standard for pain management.

RANI HAJELA SRIVASTAVA, RN, BN, MScN, PhD (cand), is a nursing professional with more than twenty years' healthcare experience, reflecting a blend of academia and practice. She has held academic appointments at University of Toronto and Memorial University of Newfoundland. Her practice background includes experience as a staff nurse, advanced practice nurse, director of nursing, and professional leader for nursing. Rani's research interests are in the area of stress and coping, the influence of culture on health practices, and cultural competence. Her doctoral work examines the influence of organizational factors on clinical cultural competence. She has worked closely with the College of Nurses of Ontario in the development of the professional standards for providing culturally sensitive care, and is currently serving as panel chair for a Healthy Work Environment Best Practice Guideline, "Embracing Cultural Diversity: Developing Cultural Competence," a collaborative initiative of the Registered Nurses Association of Ontario, the Ontario Ministry of Health and Long-Term Care, and Health Canada. Rani has also been a speaker at several national and international conferences and workshops.

NANCY WATTS, RN, MN, PNC(c), works as a clinical nurse specialist in the Perinatal Program at London Health Sciences Centre. Her background includes many years as a staff nurse in single-room maternity care, public health, and prenatal class teaching. In her current role, she integrates culture into all aspects of orientation with new nurses and continuing education with other staff members. She is involved with women/families with complex needs as well as perinatal nursing practice.

Index

Page numbers followed by f indicate figures; t, tables; b, boxes